Oncology

Theory & Practice

Oncology – Theory & Practice

Publisher: iConcept Press Ltd.
Cover design: Pineapple Design Ltd.
Interior design: iConcept Press Ltd.
Typesetting and copy editing: iConcept Press Ltd. and Pineapple Design Ltd.

ISBN: 978-1-922227-80-5

Printed in the United States of America

Copyright © iConcept Press 2014

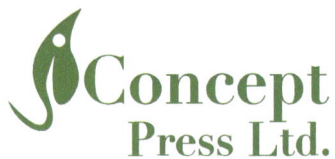

❦Concept
Press Ltd.

www.iconceptpress.com

Contents

Preface

Oncology is a branch of medicine that deals with cancer. "Onco" means bulk, mass, or tumor while "logy" means study. Each of the cells of the body have a tightly regulated system that controls their growth, maturity, reproduction and eventual death. Cancer begins when cells in a part of the body start to grow out of control. There are many kinds of cancer, but they all start because of out-of-control growth of abnormal cells. This book focus on the recent progress and research on oncology and serves as an essential guide for oncologists. Oncologists are medical professionals who practice oncology. These oncologists have several specific roles. They help in diagnosis of the cancer, help in staging the cancer and grading the aggressive nature of the cancer.

There are totally 10 chapters in this book. Chapter 1 shows that chronic IGF-1 stimulation can bypass chemoresistance and support Ewing sarcoma cell apoptosis in combination with the death ligand Apo2L/TRAIL. The findings may have important implications for the biology as well as the clinical management of the Ewing sarcoma family of tumor. Chapter 2 tests total cfDNA concentration, cfDNA integrity, BRAFV600E mutation and RASSF1A promoter methylation associated to cfDNA in melanoma patients and healthy controls in order to identify a sequential multi-marker panel in cfDNA able to increase the predictive capability in the diagnosis of cutaneous melanoma. Chapter 3 overviews transforming growth factor-β (TGFβ)-mediated tumour suppressive pathways and outlines the molecular mechanisms of these effects. The studies presented here propose a pivotal function for E2F transcription factors as potent co-transducers of TGFβ signalling and highlight the central role for the pRb-E2F pathway in regulating TGFβ tumour suppressive effects. Chapter 4 reviews the contribution of urokinase-type plasminogen activator system in breast cancer; the most common cancer in women worldwide. Better understanding of the molecular biology of this malignancy leads to efficient prognosis and therapies for the disease.

Chapter 5 describes how non coding RNA families can influence the development of neuroblastoma and also possibly give further insights to new diagnostic procedures and therapies for this devastating paediatric cancer. The discovery of the utility of non coding RNA families, such as miRNAs and lncRNAs in the past 16 years has led to an astonishing new realm regarding the understanding of disease progression at the molecular level and can also serve to develop novel diagnostic and therapeutic measures within the clinical setting. Chapter 6 reviews the current knowledge of Thymidine Kinase 1 a clinically relevant cancer biomarker which is significantly elevated in serum and tissue of cancer patients. Measurement of Thymidine Kinase 1 is useful as an aid in diagnosis and prognosis of many different cancer types and has recently been shown to have vast clinical potential especially as a screening and monitoring tool for cancer patients. Chapter 7 discusses the characteristic pathological, immunophenotypic, and genetic features of different GI lymphomas categorized according to World Health Organization (WHO) classification. The epidemiological, clinical, and pathological features as well as diagnosis of lymphomas occurring in each part of the GI tract are summarized and the key points regarding lymphomas at each site are emphasized. Chapter 8 provides an overview of the chemokine system in homeostasis and cancer, with a focus on the CX3CL1/CX3CR1 axis to illustrate the complex interplay between the chemokines and other molecules that shape tumor's microenvironment and its progression.

Chapter 9 reviews the recent advances in cohesin and its associate proteins and discusses the relation between their deregulation and tumorigenesis. Cohesin plays a critical role in regulating sister chromatid cohesion and separation, DNA damage signaling and repair, gene expression, as well as centrosome biogenesis, etc. Chapter 10 reviews the current diagnostic issues that are focused on the identification of the thyroid biomarkers. It shows that thyroid biomarkers has a potential to improve the diagnostic accuracy.

Editing and publishing a book is never an easy task. Each chapter in this book has gone through a peer review, a selection and an editing process so as to guarantee its quality. Without the supports and contributions of the authors and reviewers, this book can never be able to complete. We would like to thank all of the authors in this book and all of the reviewers who participated in the reviewing process: Fawzi Aoudjit, Venkata Satya Suresh Attili, Swati Biswas, Elisa Caffarelli, Javier Camacho, Jose A. Costoya, Yao Dai, S de Jong, Petra Barros dos Santos, Giulia Ferrari-Toninelli, Junjiang Fu, Peter Brian Gahan, Jiangping Gong, James D. Griffin, OKIO HINO, Zhuo-Wei Hu, Heba M. S. Ismail, Hongbin Ji, Santosh Kesari, YAMING LI, Jun-Yang Liou, Jyothi B Lngegowda, Keivan Majidzadeh-A, Giorgio Malpeli, Olivier Micheau, S. David Nathanson, Eric O'Neill, Rimas J. Orentas, Sang-Youel Park, Giuliana Pelicci, Phuc Pham, Amit Sengupta, Takehiko Shiraishi, Marcelo B. Soares, Laura Soucek, Josena K. Stephen, Takuji Tanaka, Satoshi Tanida, Diana O. Treaba, Fabrizio Vinante, Paul Zarogoulidis and Yitzhak Zimmer. We hope that you, the reader, will find this book interesting and useful. Any advices please feel free and are always welcome to tell us.

iConcept Press Ltd
September 2014

Insulin-like Growth Factor-1 (IGF-1): A Double-Edged Sword In Ewing Tumour Cell Death

Frans Van Valen
Institute of Experimental Musculoskeletal Medicine
University Hospital Münster, Germany

Henning Harrer
Institute of Food Chemistry
University Münster, Germany

Marc Hotfilder, Uta Dirksen
Department of Paediatric Haematology and Oncology
University Children's Hospital Münster, Germany

Borna Truckenbrod, Thomas Pap
Institute of Experimental Musculoskeletal Medicine
University Hospital Münster, Germany

George Gosheger
Department of Orthopaedic Surgery
University Hospital Münster, Germany

Hans-Ulrich Humpf
Institute of Food Chemistry
University Münster, Germany

Herbert Jürgens
Department of Paediatric Haematology and Oncology
University Children's Hospital Münster, Germany

1   Introduction

The Ewing sarcoma family of tumour (ESFT) of bone and soft tissue includes Ewing sarcoma, peripheral primitive neuroectodermal tumour (pPNET) and Askin tumour, which are amongst the most aggressive of malignancies encountered in children and young adults. Despite intensive multiple-agent chemo-therapy in combination with surgery and/or radiation, the survival rate for patients with metastatic and recurrent disease is still low, approximately 25% at 5 years (Dirksen & Jürgens, 2010). Improved insight into mechanisms of malignancy remains a high priority in ESFT research and is a prerequisite for the identification of new targeted therapies.

Several lines of evidence suggest that the insulin-like growth factor-1 (IGF-1)–IGF-1 receptor (IGF-1R) axis plays critical roles in the proliferation, metastasis, and survival of ESFT (Toomey *et al.*, 2010). As a consequence, the IGF-1 signalling pathway has been studied as a potential therapeutic target in patients with ESFT by selectively inhibiting the activity of IGF-1R (Wagner & Maki, 2013). IGF-1R belongs to the tyrosine kinase family of receptors and consists of two extracellular α-subunits and two β-subunits that have transmembrane domains and cytoplasmic tails (Samani *et al.*, 2007). The β-subunits contain intrinsic tyrosine kinase domains, which when activated results in autophosphorylation of the β-subunits on key tyrosine residues that serve as docking sites for effector molecules. High-affinity IGF-1R and IGF-2R are expressed in ESFT cells and metabolic actions such as stimulation of glucose transport, glycogen synthesis and thymidine incorporation into DNA by both IGF-1 and IGF-2 are transmitted through IGF-1R (Van Valen *et al.*, 1992). An IGF-1–IGF-1R autocrine circuit was suggested in some ESFT cells because addition of IGF-1R antibody caused inhibition of cell proliferation (Yee *et al.*, 1990). IGF-1 release can be induced and IGF-binding protein-3 (IGFBP-3) formation can be repressed in ESFT cells by oncogenic fusion proteins that may allow for IGF-1R activation through increased ligand binding (Prieur *et al.*, 2004; Cironi *et al.*, 2008). Most importantly, IGF-1 reputedly opposes chemotoxicity in ESFT cells. Hofbauer *et al.* (1993) noticed that the cytotoxicity of various chemotherapeutic agents such as doxorubicin (DOX) and etoposide (VP16) can be suppressed by serum IGF-1. Toretsky *et al.* (1999) reported that recombinant human IGF-1 can protect ESFT cells from chemotherapy-induced cell death through activation of AKT (also known as protein kinase B), a phosphatidylinositol-3-kinase (PI3K)-regulated serine/threonine protein kinase that has several downstream substrates including mammalian target of rapamycin (mTOR) and glycogen synthase kinase-3 (GSK-3). However, there have been no studies investigating the activity of IGF-1 in ESFT cells in response to treatment with apoptosis ligand 2 (Apo2L)/tumour necrosis factor (TNF)-related apoptosis-inducing ligand (TRAIL).

Apo2L/TRAIL is a TNF family member with highest homology to Fas ligand. Unlike TNF-α and Fas ligand, Apo2L/TRAIL represents a most valuable candidate for cancer therapy because it initiates programmed cell death (apoptosis) preferably in tumour cells over non-malignant cells, both *in vitro* and *in vivo* in non-human primates and mice (Wiley *et al.*, 1995; Pitti *et al.*, 1996; Ashkenazi *et al.*, 1999). The possible use of Apo2L/TRAIL in cancer treatment has been reconsidered because *in vitro* studies documented that the cytokine can elicit apoptosis in non-malignant human hepatocytes and brain tissue (Jo *et al.*, 2000; Nitsch *et al.*, 2000). However, different recombinant preparations of Apo2L/TRAIL may differ in biological potential for lethality in non-malignant human cells. *In vivo* and *in vitro* studies revealed that histidine-tagged and leucine zipper-fused versions of Apo2L/TRAIL are toxic to non-malignant hepatocytes and keratinocytes, whereas native Apo2L/TRAIL is innocuous to these cell types (Lawrence *et al.*, 2001; Qin *et al.*, 2001). The native version of Apo2L/TRAIL therefore is still seriously considered for the clinical management of cancer and studies are ongoing to evaluate its safety and anti-tumour activity (Herbst *et al.*, 2010).

To date, the cells most sensitive to Apo2L/TRAIL originate from ESFT with apoptotic responsiveness reported in the majority of established cell lines *in vitro* and patient-derived cells *ex vivo* thus indicating the eminence of this therapeutic concept (Van Valen *et al.*, 2000; Kontny *et al.*, 2001; Kumar *et al.*, 2001; Mitsiades *et al.*, 2001). Apo2L/TRAIL triggers apoptosis by interacting with specific death receptors (TRAIL-R1/DR4 and/or TRAIL-R2/DR5) followed by activation of initiator caspase-8 and subsequent activation of effector caspases 3 and 7 (extrinsic or death receptor signalling pathway of apoptosis) (Ashkenazi *et al.*, 2008). Apo2L/TRAIL can also initiate caspase-8-dependent mitochondrial dysfunction leading to activation of caspase-9 (intrinsic or mitochondrial signalling pathway of apoptosis). Intrinsic apoptosis can be regulated both negatively and positively by mitochondria-associated anti-apoptotic, respectively, pro-apoptotic members of the Bcl-2 family, whereas extrinsic apoptosis is primarily blocked by inhibitor of apoptosis protein (IAP) family members including X chromosome-linked IAP (XIAP) that binds directly to the catalytically active sites of effector caspases (Ola *et al.*, 2011; Schimmer *et al.*, 2004; Varfolomeev *et al.*, 2009; Sensintaffar *et al.*, 2011). XIAP is a direct downstream target of AKT and an important mediator of IGF-1 on cell survival (Dan *et al.*, 2004; Liu *et al.*, 2011). Increased levels of XIAP protein and/or AKT activity have been correlated with resistance to Apo2L/TRAIL in many cancer cell types (Chen *et al.*, 2001; Poulaki *et al.*, 2002; Asakuma *et al.*, 2003; Fakler *et al.*, 2009).

The goal of this report[1] was to examine the role of the IGF-1–IGF-1R axis in regulating apoptosis induction by native human Apo2L/TRAIL (dulanermin) in ESFT cells. Our study unveils that depending on treatment duration IGF-1 is a life-to-death switch in the context of apoptosis triggered by Apo2L/TRAIL. Interestingly α-IR3, a specific IGF-1R antibody, is functionally equivalent to IGF-1. Short term IGF-1 treatment stimulates AKT kinase and increases XIAP protein that is associated with inhibition of Apo2L/TRAIL-mediated apoptosis. In contrast, long term IGF-1 treatment results in repression of XIAP protein through ceramide formation derived from *de novo* synthesis that is associated with stimulation of Apo2L/TRAIL-mediated apoptosis. During the process, IGF-1 induces down-regulation of IGF-1R well before the onset of its pro-apoptotic effects. Noteworthy, resistance to conventional chemotherapeutic agents is maintained in cells following long term IGF-1 treatment. Collectively, the results suggest that chronic IGF-1 exposure selectively renders ESFT cells susceptible to Apo2L/TRAIL-induced apoptosis and may have important implications for the biology as well as the clinical management of refractory ESFT.

2   Materials and Methods

2.1   Reagents

Recombinant human IGF-1 (PreproTech, Rocky Hill, NJ, USA), mouse IGF-1R antibody α-IR3, doxorubicin, z-VAD-fmk, z-DEVD-fmk, wortmannin, AKTi-1/2, TDZD-8 (Merck Chemicals, Darmstadt, Germany), fumonisin B1, Ro-31-8425 (Biomol, Hamburg, Germany), rapamycin, and fatty acid-free bovine serum albumin (Sigma-Aldrich, Taufkirchen, Germany) were purchased from the indicated suppliers. The

---

[1] This paper is an updated and expanded version of 'Van Valen, F., Harrer, H., Hotfilder, M., Dirksen, U., Pap, T., Gosheger, G., Humpf, H.U., & Jürgens, H. (2012). A novel role of IGF1 in Apo2L/TRAIL-mediated apoptosis of Ewing tumor cells' previously published in Sarcoma, 2012, 782970, Hindawi Publishing Corporation.

sphingolipids d17:0-sphinganine, d17:1-sphingosine, d18:1/C17:0-ceramide, and d18:1/C17:0-sphingomyelin were obtained from Avanti Polar Lipids (Alabaster, AL, USA). Etoposide was liberally supplied by Cipla (Mumbai, India) through Medac (Wedel, Germany). Recombinant human Apo2L/TRAIL (dulanermin) was generously provided by Genentech (San Francisco, CA, USA).

2.2   Cell Culture and Incubation Conditions

Human ESFT cell lines studied were A9423 (provided by Timothy Triche, Los Angeles, CA, USA), ES-2 (provided by Thomas Look, Memphis, TN, USA), LAP-35 (provided by Katia Scotlandi, Bologna, Italy), and A17/95 (provided by Ursula Anderer, Berlin, Germany). ESFT cell lines RD-ES and SK-ES-1 were obtained from the American Type Culture Collection (ATCC, Rockville, MD, USA), and CADO-ES-1 and MHH-ES-1 were from the Leibniz Institute-German Collection of Microorganisms and Cell Cultures (Leibniz Institut-DSMZ, Braunschweig, Germany). ESFT cell lines VH-64 and WE-68 were previously established in our laboratory (Van Valen *et al.*, 1992). The clinical data and the cytogenetic features of all cell lines have been reviewed (Van Valen, 1999). Cells were maintained in RPMI-1640 medium supplemented with 10% foetal calf serum (FCS), 1% antibiotic-antimycotic mixture (10 mg/mL streptomycin, 10,000 U/mL penicillin, and 25 μg/mL amphotericin B) and 2 mM *L*-glutamine (Gibco, Grand Island, NY, USA) (*i.e.*, serum-containing medium) at 37°C in a humidified atmosphere with 5% CO_2. Cells were passaged in 25-cm^2 tissue culture flasks using 0.05% trypsin/0.02% EDTA in Puck's saline (Gibco). Cells (8 x 10^4/cm^2) were seeded in 96-well plates for cell viability, in white-walled 96-well luminometer plates for caspase assays, in 12-well plates for apoptosis assays, in 6-well plates for protein extraction, in 25-cm^2 tissue culture flasks for IGF-1R analysis and receptor tyrosine kinase arrays, and in 75-cm^2 tissue culture flasks for sphingolipid extraction. All synthetic culture ware (Falcon Plastics, Oxnard, CA, USA) was collagen-coated (5 μg/cm^2; BioConcept, Salem, NH, USA) as described (Van Valen *et al.*, 2000). For analysis of the effects of IGF-1, cultures were washed and maintained in serum-free medium substituting serum by 0.2% fatty acid-free bovine serum albumin (BSA) for 24 hours until experimentation. Cells were pretreated with IGF-1 followed by incubation with Apo2L/TRAIL for the indicated times. To assess the effects of pharmacological inhibitors, these agents were added to the cultures at the indicated concentrations 30 min prior to treatment with IGF-1 and/or Apo2L/TRAIL.

2.3   Apoptosis and Cell Viability Assays

For fluorescence-activated cell sorting (FACS) analysis of apoptosis, cells were detached with 5 mM EDTA in PBS and washed in PBS containing 0.2% BSA. Cells were incubated with R-phycoerythrin-conjugated annexin-V (1:100) and 7-amino-actinomycin D (1:200; Invitrogen, Darmstadt, Germany) at room temperature in the dark. After 20 min cells were washed in ice-cold PBS containing 0.5% sodium azide and analysed by flow cytometry using FACS-Calibur (BD Biosciences, Heidelberg, Germany) and accompanying CellQuest Pro software (BD Biosciences). Specific apoptosis was calculated as follows: 100 x (experimental apoptosis [%] - spontaneous apoptosis [%] / 100% - spontaneous apoptosis [%]). For assessment of cell viability, the spectrophotometric conversion of 3-(4,5-dimethylthiazol-2-yl)-2,5-diphenyltetrazolium bromide (MTT; Sigma-Aldrich) was measured using a Victor^3 1420 Multilabel Counter (PerkinElmer, Rodgau, Germany) at 550 nm. Percentage of cell viability was calculated by the formula: 100 x (absorbance of experimental wells / absorbance of control wells).

2.4 Caspase Activity Assays

Caspase-8, caspase-9 and caspase-3/-7 activities were analysed by the Caspase-Glo-8, Caspase-Glo-9, respectively, Caspase-Glo-3/7 assays (Promega, Madison, WI, USA). Cells (2.5×10^4/well) in serum-free medium (100 μL) were exposed to IGF-1 for the times indicated and subsequently incubated for 4 hours with Apo2L/TRAIL. Thereafter, an equal volume of Caspase-Glo-8, Caspase-Glo-9 or Caspase-Glo-3/7 reagent was added to the cells and cultures were incubated for an additional 45 min. The aminoluciferin released by caspase-mediated cleavage of proluminogenic substrate was determined using Victor[3] plate reader (PerkinElmer). Background luminescence was determined using reactions lacking cells. Caspase activity was expressed as fold increase in relative light unit ratio between the caspase activities of treated cells *versus* untreated cells (normalized to relative unit of 1.0).

2.5 Western Blot Analysis

Harvested cells were rinsed in PBS containing 100 μM Na_3VO_4 and lysed for 30 min at 4°C in Triton X-100 buffer (20 mM Tris, pH 7.5, 150 mM NaCl, 1 mM EDTA, 1 mM EGTA, 2.5 mM $Na_4P_2O_7$, 1 mM β-glycerophosphate, 1 mM Na_3VO_4, 1 μg/mL leupeptin, 1 mM PMSF (phenylmethylsulfonyl fluoride), 1% Triton X-100) (Van Valen et al., 2003). Protein expression was determined in whole-cell lysates (50-100 μg) using detergent compatible Bio-Rad protein assay. Proteins were dissolved in Laemmli buffer, resolved on 12% SDS-PAGE gels, and transferred to PVDF membranes. After treatment with 5% Western blot blocking buffer, membranes were incubated with the appropriate antibodies. Primary antibodies used were rabbit anti-AKT polyclonal antibody (1:500), rabbit anti-phosphorylated AKT(Ser473) polyclonal antibody (1:100), rabbit anti-Mcl-1 polyclonal antibody (1:500; Santa Cruz Biotechnology, Santa Cruz, CA, USA), rabbit anti-GSK-3α/β mAb (1:1,000), rabbit anti-phosphorylated GSK-3α/β(Ser21/9) polyclonal antibody (1:1,000; Cell Signaling Technology, Beverly, MA, USA), mouse anti-XIAP mAb (1:250), and rabbit anti-Bax polyclonal antibody (1:1,000; BD Biosciences). The secondary antibodies used were goat anti-mouse IgG (1:5,000) and goat anti-rabbit IgG (1:5,000; DakoCytomation, Hamburg, Germany). Enhanced chemiluminescence (GE Healthcare, Freiburg, Germany) was used for signal detection. Equal protein loading was monitored by immunodetection of β-actin using mouse anti-β-actin mAb (1:25,000; Sigma-Aldrich).

2.6 Receptor Tyrosine Kinase (RTK) Array

Cells in serum free-medium were incubated with IGF-1 (50 ng/mL; 30 min). Thereafter, cells were washed with PBS containing 100 μM Na_3VO_4, solubilized in lysis buffer, and then 300 μg of total protein were incubated with human proteome profiler phosphorylated-RTK antibody arrays (R&D Systems, Wiesbaden, Germany) following the manufacturer's instructions. Briefly, array membranes coated with 42 different RTK antibodies were incubated with whole-cell lysate overnight at 4°C while shaking. After washing with the supplied washing buffer, membranes were incubated with anti-phosphotyrosine-horseradish peroxidase-conjugated antibodies for 2 hours at room temperature prior to incubation with chemiluminescent reagent (GE Healthcare) and film exposure.

2.7 Enzyme-Linked Immunosorbent Assay (ELISA) and Enzyme Immunometric Assay (EIA)

Expression of phosphorylated AKT(Ser473) and total AKT in cell lysates was validated by PathScan Sandwich ELISA (Cell Signaling Technology). Determination of phosphorylated GSK-3β(Ser9), total GSK-3β, and XIAP was conducted by TiterZyme EIA (Assay Designs, Ann Arbor, MI, USA). Cell lysis buffer was supplemented with protease inhibitor cocktail (P-8340; Sigma-Aldrich). Optical density was determined at 450 nm and 570 nm employing Victor^3 plate reader (PerkinElmer). Data were expressed as pAKT/AKT and pGSK-3/GSK-3 ratios. XIAP protein concentration was expressed as nanogram per 10^6 viable cells. Number of viable cells was determined using CASY Counter (Roche Applied Science, Penzberg, Germany) per the manufacturer's protocol.

2.8 Sphingolipid Identification and Quantitation

Cells were harvested by trypsinization and washed in ice-cold PBS. Final cell pellets were stored under liquid nitrogen. For lipid extraction, cell pellets were lyophilized and extracted using a mixture of ethyl acetate:isopropanol:water (60:30:10, v/v/v) (Shaner *et al.*, 2009). The samples were spiked with a sphingolipid internal standard mixture consisting of d17:0-sphinganine (50 pmol), d17:1-sphingosine (150 pmol), d18:1/C17:0-ceramide (250 pmol), and d18:1/C17:0-sphingomyelin (500 pmol). Sphingolipids were quantitated by high performance liquid chromatography coupled to electrospray ionization tandem mass spectrometry (HPLC-ESI-MS/MS) on an API 4000 triple quadrupole mass spectrometer (Applied Biosystems, Darmstadt, Germany) (Shaner *et al.*, 2009). Cellular sphingolipid levels were normalized to viable cell number.

2.9 Cells-Surface IGF-1R Analysis

Cells in serum-free medium were incubated with IGF-1 (50 ng/mL) at 37°C for the times indicated and detached in PBS-5 mM EDTA. For staining of cell-surface IGF-1R, cells (1×10^6) in 100 μL of PBS-0.2% BSA were incubated with 10 μL of Alexa Fluor®488-conjugated mouse anti-human IGF-1R (CD221, IgG1, 0.05 mg/mL, clone 1H7) (AbD Serotec, Oxford, UK) at 4°C in the dark. Alexa Fluor®488-conjugated mouse IgG1 (AbD Serotec) was used as isotype control. After 20 min cells were washed in ice-cold PBS-0.5% sodium azide and analysed by flow cytometry using Cytomics FC500 (Beckman Coulter, Krefeld, Germany) and accompanying CXP software (BD Biosciences).

2.10 Statistical Analysis

Differences between experimental groups were evaluated by ANOVA and Tukey's *post-hoc* test using SigmaStat 3.5 software (Systat Software Inc., San Jose, CA, USA). A P value < 0.05 was regarded as statistically significant.

3 Results

We first examined the temporal effect of IGF-1 on Apo2L/TRAIL lethality in ESFT cells. As revealed in Figure 1A, incubation of VH-64 cells with IGF-1 (50 ng/mL) resulted in gradual protection from apoptosis induced by Apo2L/TRAIL (50 ng/mL), with significant resistance observed 24 hours after IGF-1 addition. However, as time of incubation continued, IGF-1 caused a marked amplification of apoptosis induced by Apo2L/TRAIL, beginning 48 hours after IGF-1 addition. After 72 hours, IGF-1 elicited a 3-fold ($P < 0.02$) increase in the percentage of apoptotic cells compared with untreated control. IGF-1 as a single agent did not induce apoptosis in VH-64 cells, not even when cells were incubated for up to 72 hours with IGF-1 (Figure 1A).

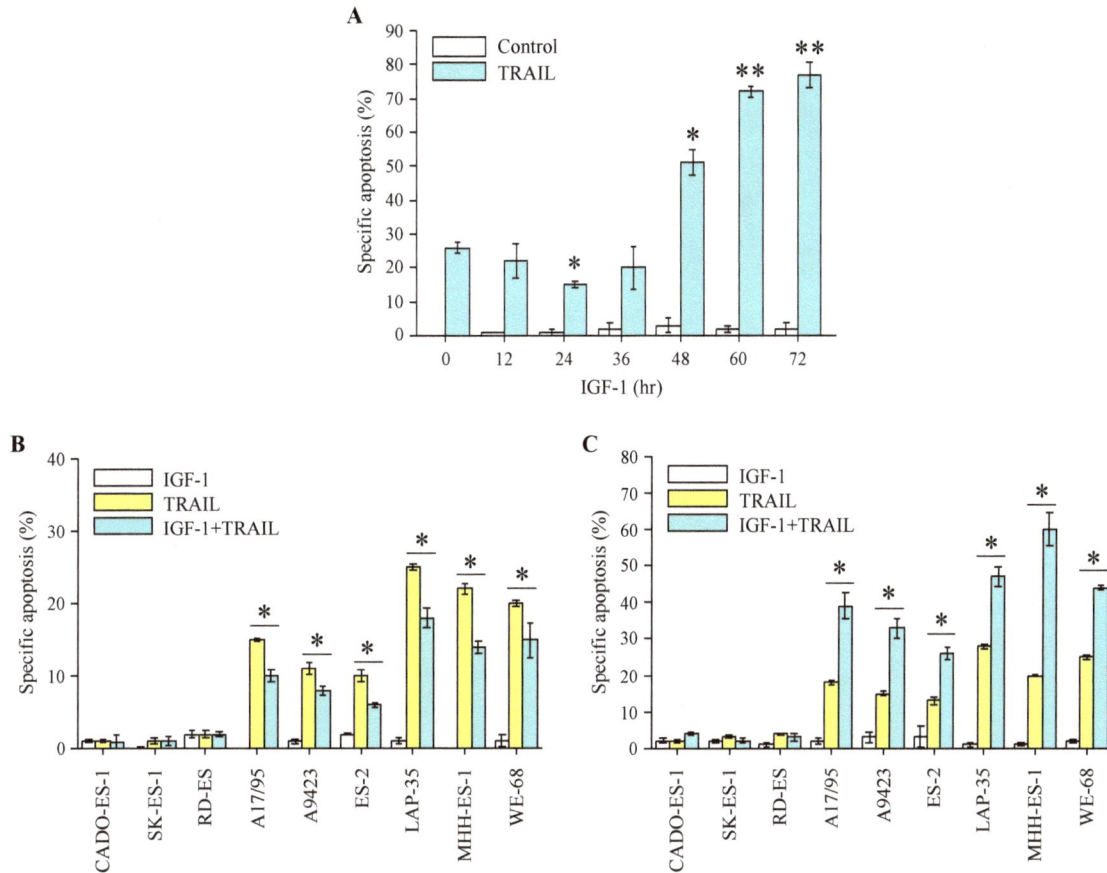

Figure 1: Time-dependency of IGF-1 on Apo2L/TRAIL-induced apoptosis. *A.* Percentage specific apoptosis in VH-64 cells treated for the times indicated with IGF-1 (50 ng/mL), followed by incubation with Apo2L/TRAIL (*TRAIL*; 50 ng/mL; 8 hours) or serum-free medium alone (*Control*). Percentage specific apoptosis in cells from different ESFT lines treated for (*B*) 24 hours and (*C*) 72 hours in the absence and presence of IGF-1 (50 ng/mL), followed by incubation with Apo2L/TRAIL (*TRAIL*; 50 ng/mL; 8 hours) or serum-free medium alone. Asterisks: * $P < 0.05$; ** $P < 0.02$; error bars: mean $\pm$ SD of triplicate determinations from 3 independent experiments.

Besides cell line VH-64, additional ESFT cell lines also displayed time-dependent dual regulation of Apo2L/TRAIL-induced apoptosis by IGF-1. The results are summarized in Figures 1B and 1C. While 24 hours of IGF-1 treatment caused suppression of Apo2L/TRAIL lethality (Figure 1B), 72 hours of IGF-1 treatment caused amplification of Apo2L/TRAIL lethality (Figure 1C) in ESFT cell lines A17/95, A9423, ES-2, LAP-35, MHH-ES-1, and WE-68, which like VH-64 are all sensitive to Apo2L/TRAIL (Van Valen *et al.*, 2000). In contrast, IGF-1 treatment for 24 hours and 72 hours did not affect the Apo2L/TRAIL response in ESFT cell lines CADO-ES-1, SK-ES-1 and RD-ES (Figures 1B and 1C), which are all resistant to Apo2L/TRAIL (Van Valen *et al.*, 2000). IGF-1 (50 ng/mL) alone provoked minimal, if at all, apoptosis in the ESFT cell lines examined (Figures 1B and 1C).

Together, these data suggest that depending on the duration of treatment IGF-1 initially inhibits apoptosis and subsequently promotes apoptosis induced by Apo2L/TRAIL.

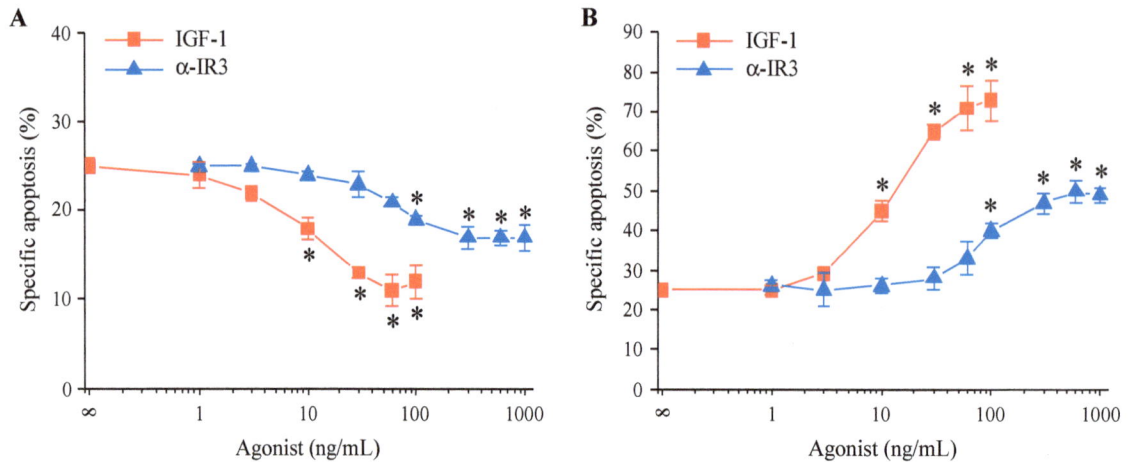

Figure 2: Concentration-dependency of IGF-1 and IGF-1R antibody α-IR3 on Apo2L/TRAIL-induced apoptosis. Percentage-specific apoptosis in VH-64 cells treated for (*A*) 24 hours and (*B*) 72 hours with the indicated concentrations of IGF-1 and α-IR3, followed by incubation with Apo2L/TRAIL (50 ng/mL; 8 hours). All incubations contained non-specific isotype IgG at a final concentration of 3 μg/mL. Asterisks: * *P* < 0.05; error bars: mean ± SD of triplicate determinations from 3 independent experiments.

Next, IGF-1 concentration response experiments were performed. As shown in Figure 2A, IGF-1 in the range 10-100 ng/mL induced apoptosis resistance to Apo2L/TRAIL in VH-64 cells (IC$_{50}$ of IGF-1 ~1.3 nM [~10 ng/mL]) during 24-hour incubation periods. Equivalent IGF-1 concentrations (10-100 ng/mL) and IC$_{50}$ (~1.3 nM IGF-1) amplified Apo2L/TRAIL lethality during 72-hour incubation periods (Figure 2B). α-IR3, a specific IGF-1R antibody (Kato *et al.*, 1993), in the range 100-1000 ng/mL also elicited biphasic effects on Apo2L/TRAIL-induced apoptosis causing suppression during 24-hour and amplification during 72-hour incubation periods (Figures 2A and 2B). Under each incubation condition, the antibody was 2.2 times more efficient (IC$_{50}$ of α-IR3 ~0.6 nM [~100 ng/mL]) than IGF-1. When used at peak concentrations, α-IR3 was ~2 times less potent compared with IGF-1. This finding suggests that IGF-1R binding sites with similar affinities for a given agonist are responsible for the transduction of opposite biological responses.

To gain further insight into the mechanism by which IGF-1 modulates Apo2L/TRAIL lethality in ESFT cells, we investigated whether caspase-like proteases were involved in Apo2L/TRAIL-induced apoptosis. As shown in Figure 3A, the caspase-3/-7 antagonist z-DEVD-fmk prevented Apo2L/TRAIL lethality in a dose-dependent fashion in both IGF-1-treated and untreated cells.

We then examined the effect of IGF-1 on different components of the caspase cascade. The activation of caspase-8, a key upstream mediator of extrinsic and intrinsic apoptosis, caspase-9, a downstream mediator of intrinsic apoptosis, and caspase-3/-7, key effector caspases of extrinsic and intrinsic apoptosis, was monitored by luminescence assay. IGF-1 treatment suppressed the activation of caspase-8 and caspase-3/-7 by Apo2L/TRAIL after 24 hours but increased their activities after 48-72 hours (Figure 3B). IGF-1 failed to modify the activation of caspase-9 by Apo2L/TRAIL. During the entire incubation period, IGF-1 as a single agent did not significantly affect caspase activity.

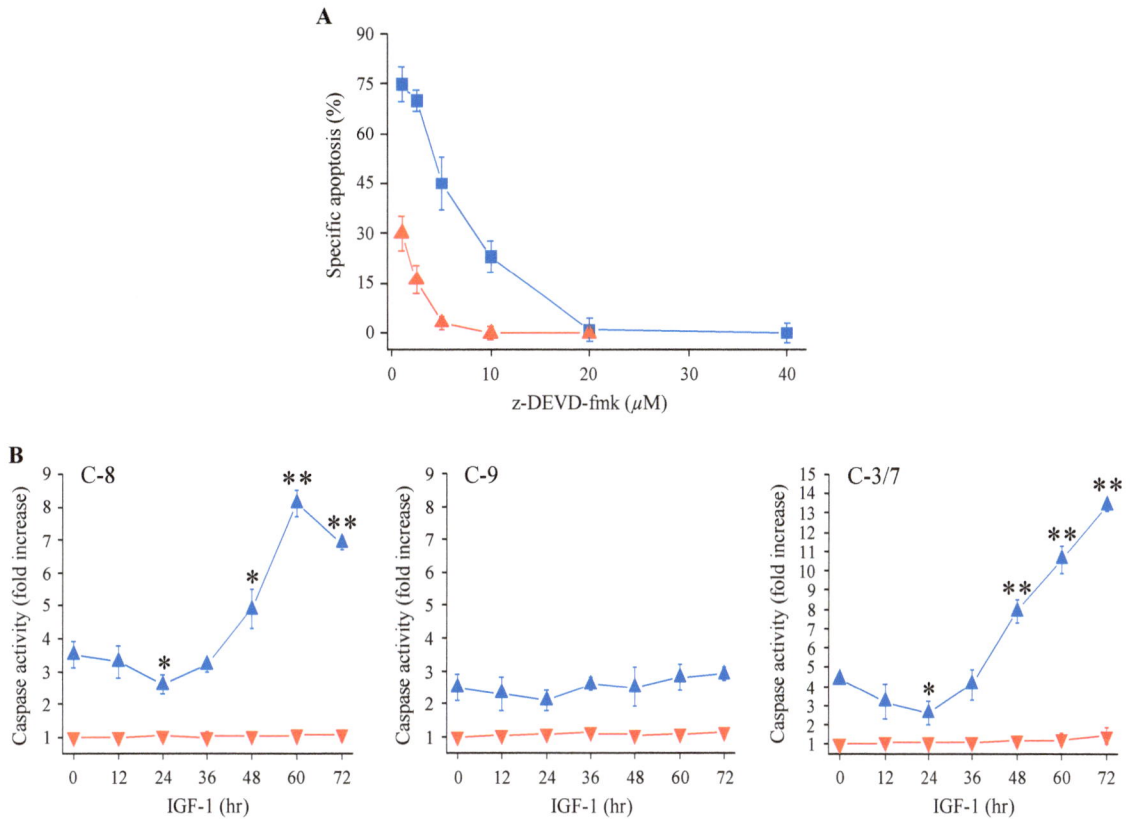

Figure 3: Involvement of caspase-like proteases in Apo2L/TRAIL-induced apoptosis. *A.* Percentage-specific apoptosis in VH-64 cells treated for 72 hours in the absence (▲) and presence (■) of IGF-1 (100 ng/mL), and subsequently for 30 min with varying concentrations of caspase-3/-7 inhibitor (*z-DEVD-fmk*), followed by incubation with Apo2L/TRAIL (50 ng/mL; 8 hours). Error bars: mean $\pm$ SD of triplicate determinations from 2 independent experiments. *B.* Fold increase in the activity of caspase-8 (*C-8*), caspase-9 (*C-9*) and caspase-3/-7 (*C-3/7*) in cells treated for the indicated times with IGF-1 (100 ng/mL), followed by incubation in the absence (▼) and presence (▲) of Apo2L/TRAIL (50 ng/mL; 4 hours). Values of vehicle-treated controls for caspase-8, caspase-9, and caspase-3/-7 activity were set to 1. Asterisks: * $P < 0.05$, ** $P < 0.02$; error bars: mean $\pm$ SD of triplicate determinations from 3 independent experiments.

We next investigated whether IGF-1 could modulate the expression of specific anti-apoptotic and pro-apoptotic proteins that may regulate Apo2L/TRAIL signalling in ESFT cells. IGF-1 stimulated the expression of XIAP protein within 12-24 hours (Figure 4A). However, prolonged incubation of cells with IGF-1 revealed that the increase in XIAP expression was only temporary and was inhibited 48 hours after IGF-1 addition. Mitochondria-related pro-apoptotic Bax appeared somewhat less at 24-48 hours and anti-apoptotic Mcl-1 appeared more at 24-48 hours than at time zero. Immunoassay evaluation of XIAP affirmed that IGF-1 exhibited a biphasic effect on XIAP expression; 12-24 hours after IGF-1 incubation XIAP protein level was increased, followed by its reduction to below basal level at 48-72 hours (Figure 4B).

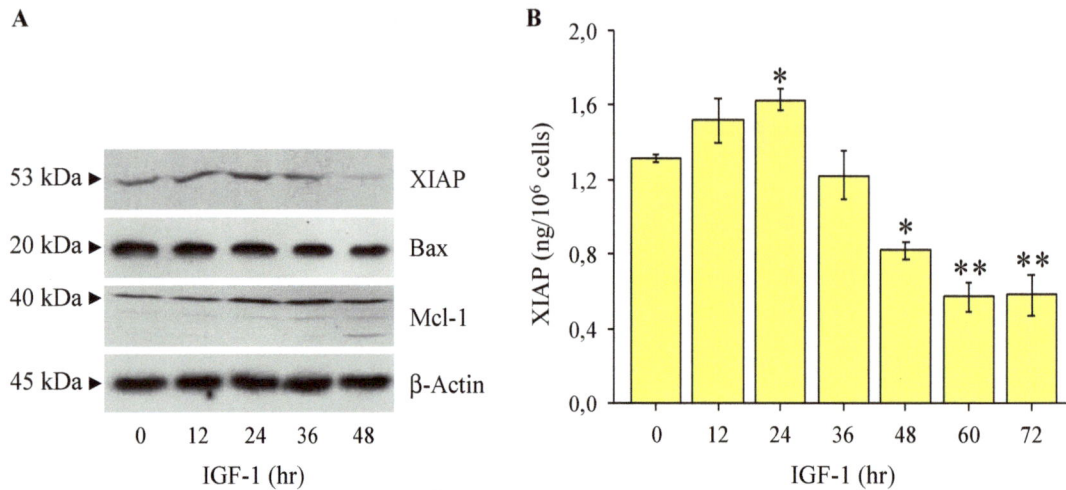

Figure 4: IGF-1 has biphasic effects on XIAP protein expression. *A.* Western blot assays of VH-64 cell lysates with antibodies to XIAP, Bax and Mcl-1. Cells were treated for the indicated times with IGF-1 (100 ng/mL). Representative non-stripped blots separately probed with the different antibodies are shown. Expression of β-actin was used to control equal protein loading. *B.* EIA analysis of XIAP in cells incubated for the indicated times with IGF-1 (100 ng/mL). Asterisks: * $P < 0.05$, ** $P < 0.02$; error bars: mean $\pm$ SD of triplicate determinations from 4 independent experiments.

AKT mediates survival of ESFT cells induced by IGF-1 (Toretsky *et al.*, 1999). Moreover, XIAP is a direct target of AKT (Dan *et al.*, 2004). We first investigated the effect of IGF-1 on AKT and its downstream serine/threonine protein kinase, GSK-3. As shown in Figure 5A, incubation of cells with IGF-1 resulted in increased phosphorylation (*i.e.*, activation) of pAKT and phosphorylation (*i.e.*, inhibition) of pGSK-3 within 6 hours. However, continuous incubation of cells with IGF-1 led to gradual inhibition of AKT activity and stimulation of pGSK-3 activity, as demonstrated by the hypophosphorylation of pAKT and pGSK-3 at 48 hours. Analysis of the pAKT/AKT and pGSK-3/GSK-3 ratios by immunoassays also revealed dual regulation of AKT and GSK-3 activities by IGF-1; 6 hours after IGF-1 addition the ratios were increased, followed by their decrease to below basal values at 48-72 hours (Figure 5B). Treatment of cells with 500 nM wortmannin (WM), a specific PI3K inhibitor, reduced the basal pAKT/AKT ratio from $0{,}321 \pm 0{,}019$ to $0{,}123 \pm 0{,}011$, which is comparable to the ratio obtained after incubation of cells for 72 hours with IGF-1 (50 ng/mL) alone (*i.e.*, $0{,}121 \pm 0{,}009$). Moreover, WM completely prevented the increase in pAKT/AKT ratio upon treatment of cells with IGF-1 for up to 24 hours (data not shown). Noteworthy, WM partially reduced the basal pGSK-3/GSK-3 ratio but failed to inhibit its stimulation by IGF-1. Instead Ro-31-8425 (2 μM), a specific protein kinase C inhibitor, potently reduced the basal pGSK-3/GSK-3 ratio and partially prevented its stimulation by IGF-1 (data not shown).

We then examined whether inhibition of AKT activity by WM could alter apoptosis induced by Apo2L/TRAIL in ESFT cells. Treatment of cells with WM augmented Apo2L/TRAIL-mediated apoptosis in a concentration-dependent manner. Sensitization to Apo2L/TRAIL was more efficient in untreated cells, compared to cells that had been treated with IGF-1 for 24 hours (Figure 5C). TDZD-8 (10 μM), a specific GSK-3 inhibitor, and rapamycin (20 ng/mL), a specific mTOR inhibitor, did not significantly affect Apo2L/TRAIL-induced apoptosis in IGF-1-treated and untreated cells (data not shown).

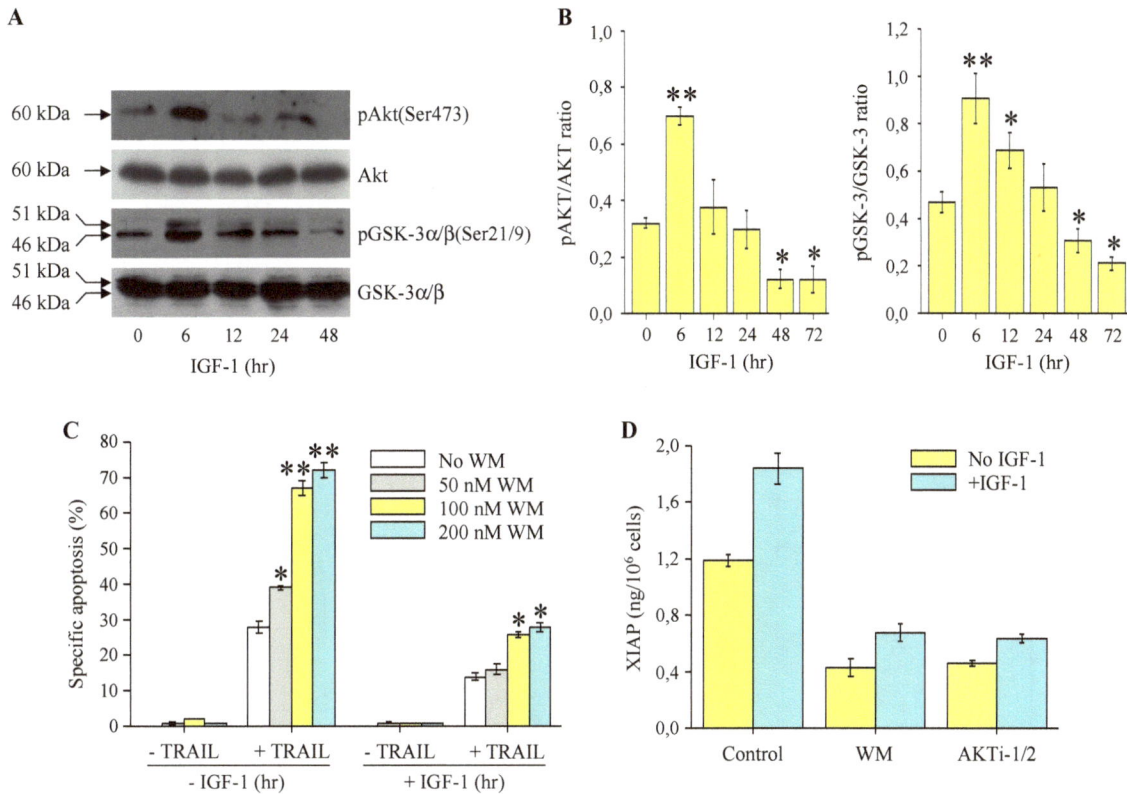

Figure 5: Activation of AKT is associated with increased XIAP protein expression and Apo2L/TRAIL resistance. *A.* Western blot assays of VH-64 cell lysates with antibodies to phosphorylated AKT (*pAKT(Ser473)*) and GSK-3 (*pGSK-3α/β(Ser21/9)*), and total AKT (*AKT*) and GSK-3 (*GSK-3α/β*). Cells were treated for the indicated times with IGF-1 (100 ng/mL). Representative non-stripped blots separately probed with the different antibodies are shown. *B.* Ratio of phosphorylated AKT to total AKT (*pAKT/AKT*) and of phosphorylated GSK-3β to total GSK-3β (*pGSK-3/GSK-3*) determined by immunoassay in cells treated for the indicated times with IGF-1 (100 ng/mL). *C.* Percentage-specific apoptosis in VH-64 cells treated with the indicated concentrations of wortmannin (*WM*) in the absence and presence of IGF-1 (50 ng/mL; 24 hours), followed by incubation without and with Apo2L/TRAIL (*TRAIL*; 50 ng/mL; 8 hours). *D.* EIA analysis of XIAP in cells treated with wortmannin (*WM*; 500 nM), AKTi-1/2 (2 μM) or serum-free medium alone (*Control*), followed by incubation in the absence and presence of IGF-1 (100 ng/mL; 24 hours). Asterisks: * $P < 0.05$, ** $P < 0.02$; error bars: mean ± SD of triplicate determinations from 3 independent experiments.

To evaluate the importance of AKT activity in XIAP expression induced by IGF-1, we measured XIAP protein levels in cells treated with WM and the specific AKT inhibitor, AKTi-1/2. As shown in Figure 5D, WM (500 nM) and AKTi-1/2 (2 μM) reduced constitutive XIAP levels and partially inhibited the increase in XIAP expression stimulated by IGF-1 at 24 hours.

Together, these data suggest that activation of PI3K–AKT is associated with stimulation of XIAP expression and Apo2L/TRAIL resistance in ESFT cells in response to short term IGF-1 exposure.

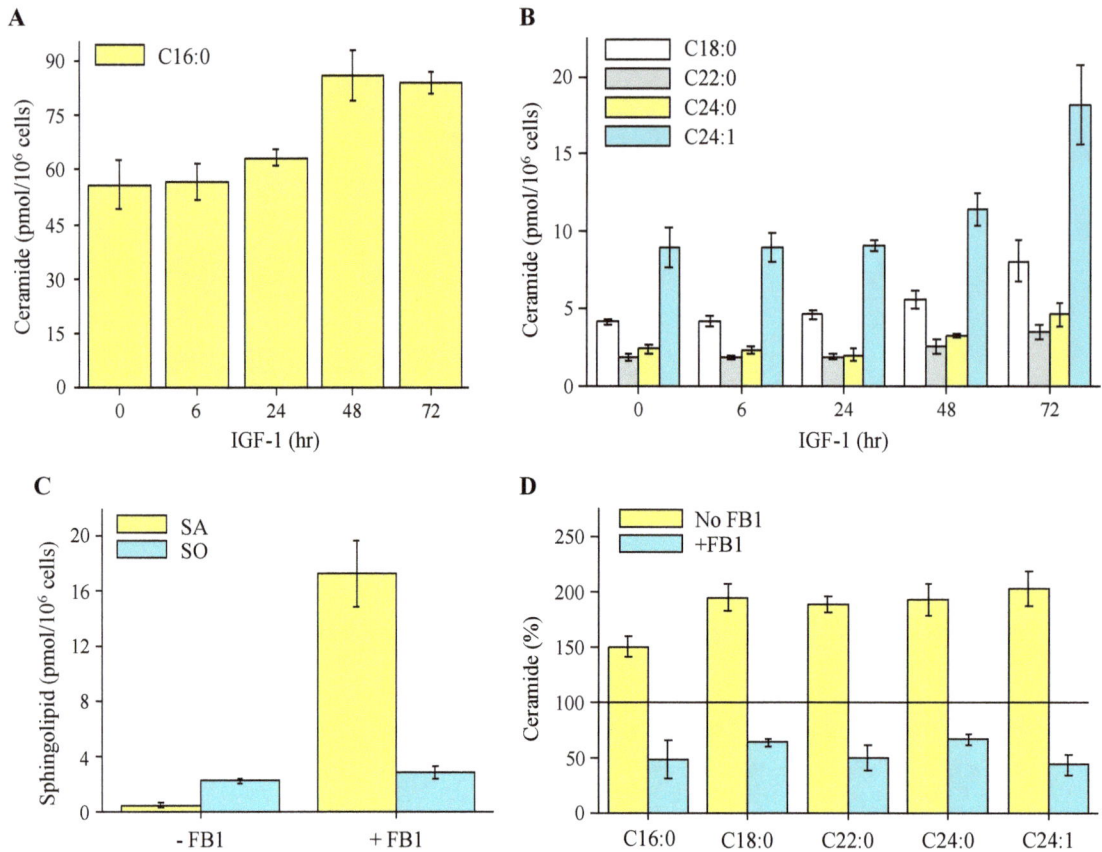

Figure 6: IGF-1 increases *de novo* ceramide (CER) formation. Levels of (*A*) C16:0-CER and (*B*) C18:0-, C22:0-, C24:0-, and C24:1-CER in VH-64 cells incubated for the indicated times with IGF-1 (100 ng/mL). *C*. Levels of sphinganine (*SA*) and sphingosine (*SO*) in VH-64 cells treated for 72 hours with IGF-1 (100 ng/mL) in the absence and presence of fumonisin B1 (*FB1*; 30 μM). *D*. Percentage of different CER species in VH-64 cells treated for 72 hours with IGF-1 (100 ng/mL) in the absence and presence of fumonisin B1 (*FB1*; 30 μM). Values of vehicle-treated controls for the different CER species were set to 100 %. Error bars: mean $\pm$ SD of triplicate determinations.

The sphingolipid molecule ceramide (CER) has been implicated in long term IGF-1 signalling (Chi *et al.*, 2000; Costantini *et al.*, 2006). Furthermore, CER formation has been linked to inhibition of AKT activity and down-regulation of XIAP protein expression (Schmitz-Peiffer *et al.*, 1999; Kroesen *et al.*, 2003). To investigate the extent to which CER synthesis is involved in Apo2L/TRAIL sensitization, XIAP suppression and AKT inhibition induced by long term IGF-1 stimulation, we first measured intracellular CER expression in VH-64 cells and its regulation by IGF-1. Several CER species were detected particularly C16:0-, C18:0-, C22:0-, C24:0-, and C24:1-CER of which C16:0-CER was the most abundant compound determined by HPLC-ESI-MS/MS (Figures 6A and 6B). CER levels were not changed after 24 hours exposure to IGF-1. However, treatment of cells with IGF-1 for 48-72 hours induced a 1.5- to 2-fold increase in CER levels.

A

B

C

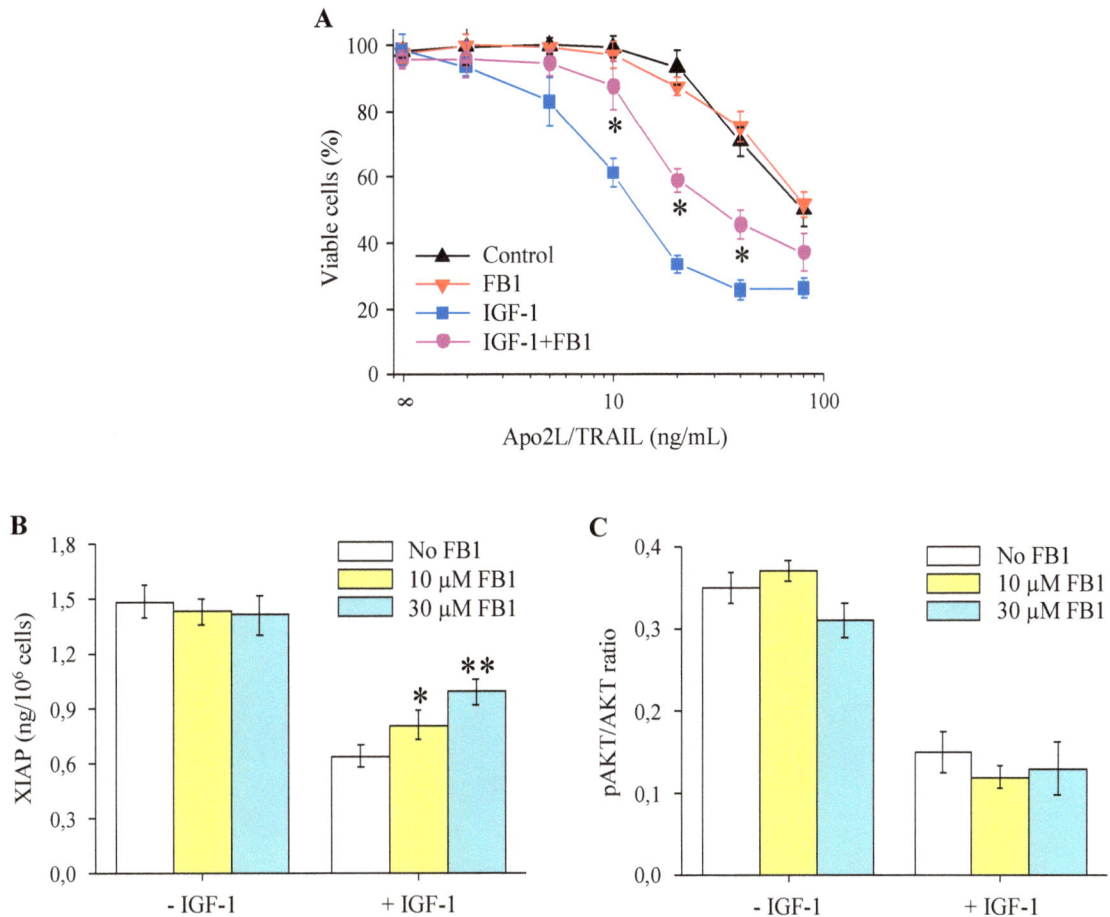

Figure 7: Functional consequences of *de novo* CER formation. *A.* Percentage of viable VH-64 cells treated for 72 hours without (▲, ▼) and with (•, ■) IGF-1 (100 ng/mL) in the absence (▲, ■) and presence (▼, •) of fumonisin B1 (*FB1*; 30 μM), followed by incubation for 18 hours with the indicated concentrations of Apo2L/TRAIL. *B.* EIA analysis of XIAP in VH-64 cells treated for 72 hours without and with IGF-1 (100 ng/mL), in the presence of the indicated concentrations of fumonisin B1 (*FB1*). *C.* Ratio of phosphorylated AKT to total AKT (*pAKT/AKT*) determined by ELISA in cells treated for 72 hours without and with IGF-1 (100 ng/mL) in the presence of the indicated concentrations of fumonisin B1 (*FB1*). Asterisks: * $P < 0.05$, ** $P < 0.02$; error bars: mean $\pm$ SD of quadruplicate determinations from 3 indepen-dent experiments.

Intracellular CER formation is derived from two main pathways: the ceramide synthase (CerS)-dependent CER *de novo* pathway and the CerS-dependent CER salvage pathway (Mullen et al., 2012). To delineate the pathway that is utilized by IGF-1 to increase CER generation, we measured the expression of sphinganine (SA), a precursor in the *de novo* CER pathway, and sphingosine (SO), a precursor in the CER salvage pathway. As demonstrated in Figure 6C, addition of the specific CerS inhibitor fumonisin B1 (FB1) during IGF-1 treatment resulted in the accumulation of SA but not SO. Moreover, treatment of cells with FB1 completely blocked the stimulation of CER formation by IGF-1 (Figure 6D).

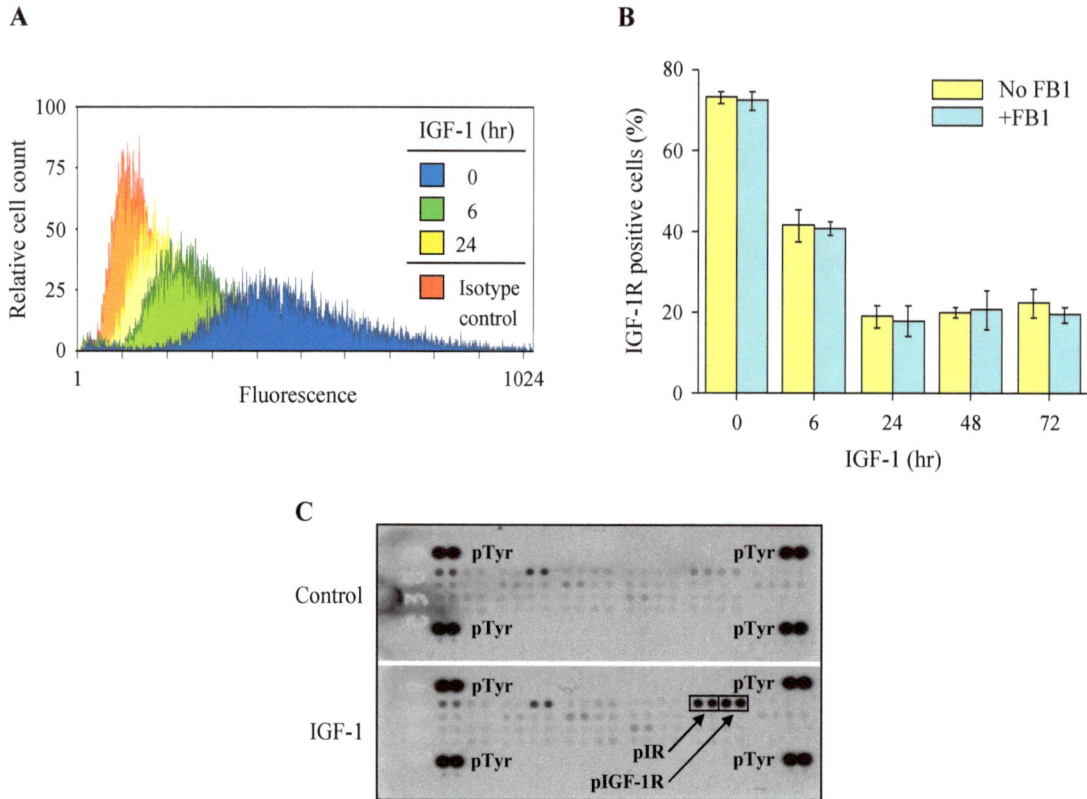

Figure 8: IGF-1 induces activation and down-regulation of IGF-1R. *A.* Histogram showing cell-surface expression of IGF-1R in VH-64 cells treated for the indicated times with IGF-1 (50 ng/mL). *B.* Percentage IGF-1R-positive cells determined by density blots in VH-64 cultures treated for the indicated times with IGF-1 (50 ng/mL) in the absence and presence of fumonisin B1 (*FB1*; 30 μM). Cells were stained with Alexa Fluor®488-conjugated mouse anti-human IGF-1R. Alexa Fluor®488-conjugated mouse IgG1 was used as isotype control. *C.* Human proteome profiler phosphorylated-RTK antibody arrays were employed to screen for activation of specific tyrosine kinases in VH-64 cells treated with IGF-1 (50 ng/mL; 30 min) or serum-free medium alone (*Control*). *pIGF-1R*, tyrosine-phosphorylated IGF-1R; *pIR*, tyrosine-phosphorylated insulin receptor; *pTyr*, tyrosine-phosphorylated control duo spots. *Columns*, means of duplicate determinations from two independent experiments; *bars*, SD.

We then investigated the functional consequences of CER formation by IGF-1 using FB1. As shown in Figure 7A, addition of FB1 suppressed Apo2L/TRAIL lethality in IGF-1-treated but not untreated cells. To assess whether CER formation amplifies Apo2L/TRAIL-induced apoptosis through inhibition of XIAP levels, we investigated the effect of FB1 on XIAP expression in long term IGF-1-stimulated cells. As demonstrated in Figure 7B, FB1 reversed the repression of XIAP protein in a concentration-dependent manner in IGF-1-treated but not untreated cells. Under these conditions, FB1 did not modulate the inhibition of AKT activity induced by IGF-1 at 72 hours (Figure 7C).

These results suggest that CER generation via *de novo* synthesis mediates XIAP repression and Apo2L/TRAIL amplification in ESFT cells in response to long term IGF-1 exposure.

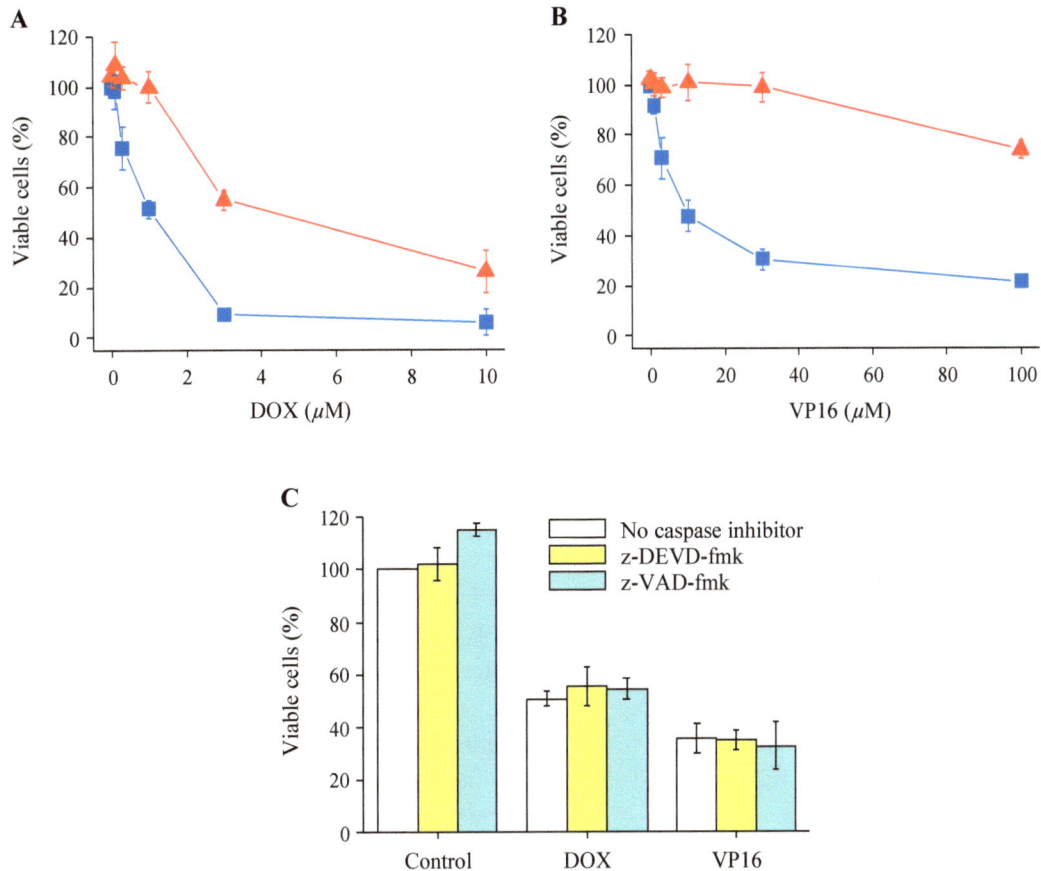

Figure 9: Long term IGF-1 treatment induces resistance to conventional chemotherapeutic agents doxorubicin (DOX) and etoposide (VP16). Percentage of viable VH-64 cells incubated for 72 hours in the absence (■) and presence (▲) of IGF-1 (100 ng/mL), followed by incubation for 18 hours with the indicated concentrations of *(A)* DOX and *(B)* VP16. *C.* Percentage of viable VH-64 cells incubated for 30 min with caspase-3/-7 inhibitor (*z-DEVD-fmk*; 20 μM), general caspase inhibitor (*z-VAD-fmk*; 20 μM) or vehicle (*no caspase inhibitor*), followed by incubation for 18 hours with DOX (1.5 μM), VP16 (20 μM) or serum-free medium alone (*Control*). Error bars: mean ± SD of triplicate determinations from 4 independent experiments.

We next examined the expression of IGF-1R and its regulation by IGF-1. VH-64 cells constitutively express IGF-1R and IGF-1 treatment induced a reduction in cell-surface IGF-1R within 6 hours and with maximal effect observed at 24-72 hours (Figures 8A and 8B). Basal expression of IGF-1R and its decrease by IGF-1 were insensitive to FB1 (Figure 8B). Screening for activation of RTKs in serum-free conditions revealed that treatment of VH-64 cells with IGF-1 resulted in tyrosine phosphorylation of the IGF-1R and the insulin receptor (IR) determined by human phosphorylated-RTK antibody arrays (Figure 8C).

Studies in ESFT cells have shown that short term IGF-1 treatment (≤ 24 hours) provides resistance to chemotherapeutic agents DOX and VP16 (Hofbauer et al., 1993; Toretsky et al., 1999), and this was confirmed by us (data not shown). We then assessed the effect of long term IGF-1 treatment on chemotoxicity. As shown in Figures 9A and 9B, exposure of VH-64 cells to IGF-1 (100 ng/mL) for 72 hours induced resistance to DOX (0.3-10 μM) and VP16 (3-100 μM). Evaluation of the mode of chemo-therapy-mediated cytotoxicity revealed that the caspase-3/-7 inhibitor z-DEVD-fmk and the pan-caspase inhibitor z-VAD-fmk did not prevent DOX- and VP16-induced cell death (Figure 9C).

4   Discussion

Very few studies in human cells have documented cell degenerating activity of IGF-1 in the context of death ligand-mediated cytotoxicity. Thus, in addition to its stimulatory effect on cell survival, IGF-1 has been shown to amplify Fas antibody-induced apoptosis in normal and malignant osteoblastic cells (Ka-wakami *et al.*, 1998), and to enhance Apo2L/TRAIL-mediated apoptosis in some colon carcinoma cell lines (Remacle-Bonnet *et al.*, 2005). The mechanisms by which IGF-1 can have opposite effects on cell death are incompletely understood and may be cell type-specific.

In this study, we investigated the role of the IGF-1–IGF-1R axis in regulating the responsiveness of ESFT cells to apoptosis induced by Apo2L/TRAIL. The findings show that time is an important factor in deciding whether IGF-1 may act as pro-survival factor or pro-death factor. The results demonstrate that opposite to the temporary survival effect of acute IGF1 treatment, chronic IGF1 treatment amplifies Apo2L/TRAIL lethality. Dual regulation of cell fate by IGF-1 is observed in Apo2L/TRAIL-responsive but not resistant cell lines, suggesting that IGF-1 operates by modifying Apo2L/TRAIL-responsiveness rather than by reversing resistance *per se*. The ability of IGF-1 at physiological range to facilitate Apo2L/TRAIL-mediated apoptosis could be an explanation for the exquisite Apo2L/TRAIL-sensitivity encountered in the majority of established ESFT cell lines *in vitro* and primary patient-derived ESFT cells *ex vivo* when maintained in culture media supplemented with serum (Van Valen *et al.*, 2000; Kontny *et al.*, 2001; Kumar *et al.*, 2001; Mitsiades *et al.*, 2001).

Our results concord with previous accounts of PI3K–AKT-dependent protection from death-inducing stimuli in ESFT cells (Toretsky *et al.*, 1999; Hotfilder *et al.*, 2005). The data show that inhibi-tion of PI3K–AKT by WM and AKTi-1/2 results in sensitization to Apo2L/TRAIL, indicating that PI3K–AKT signalling prevents efficient induction of apoptosis by Apo2L/TRAIL. The results demonstrate that WM and AKTi-1/2 inhibit constitutive XIAP levels. However, WM and AKTi-1/2 do not completely prevent the up-regulation of XIAP levels by IGF-1, implying that alternative survival signal transduction pathways are also involved in IGF-1-mediated stimulation of XIAP expression. Incubation with WM for 24 hours does not affect ESFT cell viability, suggesting that PI3K–AKT inactivation itself does not in-duce apoptosis. Collectively, the findings indicate that increased XIAP protein expression by PI3K–AKT pathway is one mechanism responsible for inhibition of Apo2L/TRAIL-induced apoptosis in ESFT cells following acute IGF-1 treatment.

The results showed that long term IGF-1 treatment induces inactivation of AKT and down-regulation of XIAP protein levels. Meanwhile, the same treatment results in *de novo* CER formation that correlated well with the progression of Apo2L/TRAIL sensitivity. Although we demonstrated that AKT activation is associated with XIAP up-regulation by early IGF-1 stimulation, the inhibition of AKT does not account for XIAP down-regulation by IGF-1 at later stages. We find that *de novo*-generated CER me-diates repression of XIAP at a level downstream or independent of AKT. The mechanism by which CER may cause down-regulation of XIAP in ESFT cells is presently unknown. Studies in B-cell receptor-activated lymphoma cells have shown that *de novo* CER formation can induce degradation of XIAP in a proteasome-dependent manner (Kroesen *et al.*, 2003). Also, the mechanism for inactivation of AKT in response to long term IGF-1 stimulation is unclear. In many cell types, Rui *et al.* (2001) have found that chronic IGF-1 stimulation of mTOR can result in feedback inhibition of PI3K–AKT signalling through phosphorylation and subsequent proteasomal degradation of insulin receptor substrate-2 (IRS-2).

Evidence indicates that *de novo*-generated CER can trigger cell death, *e.g.*, by stimulation of caspases (Ogretmen & Hannun, 2004). In this study, *de novo* CER formation upon treatment of cells for 72 hours with IGF-1 does not result in apoptosis. This finding differs from CER species accumulated *de novo* in other human cell systems in response to various stress stimuli. For example, *de novo*-generated C16- and/or C24-CER provoked apoptosis in lymphoma cells in response to B-cell receptor activation (Kroesen et al., 2003), in prostate carcinoma cells by androgen deprivation and interleukin-24 stimulation (Eto *et al.*, 2003; Sauane *et al.*, 2010), and in neutrophils by cell autonomous mechanisms (Seumois *et al.*, 2007). Alternatively, apart from its biological effects as intracellular second messenger, CER may also have biophysical effects through the formation of membrane lipid raft microdomains (caveolae) affecting the localization of receptors and their function (van Blitterswijk *et al.*, 2003). In relation to this option, it is of interest that membrane lipid rafts have been reported to segregate pro-apoptotic from anti-apoptotic IGF-1R signal transduction pathways (Remacle-Bonnet *et al.*, 2005). Furthermore, recent studies have pointed out that the redistribution of Apo2L/TRAIL death receptors DR4 and DR5 to membrane lipid rafts constitutes an important regulatory event for optimal activation of the apoptotic death programme (Pennarun *et al.*, 2010).

The findings revealed that IGF-1 stimulates IGF-1R down-regulation prior to the onset of its pro-apoptotic effects such as *de novo* CER formation and support the view that IGF-1R signalling can continue and also change after receptor down-regulation (Sorkin & von Zastrow, 2009). Previously, Martins *et al.* (2011) showed that IGF-1R undergoes ligand-dependent down-regulation through internalization in ESFT cells. Taking into account these observations, our findings are most consistent with a spatio-temporal model of IGF-1R signalling, with a role of IGF-1R internalization in transmitting CER-dependent pro-death signals from intracellular compartments and AKT-dependent pro-survival signals from IGF-1R at the cell surface (Figure 10). We find that IR is also phosphorylated by IGF-1, implying that part of IGF-1 signal transduction could be via IR homodimeric and/or IGF-1R–IR heterodimeric receptors (Samani *et al.*, 2007). Obviously, the mechanisms for regulation of Apo2L/TRAIL-mediated apoptosis by IGF-1 are complex. Nevertheless, it is reasonable to assume that CER–XIAP signalling represents a key pathway for sensitization to Apo2L/TRAIL-induced apoptosis in ESFT cells following chronic IGF-1 treatment.

IGF-1 regulates Apo2L/TRAIL-mediated caspase-3/-7 activation in a biphasic fashion, whereas IGF-1 does not affect caspase-9 activation. The undulating modulation of caspase-3/-7 activation inversely correlates with changes in XIAP expression by IGF-1 treatment, a finding in agreement with studies reported previously on the critical function of XIAP in regulating caspase-3/-7 activation during apoptosis (Scott *et al.*, 2005; Varfolomeev *et al.*, 2009; Sensintaffar *et al.*, 2010). We also showed that IGF-1 displays biphasic effects on caspase-8 activation, suggesting that IGF-1 oppositely regulates expression of apoptotic molecules of the Apo2L/TRAIL signalling pathway upstream of caspase-3/-7. Preliminary experiments demonstrated that IGF-1 does not change the expression profile of death receptors for Apo2L/TRAIL (unpublished data). Interestingly, several reports have indicated that caspase-3/-7 can mediate feedback regulation of caspase-8 activation in death receptor-induced apoptosis (Yang *et al.*, 2006; Ferreira *et al.*, 2012). Together, the data suggest that the dual effect of IGF-1 on Apo2L/TRAIL-mediated cell death relies to a large extent on modulation of the extrinsic rather than the intrinsic signalling pathway of apoptosis.

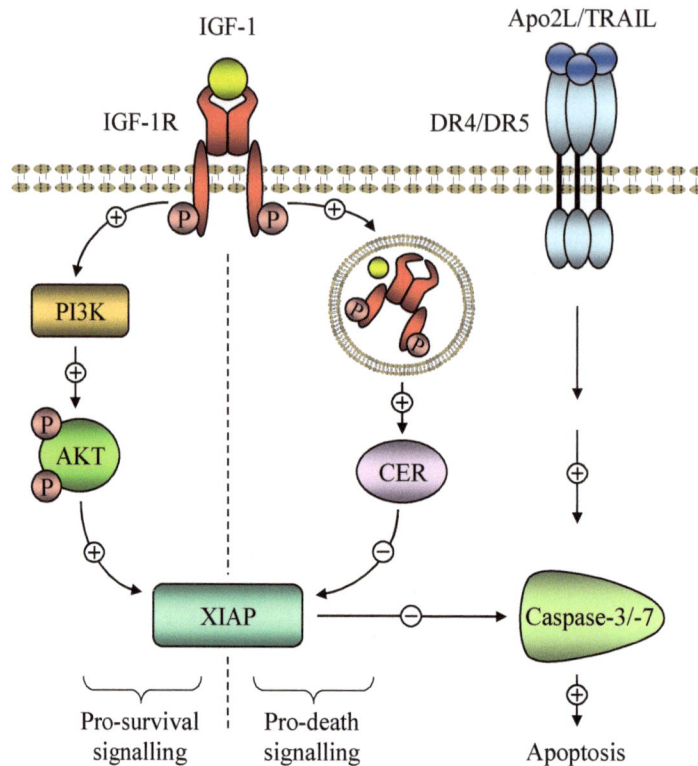

Figure 10: Spatio-temporal model of IGF-1–IGF-1R regulation of Apo2L/TRAIL-induced apoptosis. Short term IGF-1 stimulation results in activation of IGF-1R–PI3K–AKT–XIAP signalling
pathway that is associated with reduced Apo2L/TRAIL lethality, whereas long term IGF-1 stimulation results in activation of IGF-1R–CER–XIAP signalling pathway that is associated with increased Apo2L/TRAIL lethality. IGF-1 induces IGF-1R down-regulation presumably through internalization (Martins *et al.*, 2011), prior to stimulation of CER formation.

We showed that while Apo2L/TRAIL-insensitive VH-64 cells can be converted to sensitive, their
sensitiveness to DOX and VP16 is hampered by long term IGF-1 stimulation. The latter event occurred in
spite of the inactivation of AKT. As far as the resistance to DOX and VP16 is concerned, the early stimulation of AKT by IGF-1 could be the point of no return. However, alternative survival signalling pathways activated by IGF-1 may as well promote resistance to conventional chemotherapeutic agents, as
discussed by Toretsky *et al.* (1999). Using ESFT cells stably expressing a myristoylated version of AKT,
these authors showed that constitutively active AKT only partially accounted for the suppression of
chemotoxicity.

We also demonstrated that DOX- and VP16-mediated cytotoxicity is not obstructed by caspase inhibitor at a concentration (20 μM) that readily prevented Apo2L/TRAIL lethality, indicating that the main
mode of DOX- and VP16-induced cell death is caspase-independent. Although a previous study in ESFT
cells reported inhibition of VP-16-induced cytotoxicity by caspase inhibitors z-DEVD-fmk and z-VAD-
fmk (Mauz-Körholz *et al.*, 2004), it must be pointed out that the caspase inhibitor concentration used in
that study was high enough (100 μM) to block non-caspase proteases in a non-specific manner (Schotte *et*

al., 1999). It is apparent from our findings that beyond its role in resistance to conventional chemotherapy, IGF-1 can bypass this resistance and selectively sensitize ESFT cells to caspase-dependent apoptosis induction by Apo2L/TRAIL.

The physiological significance of our results has yet to be shown. Apo2L/TRAIL is considered the prime host-defence mechanism against incipient cancers and can be expressed by various cells of the immune system such as natural killer cells, dendritic cells, macrophages, and T lymphocytes (Falschlehner *et al.*, 2009). A growing body of evidence points to a pronounced influence of IGF-1 on the maintenance of normal immune function (Smith, 2010). As lymphohaematopoietic factor, IGF-1 has been reported previously to stimulate lymphocyte proliferation and survival, to accelerate cytokine-stimulated natural killer cell activity, and to support monocyte-derived dendritic cell maturation *in vivo* and *in vitro* (Clark *et al.*, 1993; Auernhammer *et al.*, 1996; van Buul-Offers & Kooijman, 1998; Liu *et al.*, 2003). Recently, studies have indicated that lymphocyte recovery is an independent prognostic indicator for high-risk ESFT (De Angulo *et al.*, 2007), and that ESFT cells are highly sensitive to killing by autologous dendritic cells and allogeneic natural killer cells *in vivo* and *in vitro* (Suminoe *et al.*, 2009; Cho *et al.*, 2010). Hence, it is worth considering the extent to which IGF-1 may facilitate Apo2L/TRAIL-mediated ESFT cytotoxicity *in vivo* not only directly but also indirectly through stimulation of an innate immune response.

Another intriguing aspect of the present study relates to α-IR3. This specific IGF-1R antibody has been employed to modulate ESFT cell growth *in vitro* and *in vivo* (Yee *et al.*, 1992; Scotlandi *et al.*, 1996; Scotlandi *et al.*, 1998). The inhibition of cell proliferation by α-IR3 has been interpreted to result from obstructing the activation of IGF-1R by growth factor released by the tumour cells in an autocrine manner. The current study reveals that α-IR3 behaves like a protagonist, mimicking the short term Apo2L/TRAIL-inhibitory and long term Apo2L/TRAIL-stimulatory effects of IGF-1 thus contradicting the antagonist concept. Furthermore, the data show that constitutive levels of phosphorylated IGF-1R (and IR) in serum-free conditions are extremely low, implying that an autocrine mechanism is essentially absent in the cells. With respect to α-IR3 displaying protagonist features, numerous studies in malignant and non-malignant cells have documented that α-IR3 can operate as an activating IGF-1R antibody and substitute for a plethora of biochemical and biological effects of IGF-1 and IGF-2 on IGF-1R including phosphorylation/activation and down-regulation/internalization of IGF-1R, synthesis and release of IGFBPs, production of vascular endothelial growth factor (VEGF), stimulation of cell proliferation, cell differentiation and cell contractility, and stimulation and inhibition of apoptosis (Bergmann *et al.*, 1995; Chi *et al.*, 2000; De Leon *et al.*, 1992; Duan *et al.*, 1996; Kato *et al.*, 1993; Katz *et al.*, 1995; Kinugawa *et al.*, 1999; Lee *et al.*, 2003; Li *et al.*, 1993; Pommier *et al.*, 1992; Remacle-Bonnet *et al.*, 2000; Reynolds *et al.*, 1996; Soos *et al.*, 1992; Steele-Perkins & Roth, 1990; Warren *et al.*, 1996; Zhang *et al.*, 2006).

Recently, studies have been focusing on the use of IGF-1R antibody as potential therapy in ESFT patients (Ho & Schwartz, 2011; Malempati *et al.*, 2012; O'Neill *et al.*, 2013; Wagner & Maki, 2013). Apparently, the ability to initiate down-regulation and nuclear localization of IGF-1R rather than to inhibit IGF-1R activity or to compete with the ligand is required for the anti-ESFT activity of several humanized IGF-1R antibodies including those developed by Pfizer (CP-751,871) and Hoffmann-La Roche (R1507) (Asmane *et al.*, 2012; Zheng *et al.*, 2012). Jürgens *et al.* (2011) reported preliminary data from a phase I/II trial evaluating the efficacy of CP-751,871 (figitumumab), in which treatment of 106 patients with advanced ESFT resulted in a modest overall response rate of 14.2% and median survival of 8.9 months. Disappointing response rates of 10% and median survival of 7.6 months were also recorded in a phase II study involving 109 patients with recurrent or refractory ESFT following treatment with R1507 (teprotumumab) (Pappo *et al.*, 2011). Clearly, the results of these and other clinical trials (Baserga, 2013) have blunted excitement for using IGF-1R antibody as a single agent for the management of ESFT. However, in view of our *in vitro* data demonstrating the apoptosis-sensitizing effects of α-IR3 in ESFT cells, it is tempting to speculate that the clinical benefit of IGF-1R antibody therapy could extend to more patients when it is combined with Apo2L/TRAIL-based regimens.

5   Conclusions

Despite improvements over the past two decades in the therapy of ESFT, the survival expectancy for patients with recurrent or metastatic disease is still dismal. It is recognized that IGF-1 is associated with ESFT cell survival and chemoresistance. However, the present study paradoxically suggests that chronic IGF1 stimulation can bypass chemoresistance and support cell death in combination with Apo2L/TRAIL. Thus this study provides novel insight into the dynamic role of the IGF-1–IGF-1R system in regulating ESFT cell fate. Our findings showing that IGF-1R antibody displays IGF-1 mimicry may have important implications for the design of Apo2L/TRAIL-based therapies to treat refractory ESFT.

Conflict of Interests

The authors state that they have no conflict of interests.

Acknowledgements

This work was funded by the European Community's Sixth Framework Programme *Specific Targeted Research Project* (PROTHETS, 503036) to F. Van Valen, and by BMBF (TranSaRNet, 01GM0869) to M. Hotfilder, U. Dirksen and H. Jürgens.

References

Asakuma, J., Sumitomo, M., Asano, T., Asano, T., & Hayakawa, M. (2003). Selective Akt inactivation and tumor necrosis factor-related apoptosis-inducing ligand sensitization of renal cancer cells by low concentrations of paclitaxel. Cancer Research, 63(6), 1365-1370.

Ashkenazi, A. (2008). Directing cancer cells to self-destruct with pro-apoptotic receptor agonists. Nature Reviews Drug Discovery, 7(12), 1001-1012.

Ashkenazi, A., Pai, R.C., Fong, S., Leung, S., Lawrence, D.A., Marsters, S.A., Blackie, C., Chang, L., McMurtrey, A.E., Hebert, A., DeForge, L., Koumenis, I.L., Lewis, D., Harris, L., Bussiere, J., Koeppen, H., Shahrokh, Z., & Schwall, R.H. (1999). Safety and antitumor activity of recombinant soluble Apo2 ligand. Journal of Clinical Investigations, 104(2), 155-162.

Asmane, I., Watkin, E., Alberti, L., Duc, A., Marec-Berard, P., Ray-Coquard, I., Cassier, P., Decouvelaere, A.V., Ranchère, D., Kurtz, J.E., Bergerat, J.P., & Blay J.Y. (2012). Insulin-like growth factor type 1 receptor (IGF-1R) exclusive nuclear staining: a predictive biomarker for IGF-1R monoclonal antibody (Ab) therapy in sarcomas. European Journal of Cancer, 48(16), 3027-3035.

Auernhammer, C.J., Feldmeier, H., Nass, R., Pachmann, K., & Strasburger, C.J. (1996). *Insulin-like growth factor I is an independent coregulatory modulator of natural killer (NK) cell activity. Endocrinology, 137(12), 5332-5336.*

Baserga, R. (2013). *The decline and fall of the IGF-I receptor. Journal of Cellular Physiology, 228(4), 675-679.*

Bergmann, U., Funatomi, H., Yokoyama, M., Beger, H.G., & Korc, M. (1995). *Insulin-like growth factor I overexpression in human pancreatic cancer: evidence for autocrine and paracrine roles. Cancer Research, 55(10), 2007-2011.*

Chen, X., Thakkar, H., Tyan, F., Gim, S., Robinson, H., Lee, C., Pandey, S.K., Nwokorie, C., Onwudiwe, N., & Srivastava, R.K. (2001). *Constitutively active Akt is an important regulator of TRAIL sensitivity in prostate cancer. Oncogene, 20(42), 6073-6083.*

Chi, M.M.Y, Schlein, A.L., & Moley, K.H. (2000). *High insulin-like growth factor 1 (IGF-1) and insulin concentrations trigger apoptosis in the mouse blastocyst via down-regulation of the IGF-1 receptor. Endocrinology, 141(12), 4784-4792.*

Cho, D., Shook, D.R., Shimasaki, N., Chang, Y.H., Fujisaki, H., & Campana, D. (2010). *Cytotoxicity of activated natural killer cells against pediatric solid tumors. Clinical Cancer Research, 16(15), 3901-3909.*

Cironi, L., Riggi, N., Provero, P., Wolf, N., Suvà, M.L., Suvà, D., Kindler, V., & Stamenkovic, I. (2008). *IGF1 is a common target gene of Ewing's sarcoma fusion proteins in mesenchymal progenitor cells. PLoS One, 3(7), e2634.*

Clark, R., Strasser, J., McCabe, S., Robbins, K., & Jardieu, P. (1993). *Insulin-like growth factor-1 stimulation of lympho-poiesis. Journal of Clinical Investigations, 92(2), 540-548.*

Costantini, C., Scrable, H., & Puglielli, L. (2006). *An aging pathway controls the TrkA to p75NTR receptor switch and amyloid beta-peptide generation. EMBO Journal, 25(9), 1997-2006.*

Dan, H.C., Sun, M., Kaneko, S., Feldman, R.I., Nicosia, S.V., Wang, H.G., Tsang, B.K., & Cheng, J.Q. (2004). *Akt phos-phorylation and stabilization of X-linked inhibitor of apoptosis protein (XIAP). Journal of Biological Chemistry, 279(7), 5405-5412.*

De Angulo, G., Hernandez, M., Morales-Arias, J., Herzog, C.E., Anderson, P., Wolff, J., & Kleinerman, E.S. (2007). *Early lymphocyte recovery as a prognostic indicator for high-risk Ewing sarcoma. Journal of Pediatric Hemato-logy/Oncology, 29(1), 48-52.*

De Leon, D.D., Wilson, D.M., Powers, M., & Rosenfeld, R.G. (1992). *Effects of insulin-like growth factors (IGFs) and IGF receptor antibodies on the proliferation of human breast cancer cells. Growth Factors, 6(4), 327-336.*

Dirksen, U. & Jürgens, H. (2010). *Approaching Ewing sarcoma. Future Oncology, 6(7), 1155-1162.*

Duan, C., Hawes, S.B., Prevette, T., & Clemmons, D.R. (1996). *Insulin-like growth factor-I (IGF-I) regulates IGF-binding protein-5 synthesis through transcriptional activation of the gene in aortic smooth muscle cells. Journal of Biological Chemistry, 271(8), 4280-4288.*

Eto, M., Bennouna, J., Hunter, O.C., Hershberger, P.A., Kanto, T., Johnson, C.S., Lotze, M.T., & Amoscato, A.A. (2003). *C16 ceramide accumulates following androgen ablation in LNCaP prostate cancer cells. Prostate, 57(1), 66-79.*

Fakler, M., Loeder, S., Vogler, M., Schneider, K., Jeremias, I., Debatin, K.M., & Fulda, S. (2009). *Small molecule XIAP inhibitors cooperate with TRAIL to induce apoptosis in childhood acute leukemia cells and overcome Bcl-2-mediated resistance. Blood, 113(8), 1710-1722.*

Falschlehner, C., Schaefer, U., & Walczak, H. (2009). *Following TRAIL's path in the immune system. Immunology, 127(2), 145-154.*

Ferreira, K.S., Kreutz, C., Macnelly, S., Neubert, K., Haber, A., Bogyo, M., Timmer, J., & Borner, C. (2012). *Caspase-3 feeds back on caspase-8, Bid and XIAP in type I Fas signaling in primary mouse hepatocytes. Apoptosis, 17(5), 503-515.*

Herbst, R.S., Eckhardt, S.G., Kurzrock, R., Ebbinghaus, S., O'Dwyer, P.J., Gordon, M.S., Novotny, W., Goldwasser, M.A., Tohnya, T.M., Lum, B.L., Ashkenazi, A., Jubb, A.M., & Mendelson, D.S. (2010). *Phase I dose-escalation study of re-combinant human Apo2L/TRAIL, a dual proapoptotic receptor agonist, in patients with advanced cancer. Journal of Clinical Oncology, 28(17), 2839-2846.*

Ho, A.L. & Schwartz, G.K. (2011). *Targeting of insulin-like growth factor type 1 receptor in Ewing sarcoma: unfulfilled promise or a promising beginning? Journal of Clinical Oncology, 29(34), 4581-4583.*

Hofbauer, S., Hamilton, G., Theyer, G., Wollmann, K., & Gabor, F. (1993). *Insulin-like growth factor-I-dependent growth and in vitro chemosensitivity of Ewing's sarcoma and peripheral primitive neuroectodermal tumour cell lines. European Journal of Cancer, 29A(2), 241-245.*

Hotfilder, M., Sondermann, P., Senss, A., Van Valen, F., Jürgens, H., & Vormoor, J. (2005). *PI3K/AKT is involved in mediating survival signals that rescue Ewing tumour cells from fibroblast growth factor 2-induced cell death. British Journal of Cancer, 92(4), 705-710.*

Jo, M., Kim, T.H., Seol, D.W., Esplen, J.E., Dorko, K., Billiar, T.R., & Strom, S.C. (2000). *Apoptosis induced in normal human hepatocytes by tumor necrosis factor–related apoptosis-inducing ligand. Nature Medicine, 6(5), 564 -567.*

Jürgens, H., Daw, N.C., Geoerger, B., Ferrari, S., Villarroel, M., Aerts, I., Whelan, J., Dirksen, U., Hixon, M.L., Yin, D., Wang, T., Green, S., Paccagnella, L., & Gualberto, A. (2011). *Preliminary efficacy of the anti-insulin-like growth factor type 1 receptor antibody figitumumab in patients with refractory Ewing sarcoma. Journal of Clinical Oncology, 29(34), 4534-4540.*

Kato, H., Faria, T.N., Stannard, B., Roberts Jr, C.T., & LeRoith, D. (1993). *Role of tyrosine kinase activity in signal transduction by the insulin-like growth factor-I (IGF-I) receptor. Characterization of kinase-deficient IGF-I receptors and the action of an IGF-I-mimetic antibody (aIR-3). Journal of Biological Chemistry, 268(4), 2655-2661.*

Katz, J., Weiss, H., Goldman, B., Kanety, H., Stannard, B., LeRoith, D., & Shemer, J. (1995). *Cytokines and growth factors modulate cell growth and insulin-like growth factor binding protein secretion by the human salivary cell line (HSG). Journal of Cellular Physiology, 165(2), 223-227.*

Kawakami, A., Nakashima, T., Tsuboi, M., Urayama, S., Matsuoka, N., Ida, H., Kawabe, Y., Sakai, H., Migita, K., Ao-yagi, T., Nakashima, M., Maeda, K., & Eguchi, K. (1998). *Insulin-like growth factor I stimulates proliferation and Fas-mediated apoptosis of human osteoblasts. Biochemical Biophysical Research Communications, 247(1), 46-51.*

Kinugawa, S., Tsutsui, H., Ide, T., Nakamura, R., Arimura, K., Egashira, K., & Takeshita, A. (1999). *Positive inotropic effect of insulin-like growth factor-1 on normal and failing cardiac myocytes. Cardiovascular Research, 43(1), 157-164.*

Kontny, H.U., Hämmerle, K., Klein, R., Shayan, P., Mackall, C.L., & Niemeyer, C.M. (2001). *Sensitivity of Ewing's sarcoma to TRAIL-induced apoptosis. Cell Death & Differentiation, 8(5), 506-514.*

Kroesen, B.J., Jacobs, S., Pettus, B.J., Sietsma, H., Kok, J.W., Hannun, Y.A., & de Leij, L.F. (2003). *BcR-induced apoptosis involves differential regulation of C16 and C24-ceramide formation and sphingolipid-dependent activation of the proteasome. Journal of Biological Chemistry, 278(17), 14723-14731.*

Kumar, A., Jasmin, A., Eby, M.T., & Chaudhary, P.M. (2001). *Cytotoxicity of tumor necrosis factor-related apoptosis-inducing ligand towards Ewing's sarcoma cell lines. Oncogene, 20(8), 1010-1014.*

Lawrence, D., Shahrokh, Z., Marsters, S., Achilles, K., Shih, D., Mounho, B., Hillan, K., Totpal, K., DeForge, L., Schow, P., Hooley, J., Sherwood, S., Pai, R., Leung, S., Khan, L., Gliniak, B., Bussiere, J., Smith, C.A., Strom, S.S., Kelley, S., Fox, J.A., Thomas, D., & Ashkenazi, A. (2001). *Differential hepatocyte toxicity of recombinant Apo2L/TRAIL versions. Nature Medicine, 7(4), 383-385.*

Lee, A.V., Schiff, R., Cui, X., Sachdev, D., Yee, D., Gilmore, A.P., Streuli, C.H., Oesterreich, S., & Hadsell, D.I. (2003). *New mechanisms of signal transduction inhibitor action: receptor tyrosine kinase down-regulation and blockade of signal transactivation. Clinical Cancer Research, 1(2), 516S-523S.*

Li, S.L., Kato, J., Paz, I.B., Kasuya, J., & Fujita-Yamaguchi, Y. (1993). *Two new monoclonal antibodies against the alpha subunit of the human insulin-like growth factor-I receptor. Biochemical Biophysical Research Communications, 196(1), 92-98.*

Liu, E., Law, H.K., & Lau, Y.L. (2003). *Insulin-like growth factor I promotes maturation and inhibits apoptosis of immature cord blood monocyte-derived dendritic cells through MEK and PI3-kinase pathways. Pediatric Research, 54(6), 919-925.*

Liu, W., D'Ercole, J.A., & Ye, P. (2011). *Blunting type 1 insulin-like growth factor receptor expression exacerbates neuronal apoptosis following hypoxic/ischemic injury. BMC Neuroscience, 12, 64.*

Malempati, S., Weigel, B., Ingle, A.M., Ahern, C.H., Carroll, J.M., Roberts, C.T., Reid, J.M., Schmechel, S., Voss, S.D., Cho, S.Y., Chen, H.X., Krailo, M.D., Adamson, P.C., & Blaney, S.M. (2012). *Phase I/II trial and pharmacokinetic study of cixutumumab in pediatric patients with refractory solid tumors and Ewing sarcoma: a report from the Children's Oncology Group. Journal of Clinical Oncology, 30(3), 256-262.*

Martins, A.S., Ordóñez, J.L, Amaral, A.T, Prins, F., Floris, G., Debiec-Rychter, M., Hogendoorn, P.C., & de Alava, E. (2011). *IGF1R signaling in Ewing sarcoma is shaped by clathrin-/caveolin-dependent endocytosis. PLoS One 6(5), e19846.*

Mauz-Körholz, C., Kachel, M., Harms-Schirra, B., Klein-Vehne, A., Tunn, P.U., & Körholz, D. (2004). *Drug-induced caspase-3 activation in a Ewing tumor cell line and primary Ewing tumor cells. Anticancer Research, 24(1), 145-149.*

Mitsiades, N., Poulaki, V., Mitsiades, C., & Tsokos, M. (2001). *Ewing's sarcoma family tumors are sensitive to tumor necrosis factor-related apoptosis-inducing ligand and express death receptor 4 and death receptor 5. Cancer Research, 61(6), 2704-2712.*

Mullen, T.D., Hannun, Y.A., & Obeid, L.M. (2012). *Ceramide synthases at the centre of sphingolipid metabolism and biology. Biochemical Journal, 441(3), 789-802.*

Nitsch, R., Bechmann, I., Deisz, R.A., Haas, D., Lehmann, T.N., Wending, U., & Zipp, F. (2000). *Human brain-cell death induced by tumour-necrosis-factor related apoptosis-inducing ligand (TRAIL). Lancet, 356(9232), 827-828.*

Ogretmen, B. & Hannun, Y.A. (2004). *Biologically active sphingolipids in cancer pathogenesis and treatment. Nature Reviews Cancer, 4(8), 604-616.*

Ola, M.S., Nawaz, M., & Ahsan, H. (2011). *Role of Bcl-2 family proteins and caspases in the regulation of apoptosis. Molecular and Cellular Biochemistry, 351(1-2), 41-58.*

O'Neill, A., Shah, N., Zitomersky, N., Ladanyi, M., Shukla, N., Uren, A., Loeb, D., & Toretsky, J. (2013). *Insulin-like growth factor 1 receptor as a therapeutic target in Ewing sarcoma: lack of consistent upregulation or recurrent mutation and a review of the clinical trial literature. Sarcoma, 2013, 450478.*

Pappo, A.S., Patel, S.R., Crowley, J., Reinke, D.K., Kuenkele, K.P., Chawla, S.P., Toner, G.C., Maki, R.G., Meyers, P.A., Chugh, R., Ganjoo, K.N., Schuetze, S.M., Jürgens, H., Leahy, M.G., Geoerger, B., Benjamin, R.S., Helman, L.J., & Baker, L.H. (2011). *R1507, a monoclonal antibody to the insulin-like growth factor 1 receptor, in patients with recurrent or refractory Ewing sarcoma family of tumors: results of a phase II Sarcoma Alliance for Research through Collaboration study. Journal of Clinical Oncology, 29(34), 4541-4547.*

Pennarun, B., Meijer, A., de Vries, E.G., Kleibeuker, J.H., Kruyt, F., & de Jong, S. (2010). *Playing the DISC: turning on TRAIL death receptor-mediated apoptosis in cancer. Biochimica et Biophysica Acta, 1805(2), 123-140.*

Pitti, R.M., Marsters, S.A., Ruppert, S., Donahue, C.J., Moore, A., & Ashkenazi, A. (1996). *Induction of apoptosis by Apo-2 ligand, a new member of the tumor necrosis factor cytokine family. Journal of Biological Chemistry, 271(22), 12687-12690.*

Pommier, G.J., Garrouste, F.L., El Atiq, F., Roccabianca, M., Marvaldi, J.L., & Remacle-Bonnet, M.M. (1992). *Potential autocrine role of insulin-like growth factor II during suramin-induced differentiation of HT29-D4 human colonic adenocarcinoma cell line. Cancer Research, 52(11), 3182-3188.*

Poulaki, V., Mitsiades, C., Kotoula, V., Tseleni-Balafouta, S., Ashkenazi, A., Koutras, D.A., & Mitsiades, N. (2002). *Regulation of Apo2L/tumor necrosis factor-related apoptosis-inducing ligand-induced apoptosis in thyroid carcinoma cells. American Journal of Pathology, 161(2), 643-654.*

Prieur, A., Tirode, F., Cohen, P., & Delattre, O. (2004). *EWS/FLI-1 silencing and gene profiling of Ewing cells reveal downstream oncogenic pathways and a crucial role for repression of insulin-like growth factor binding protein 3. Molecular and Cellular Biology, 24(16), 7275-7283.*

Qin, J., Chaturvedi, V., Bonish, B., & Nickoloff, B.J. (2001). Avoiding premature apoptosis of normal epidermal cells. Nature Medicine, 7(4), 385-386.

Remacle-Bonnet, M.M., Garrouste, F.L., Baillat, G., Andre, F., Marvaldi, J.L., & Pommier, G. (2005). Membrane rafts segregate pro- from anti-apoptotic insulin-like growth factor-I receptor signaling in colon carcinoma cells stimulated by members of the tumor necrosis factor superfamily. American Journal of Pathology, 167(3), 761-773.

Remacle-Bonnet, M.M., Garrouste, F.L., Heller, S., André, F., Marvaldi, J.L., & Pommier, G.J. (2000). Insulin-like growth factor-I protects colon cancer cells from death factor-induced apoptosis by potentiating tumor necrosis factor alpha-induced mitogen-activated protein kinase and nuclear factor kappaB signaling pathways. Cancer Research, 60(7), 2007-2017.

Reynolds, R.K., Owens, C.A., & Roberts, J.A. (1996). Cultured endometrial cancer cells exhibit autocrine growth factor stimulation that is not observed in cultured normal endometrial cells. Gynecologic Oncology, 60(3), 380-386.

Rui, L., Fisher, T.L., Thomas, J., & White, M.F. (2001). Regulation of insulin/insulin-like growth factor-1 signaling by proteasome-mediated degradation of insulin receptor substrate-2. Journal of Biological Chemistry, 276(43), 40362-40367.

Samani, A.A., Yakar, S., LeRoith, D., & Brodt, P. (2007). The role of the IGF system in cancer growth and metastasis: overview and recent insights. Endocrinology Review, 28(1), 20-47.

Sauane, M., Su, Z.Z., Dash, R., Liu, X., Norris, J.S., Sarkar, D., Lee, S.G., Allegood, J.C., Dent, P., Spiegel, S., & Fisher, P.B. (2010). Ceramide plays a prominent role in MDA-7/IL-24-induced cancer-specific apoptosis. Journal of Cell Physiology, 222(3), 546-555.

Schimmer, A.D., Welsh, K., Pinilla, C., Wang, Z., Krajewska, M., Bonneau, M.J., Pedersen, I.M., Kitada, S., Scott, F.L., Bailly-Maitre, B., Glinsky, G., Scudiero, D., Sausville, E., Salvesen, G., Nefzi, A., Ostresh, J.M., Houghten, R.A., & Reed, J.C. (2004). Small-molecule antagonists of apoptosis suppressor XIAP exhibit broad antitumor activity. Cancer Cell, 5(1), 25-35.

Schmitz-Peiffer, C., Craig, D.L., & Biden, T.J. (1999). Ceramide generation is sufficient to account for the inhibition of the insulin-stimulated PKB pathway in C2C12 skeletal muscle cells pretreated with palmitate. Journal of Biological Chemistry, 274(34), 24202-24210.

Schotte, P., Declercq, W., Van Huffel, S., Vandenabeele, P., & Beyaert, R. (1999). Non-specific effects of methyl ketone peptide inhibitors of caspases. FEBS Letters, 442(1), 117-121.

Scotlandi, K., Benini, S., Nanni, P., Lollini, P.L., Nicoletti, G., Landuzzi, L., Serra, M, Manara, M.C., Picci, P., & Baldini, N. (1998). Blockage of insulin-like growth factor-I receptor inhibits the growth of Ewing's sarcoma in athymic mice. Cancer Research, 58(18), 4127-4131.

Scotlandi, K., Benini, S., Sarti, M., Serra, M., Lollini, P.L., Maurici, D., Picci, P., Manara, M.C., & Baldini, N. (1996). Insulin-like growth factor I receptor-mediated circuit in Ewing's sarcoma/peripheral neuroectodermal tumor: a possible therapeutic target. Cancer Research, 56(20), 4570-4574.

Scott, F.L., Denault, J.B., Riedl, S.J., Shin, H., Renatus, M., & Salvesen, G.S. (2005). XIAP inhibits caspase-3 and -7 using two binding sites: evolutionarily conserved mechanism of IAPs. EMBO Journal, 24(3), 645-655.

Sensintaffar, J., Scott, F.L., Peach, R., & Hager, J.H. (2010). XIAP is not required for human tumor cell survival in the absence of an exogenous death signal. BMC Cancer, 10, 11.

Seumois, G., Fillet, M., Gillet, L., Faccinetto, C., Desmet, C., François, C., Dewals, B., Oury, C., Vanderplasschen, A., Lekeux, P., & Bureau, F. (2007). De novo C16- and C24-ceramide generation contributes to spontaneous neutrophil apoptosis. Journal of Leukocyte Biology, 81(6), 1477-1486.

Shaner, R.L., Allegood, J.C., Park, H., Wang, E., Kelly, S., Haynes, C.A., Sullards, M.C., & Merrill Jr., A.H. (2009). Quantitative analysis of sphingolipids for lipidomics using triple quadrupole and quadrupole linear ion trap mass spectrometers. Journal of Lipid Research, 50(8), 1692-1707.

Smith, T.J. (2010). Insulin-like growth factor-I regulation of immune function: a potential therapeutic target in autoimmune diseases? Pharmacological Reviews, 62(2), 199-236.

Soos, M.A., Field, C.E., Lammers, R., Ullrich, A., Zhang, B., Roth, R.A., Andersen, A.S., Kjeldsen, T., & Siddle, K. (1992). A panel of monoclonal antibodies for the type I insulin-like growth factor receptor. Epitope mapping, effects on ligand binding, and biological activity. Journal of Biological Chemistry, 267(18), 12955-12963.

Sorkin, A. & von Zastrow, M. (2009). Endocytosis and signalling: intertwining molecular networks. Nature Reviews Molecular Cell Biology, 10(9), 609-622.

Steele-Perkins, G. & Roth, R.A. (1990). Monoclonal antibody alpha IR-3 inhibits the ability of insulin-like growth factor II to stimulate a signal from the type I receptor without inhibiting its binding. Biochemical Biophysical Research Communications, 171(3), 1244-1251.

Suminoe, A., Matsuzaki, A., Hattori, H., Koga, Y., & Hara, T. (2009). Immunotherapy with autologous dendritic cells and tumor antigens for children with refractory malignant solid tumors. Pediatric Transplantation, 13(6), 746-753.

Toomey, E.C., Schiffman, J.D., & Lessnick, S.L. (2010). Recent advances in the molecular pathogenesis of Ewing's sarcoma. Oncogene, 29(32), 4504-4516.

Toretsky, J.A., Thakar, M., Eskenazi, A.E., & Frantz, C.N. (1999). Phosphoinositide 3-hydroxide kinase blockade enhances apoptosis in the Ewing's sarcoma family of tumors. Cancer Research, 59(22), 5745-5750.

van Blitterswijk, W.J., van der Luit, A.H., Veldman, R.J., Verheij, M., & Borst, J. (2003). Ceramide: second messenger or modulator of membrane structure and dynamics? Biochemical Journal, 369(2), 199-211.

van Buul-Offers, S.C. & Kooijman, R. (1998). The role of growth hormone and insulin-like growth factors in the immune system. Cellular and Molecular Life Sciences, 54(10), 1083-1094.

Van Valen, F. (1999). Ewing's sarcoma family of tumors. Human Cell Culture, volume I, 55-85, Masters, J.R.W., & Palsson, B., Eds., Kluwer Academic Publishers, London, Great Britain.

Van Valen, F., Fulda, S., Schäfer, K.L., Truckenbrod, B., Hotfilder, M., Poremba, C., Debatin, K.M., & Winkelmann, W. (2003). Selective and nonselective toxicity of TRAIL/Apo2L combined with chemotherapy in human bone tumour cells vs. normal human cells. International Journal of Cancer, 107(6), 929-940.

Van Valen, F., Fulda, S., Truckenbrod, B., Eckervogt, V., Sonnemann, J., Hillmann, A., Rödl, R., Hoffmann, C., Winkelmann, W., Schäfer, L., Dockhorn-Dworniczak, B., Wessel, T., Boos, J., Debatin, K.M., & Jürgens, H. (2000). Apoptotic responsiveness of the Ewing's sarcoma family of tumours to tumour necrosis factor-related apoptosis-inducing ligand (TRAIL). International Journal of Cancer, 88(2), 252-259.

Van Valen, F., Winkelmann, W., & Jürgens, H. (1992). Type I and type II insulin-like growth factor receptors and their function in human Ewing's sarcoma cells. Journal of Cancer Research and Clinical Oncology, 118(4), 269-275.

Varfolomeev, E., Alicke, B., Elliott, J.M., Zobel, K., West, K., Wong, H., Scheer, J.M., Ashkenazi, A., Gould, S.E., Fairbrother, W.J., & Vucic, D. (2009). X chromosome-linked inhibitor of apoptosis regulates cell death induction by proapoptotic receptor agonists. Journal of Biological Chemistry, 284(50), 34553-34560.

Wagner, M.J. & Maki, R.G. (2013). Type 1 insulin-like growth factor receptor targeted therapies in pediatric cancer. Frontiers in Oncology, 3, 9.

Warren, R.S., Yuan, H, Matli, M.R., Ferrara, N., & Donner, D.B. (1996). Induction of vascular endothelial growth factor by insulin-like growth factor 1 in colorectal carcinoma. Journal of Biological Chemistry, 271(46), 29483-29488.

Wiley, S.R., Schooley, K., Smolak, P.J., Din, W.S., Huang, C.P., Nicholl, J.K., Sutherland, G.R., Smith, T.D., Rauch, C., Smith, C.A., & Goodwin, R.G. (1995). Identification and characterization of a new member of the TNF family that induces apoptosis. Immunity, 3(6), 673-682.

Yang, S., Thor, A.D., Edgerton, S., & Yang, X. (2006). Caspase-3 mediated feedback activation of apical caspases in doxorubicin and TNF-alpha induced apoptosis. Apoptosis, 11(11), 1987-1997.

Yee, D., Favoni, R.E., Lebovic, G.S., Lombana, F., Powell, D.R., Reynolds, C.P., & Rosen, N. (1990). Insulin-like growth factor I expression by tumors of neuroectodermal origin with the t(11;22) chromosomal translocation. A potential autocrine growth factor. Journal of Clinical Investigations, 86(6), 1806-1814.

Zhang, Y.C., Wang, X.P., Zhang, L.Y., Song, A.L., Kou, Z.M., & Li, X.S. (2006). *Effect of blocking IGF-I receptor on growth of human hepatocellular carcinoma cells. World Journal of Gastroenterology, 12(25), 3977-3982.*

Zheng, H., Shen, H., Oprea, I., Worrall, C., Stefanescu, R., Girnita, A., & Girnita, L. (2012). *β-Arrestin-biased agonism as the central mechanism of action for insulin-like growth factor 1 receptor-targeting antibodies in Ewing's sarcoma. Proceedings of the National Academy of Sciences USA, 109(50), 20620-20625.*

Circulating Cell-free DNA in Melanoma Patients

Francesca Salvianti, Pamela Pinzani, Mario Pazzagli, Claudio Orlando
Department of Biomedical, Experimental and Clinical Sciences
University of Florence, Italy

Paolo Verderio, Chiara Maura Ciniselli
Unit of Medical Statistics, Biometry and Bioinformatics, Fondazione IRCCS
Istituto Nazionale dei Tumori, Milano, Italy

Daniela Massi, Vincenzo De Giorgi, Marta Grazzini
Department of Critical Care Medicine and Surgery
University of Florence, Italy

1   Introduction

Molecular features of solid tumours become central in tailoring targeted therapies, but the accessibility to tumour tissue may be sometime limited due to the size of bioptic samples or the unavailability of biological material, particularly in patient follow up after tumour removal. In this context cancer-derived cell-free DNA (cfDNA) in blood represents a promising biomarker for cancer diagnosis and an useful surrogate material for molecular characterization (Hodgson *et al.*, 2010).

The two classes of alterations detectable in cfDNA from cancer patients include quantitative and qualitative abnormalities. Concerning the former aspect, it is now evident that cancer patients have a higher concentration of cfDNA than healthy individuals (see Fleischhacker and Schmidt, 2007 for a review). The concentration of cfDNA is influenced by tumour stage, size, location, and other factors (Jung *et al.*, 2010). On the other hand, increased plasma cfDNA level is not a specific marker of carcinogenesis, as it is observed also in patients with premalignant states, inflammation or trauma (Fleischhacker and Schmidt, 2007). Total cfDNA concentration has been proposed as a marker for early cancer detection, but the studies conducted so far showed a scarce discriminatory power between patients and controls as well as limited sensitivity and specificity, not allowing to reach any final conclusion on the diagnostic impact of this parameter. Several studies report a prognostic value of total cfDNA, while conflicting results have been obtained in testing this marker for therapy monitoring (Jung *et al.*, 2010).

A higher specificity in cancer diagnosis can be achieved by detecting tumor specific alterations in cfDNA, such as DNA integrity, genetic and epigenetic modifications (Jung *et al.*, 2010). Blood cfDNA in cancer patients originates from apoptotic or necrotic cells. In solid cancers, necrosis generates a spectrum of DNA fragments with variable size, due to random digestion by DNases. In contrast, cell death in normal blood nucleated cells occurs mostly via apoptosis that generates small and uniform DNA fragments. It has generally been observed that in patients affected by several neoplastic diseases plasma DNA contains longer fragments than healthy subjects (Wang *et al.*, 2003; Umetani *et al.*, 2006; Hanley *et al.*, 2006; Hauser *et al.*, 2010 Jiang *et al.*, 2006; Tomita *et al.*, 2007).

The above mentioned parameters can obviously be considered as non-specific biomarkers, since the increase of cfDNA concentration and integrity is common to the large majority of human solid cancers. When cfDNA is used to detect genetic and epigenetic modifications in a particular neoplasia, it is necessary to select specific molecular targets, expected to be altered in affected patients.

BRAF is a serine–threonine protein kinase involved in the RAS–RAF–MEK–ERK pathway (Dhomen and Marais, 2007) which regulates cell growth, survival, differentiation and senescence (Huang *et al.*, 2009). The oncogene *BRAF* is frequently mutated in many human cancers constitutively activating the MAPK pathway. The most common BRAF mutation, which accounts for more than 90% of cases of cancer involving this gene, is the T1799A transversion, converting valine to glutamic acid at position 600 (V600E) (Davies *et al.*, 2002). *BRAF* somatic mutations have been reported in 66% of malignant melanomas and at a lower frequency in a wide range of human cancers (Davies *et al.*, 2002). *BRAF* mutations are likely to be a crucial step in the initiation of melanocytic neoplasia, as they are found also in nevi (Pollock *et al.*, 2003). *BRAF* mutations are an attractive target for therapeutic interventions, as they represent an early event in melanoma pathogenesis and are preserved throughout tumor progression (Omholt *et al.*, 2003). Specific inhibitors of mutant BRAF, such as PLX4032, were developed (Flaherty *et al.*, 2009). $BRAF^{V600E}$ mutation has been investigated as a marker in cfDNA from melanoma patients by Daniotti *et al.*, 2007 and Yancovitz *et al.*, 2007.

Finally, it is widely demonstrated that a limited number of genes is epigenetically disregulated in cutaneous melanoma. *RASSF1A* (Ras association domain family 1 isoform A) is a tumor suppressor gene, which regulates mitosis, the cell cycle and apoptosis. It is inactivated mostly by inappropriate promoter methylation in many types of cancers (Donninger *et al.*, 2007). *RASSF1A* promoter is methylated in 55% of cutaneous melanomas (Spugnardi *et al.*, 2003). Methylation of *RASSF1A* increases significantly with advancing clinical stage, suggesting that the inactivation of this gene is associated with tumor progression (Tanemura *et al.*, 2009). *RASSF1A* promoter hypermethylation has been detected in cfDNA from melanoma patients (Hoon *et al.*, 2000; Marini *et al.*, 2006) in association to a worse response to therapy and reduced overall survival (Mori *et al.*, 2005; Koyanagi *et al.*, 2006).

The aim of the present study was to identify a sequential multi-marker panel in cfDNA able to increase the predictive capability in the diagnosis of cutaneous melanoma in comparison with each single marker alone. To this purpose we tested total cfDNA concentration, cfDNA integrity, $BRAF^{V600E}$ mutation and *RASSF1A* promoter methylation associated to cfDNA in a series of 76 melanoma patients and 63 healthy controls.

2   Materials and Methods

2.1   Patients

Seventy six patients (32 females and 44 males, median age 63, range 23-94 years) affected by cutaneous melanoma (12 patients with in situ melanoma, 49 with local disease, 5 with regional metastatic disease and 10 with distant metastatic disease) were enrolled at the Department of Dermatological Sciences of the University of Florence. As a control group 63 healthy subjects (median age 62, range 25-79 years) were enrolled in the study upon a dermatological examination to exclude the presence of melanoma and to provide the number of nevi. Blood samples (5 ml) were collected in EDTA tubes during the dermatologic examination and before surgery. The research protocol was approved by the review board of the University of Florence and all the patients signed an informed consent.

2.2   DNA Extraction

Plasma was separated from blood in EDTA tubes, within three hours from blood draw by two centrifugation steps at 4 °C for 10 min: at 1600 rcf and 14000 rcf, respectively. Plasma aliquots (505 µl) were stored at −80 °C. DNA was extracted from 500 µl of plasma, by the QIAamp DSP Virus Kit (Qiagen, Italy) according to the manufacturer's instructions. RNAse digestion was included in the procedure to prevent RNA interference during the subsequent qPCR reactions.

2.3   Molecular Biomarkers in cfDNA

All the cfDNA samples from melanoma patients and healthy controls were submitted in duplicate to six qPCR assays targeting the chosen biomarkers, for a total of about 1500 determinations. All the qPCR reactions were performed using the 7900HT instrument (Applied Biosystems).

2.3.1   qPCR Assays for Total Free Circulating DNA and Integrity Indexes

Absolute quantification of the single copy gene *APP* (Amyloid Precursor protein, chr.4q11-q13) was performed on DNA from plasma to accurately measure the total amount of free circulating DNA per ml plasma, using primers and probe targeting a 67 bp sequence (Pinzani *et al.*, 2011).

Quantification of DNA concentration was obtained using an external reference curve ranging from 10 to 10^5 pg/tube of genomic DNA extracted from a blood pool of healthy donors and measured spectro-photometrically (Nanodrop ND1000, Nanodrop, USA). Results were expressed as ng circulating DNA/ml of plasma.

Three additional qPCR assays were determined by targeting longer target sequences (respectively a 180 bp or 306 bp or 476 bp) on the single copy gene *APP*, as already reported (Pinzani *et al.*, 2011). The ratio between the absolute concentration of each of the longer amplicons and the shortest one (67 bp used to quantify total cfDNA) defined the integrity indexes 180/67, 306/67 and 476/67 which were used to assess the fragmentation of cfDNA. The primers and the hydrolysis probes for the different amplicons were previously described (Lehmann *et al.*, 2000; Pinzani *et al.*, 2011) and are reported in Table 1. The reactions were carried out separately for each different-length template in a 12.5 µl mix containing 1x Quantitect® Probe PCR Master Mix (QIAgen), 300 nm primers, 200 nm probe and 1 µl sample. The thermal profile of the amplification was 50 cycles of PCR as follows: i) 15 s at 95 °C and 60 s at 60 °C for shorter amplicons (67 and 180 bps), ii) 15 s at 95 °C, 60 s at 56 °C and 60 s at 72 °C for the longer amplicons (306 and 476 bps). All the measurements were performed in triplicate on 1 µl of DNA. For cfDNA quantification targeting the 180, 306 and 476 amplicons, we used an external reference curve as reported for the 67 bp amplicon.

Forward Primer	5'-TCAGGTTGACGCCGCTGT-3'
Hydrolysis Probe	5'-FAM-ACCCCAGAGGAGCGCCACCTG-TAMRA-3'
Reverse Primer - 67 bp	5'-TTCGTAGCCGTTCTGCTGC-3'
Reverse Primer - 180 bp	5'-TCTATAAATGGACACCGATGGGTAGT-3'
Reverse Primer - 306 bp	5'-GAGAGATAGAATACATTACTGATGTGTGGAT-3'
Reverse Primer - 476 bp	5'-TAAAGTAGGACTTAATTGGGTCACAAAC-3'

Table 1 : Sequence of primers and probe.

2.3.2   Double Allele Specific qPCR to Detect $BRAF^{V600E}$ Mutation

Circulating cfDNA bearing the mutation $BRAF^{V600E}$ was quantified by an allele-specific qPCR assay, as already reported (Pinzani et al., 2010). The specificity for the mutated allele was conferred by the forward primer and the LNA probe. cfDNA was amplified in a reaction mixture containing 1× Quantitect® Probe PCR Master Mix (QIAgen), 200 nm primers and 200 nm probe in a final volume of 20 µl. The thermal profile of the reaction included a denaturation step at 95 °C for 10 min and 50 cycles of PCR (95 °C for 15 s, 64 °C for 1 min). $BRAF^{V600E}$ percentage was calculated by referring to a standard curve obtained by mixing DNA from mutant (SKMEL28) and wild type (MCF7) cell lines in the following proportions: 100%, 50%, 20%, 10%, and 1% mutated alleles. Results were expressed as percentage of mutated DNA (% $BRAF^{V600E}$) and in terms of absolute concentration of $BRAF^{V600E}$ mutated DNA (ng/ml of plasma) using the following formula:

$$BRAF^{V600E} \text{ mutated DNA (ng/ml plasma)} = (\% \ BRAF^{V600E} \times \text{total DNA})/100$$

2.3.3   qPCR Assay for *RASSF1A* Methylated form Quantification

The methylated form of *RASSF1A* promoter was quantified in plasma from melanoma patients and controls after digesting unmethylated DNA by a methylation-sensitive enzyme: 5 µl of plasma DNA were treated with 10 units of Bsh1236I (Fermentas, Canada) in a reaction volume of 25 µl at 37 °C for 16 hours. The enzyme recognizes the restriction site CGCG in the promoter of the gene *RASSF1A* and digests DNA only if the cytosines are unmethylated. The methylated DNA is then amplified by a qPCR assay targeting the promoter region of the gene comprising the restriction site of Bsh1236 I. If the digestion is complete the qPCR reaction will quantify only methylated DNA. In particular 5 µl of enzyme-treated DNA underwent a qPCR assay for *RASSF1A* promoter, in a final volume of 25 µl, according to the protocol already described by Chan et al., 2006. A reference curve obtained by serial dilutions of genomic DNA was used to quantify the methylated alleles. Results were expressed as genomic equivalents (GEQ, each corresponding to 6.6 pg DNA) per ml plasma.

2.4   Statistical Analysis

All the considered biomarkers were analysed as continuous variables in their original scale or after an appropriate transformation. Comparison of biomarkers distribution in melanoma patients (cases) and healthy subjects (controls) was performed by using the Kolmogorov-Smirnov test (KST) (Hollander & Wolfe, 1999). The relationship between each biomarker and the disease status was investigated by resorting to a logistic regression model in both univariate and multivariate fashion (Hosmer & Lemeshow, 1989). The biomarker that was statistically significant in the univariate analysis was considered in the initial model of multivariate analysis. A final more parsimonious model was then obtained using a backward selection procedure in which only the variables reaching the conventional significance level of 0.05 were retained (final model).

The predictive capability (i.e. diagnostic performance) of each biomarker was investigated by means of the area under the ROC curve (AUC) (Hanley & McNeil, 1982). This curve measures the accuracy of biomarkers when their expression is detected on a continuous scale, displaying the relationship between sensitivity (true-positive rate, y-axes) and 1-specificity (false-positive rate, x-axes) across all possible threshold values of the considered biomarker. An useful way to summarize the overall diagnostic accuracy of the biomarker is the area under the ROC curve (AUC) the value of which is expected to be 0.5 in absence of predictive capability, whereas it tends to be 1.00 in the case of high predictive capacity (Hanley & McNeil, 1982). To aid the reader to interpret the value of this statistic, we suggest that values between 0.6 and 0.7 can be considered as indicating a weak predictive capacity, values between 0.71 and 0.8 a satisfactory predictive capacity and values greater than 0.8 a good predictive capacity (Gasparini *et al.*, 1996).

Finally the contribution of each variables to the predictive capability of the final model was investigated by comparing the AUC value in the model with that of the same model without the variable itself. All statistical analyses were carried out using SAS software (Version 9.2.; SAS Institute Inc. Cary, NC).

3   Results

All the subjects enrolled in the study were tested for all the biomarkers in cfDNA.

3.1   Total cell-free DNA Concentration in Plasma

When submitted to qPCR for total cfDNA concentration in plasma, all samples from patients and controls showed positive amplification plots.

Figure 1 displays through a specific box-plot the distribution of circulating plasma cfDNA in patients with melanoma (cases) and in healthy subjects (controls) and in the table below are reported some descriptive statistics of these distributions. As shown in Figure 1, melanomas patients had an increase of about 3-fold of the amount of plasma cfDNA, since in control subjects plasma DNA level (median: 5.260 ng/ml, IQR: 6.210) was significantly lower than in melanomas patients (median:15.641 ng/ml, IQR: 19.687).

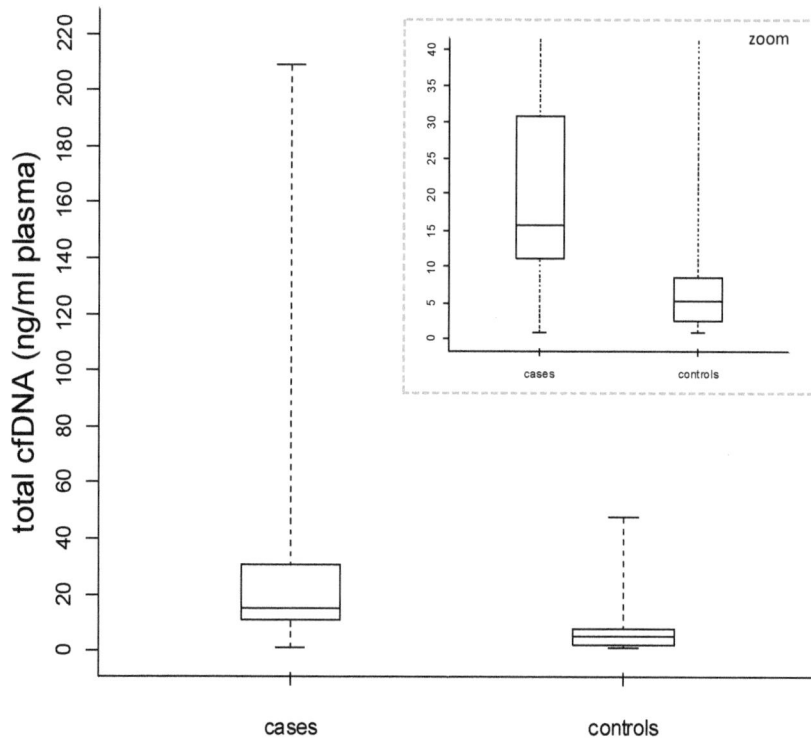

		min	25th centile	median	75th centile	max	IQR	p-value†
cfDNA	cases	0.894	11.098	15.641	30.785	208.560	19.687	
(ng/ml plasma)	controls	0.990	2.530	5.260	8.740	47.490	6.210	<0.0001

Abbreviations: IQR, Interquartile range (75th centile – 25th centile).
† p-value of the Kolmogorov-Smirnov test by comparing the distribution of cases and controls.

Figure 1: Total circulating plasma cfDNA distribution. Boxplot reflecting the free-circulating plasma DNA concentration distribution in cases and controls. The two horizontal sides of the box identify the 25th and 75th centile, the horizontal line inside the box indicates the median and the limits of the two whiskers indicates the extreme measured values. The inner box represents a zoom window to aid the visualization of the of the distribution.

3.2   Integrity Indexes 180/67, 306/67 and 473/67 of Cell-free DNA in Plasma

cfDNA integrity indexes were evaluated in plasma of our cohort of subjects. The results show a decrease of cfDNA concentration as the amplicon dimensions increase in both healthy and melanoma subjects. Moreover for each single amplicon a statistically significant difference was detected between healthy subjects and patients (Student t-Test, p-value <0.05) with constantly higher values in the melanoma group (data not shown).

Figure 2 depicts the distribution of the three integrity indexes in patients with melanoma (cases) and in healthy subjects (controls). The distribution of the integrity index 180/67 was significantly different in melanoma patients with respect to that of control subject (p-value < 0.0001). Conversely, these findings were not observed when we analysed the integrity index 306/67 (p-value = 0.981) and the integrity index 476/67 (p-value = 0.363).

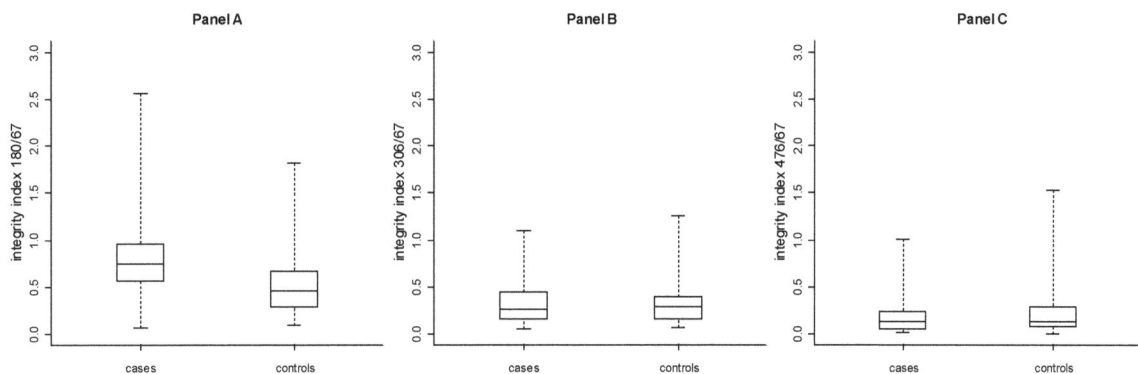

		min	25th centile	median	75th centile	max	IQR	p-value†
integrity index 180/67	cases	0.070	0.560	0.750	0.950	2.568	0.390	<0.0001
	controls	0.090	0.290	0.460	0.670	1.810	0.380	
integrity index 306/67	cases	0.050	0.150	0.260	0.440	1.100	0.290	0.981
	controls	0.070	0.150	0.290	0.400	1.260	0.250	
integrity index 476/67	cases	0.010	0.050	0.135	0.240	1.010	0.190	0.363
	controls	0.000	0.080	0.130	0.290	1.530	0.210	

Abbreviations: IQR, Interquartile range (75th centile – 25th centile).
† p-value of the Kolmogorov-Smirnov test by comparing the distribution of cases and controls.

Figure 2: Integrity index distributions. Boxplot reflecting the distribution of the integrity index 180/67 (Panel A), 306/67 (Panel B) and 476/67 (Panel C) in cases and controls. The two horizontal sides of the box identify the 25th and 75th centile, the horizontal line inside the box indicates the median and the limits of the two whiskers indicate the extreme measured values.

3.3   *BRAF*^{V600E} Percentage and Concentrations in Plasma

The median plasma percentage of *BRAF*^{V600E} DNA was higher in cases (median: 1.585, IQR: 4.655) than in control subjects (median: 1.440, IQR: 2.840). Similar results were found when evaluating the *BRAF*^{V600E} results expressed as ng/ml of plasma. In particular, a statistically difference (p-value: 0.001) in the distribution of *BRAF*^{V600E} DNA concentration (ng/ml of plasma) was observed between cases (median: 0.200 ng/ml plasma, IQR: 0.603) and controls (median: 0.080 ng/ml plasma, IQR: 0.153).

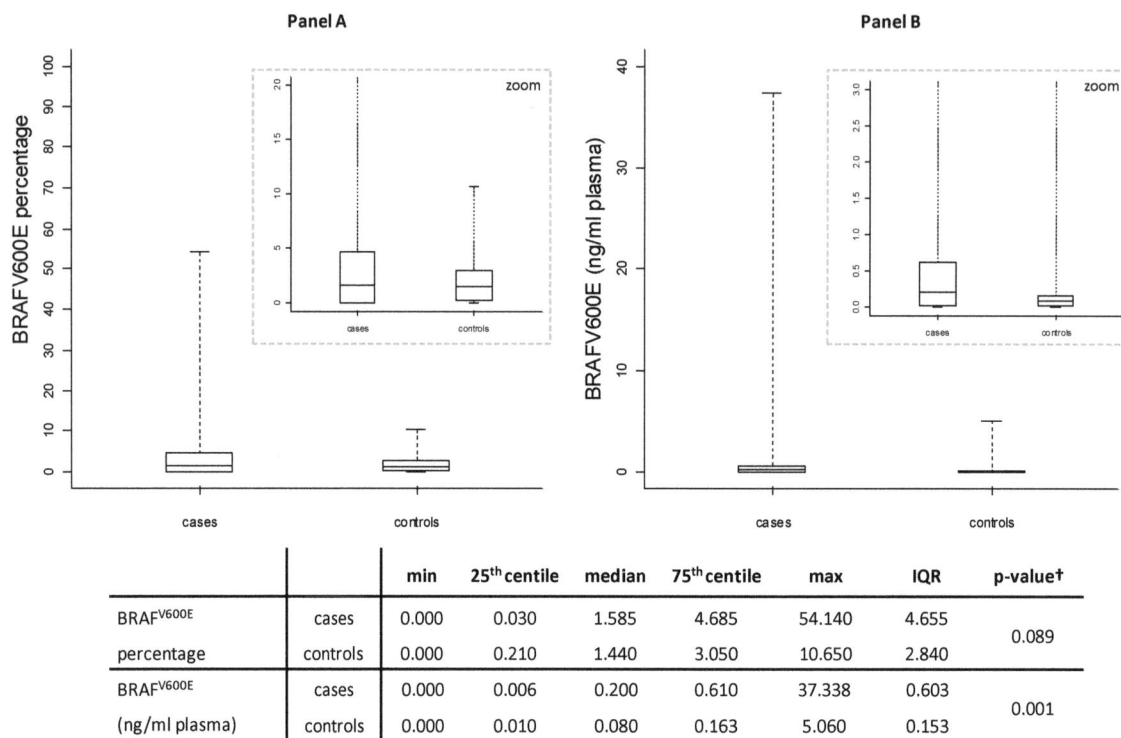

		min	25th centile	median	75th centile	max	IQR	p-value†
BRAF^{V600E}	cases	0.000	0.030	1.585	4.685	54.140	4.655	
percentage	controls	0.000	0.210	1.440	3.050	10.650	2.840	0.089
BRAF^{V600E}	cases	0.000	0.006	0.200	0.610	37.338	0.603	
(ng/ml plasma)	controls	0.000	0.010	0.080	0.163	5.060	0.153	0.001

Abbreviations: IQR, Interquartile range (75th centile – 25th centile).
† p-value of the Kolmogorov-Smirnov test by comparing the distribution of cases and controls .

Figure 3: $BRAF^{V600E}$ **distributions.** Boxplot reflecting the distribution of the plasma percentage of $BRAF^{V600E}$ DNA (Panel A) and $BRAF^{V600E}$ quantification in ng/ml of plasma (Panel B) in cases and controls. The two horizontal sides of the box identify the 25th and 75th centile, the horizontal line inside the box indicates the median and the limit of the two whiskers indicates the extreme measured values. The inner box represents a zoom window to aid the visualization of the distribution.

3.4   Methylated *RASSF1A* Concentration in Plasma

Plasma concentration of the methylated form of *RASSF1A* gene promoter were evaluated in control subjects as well as in melanoma patients. The distribution of methylated *RASSF1A* resulted significantly different in melanoma patients with respect to the control subjects (p-value: 0.0003).

3.5   Multimarker Approach

As shown in the previous paragraphs, circulating plasma total cfDNA concentration, integrity index 180/67, $BRAF^{V600E}$ and methylated *RASSF1A* showed a significant difference in the distribution of melanoma patients in comparison to that of controls, confirming the potential clinical relevance of these biomarkers for the melanoma diagnosis. For these biomarkers considered in the logistic regression model we found that a linear relationship between the log odds and their values on the original (methylated *RASSF1A*) or logarithm (total cfDNA, integrity index 180/67 and $BRAF^{V600E}$) scale was appropriate. As reported in Table 2 disease status was significantly associated with all these biomarkers in the logistic univariate analysis. Consequently all the considered biomarkers were included in the initial model of the logistic multivariate regression analysis.

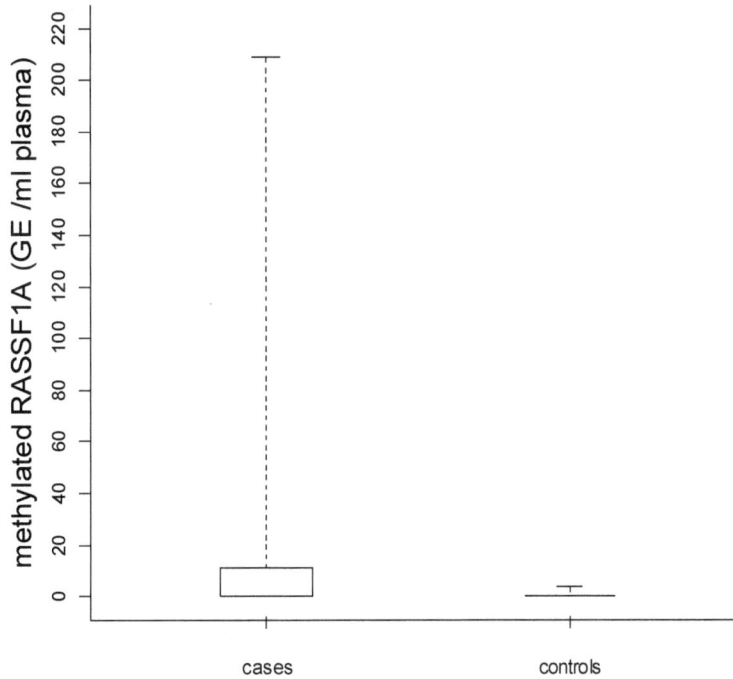

methylated RASSF1A		min	25th centile	median	75th centile	max	IQR	p-value†
methylated RASSF1A	cases	0.000	0.000	0.000	11.040	208.680	11.040	0.0003
(GE /ml plasma)	controls	0.000	0.000	0.000	0.000	4.010	0.000	

Abbreviations: IQR, Interquartile range (75th centile – 25th centile).
† p-value of the Kolmogorov-Smirnov test by comparing the distribution of cases and controls.

Figure 4: Methylated *RASSF1A* distribution. Boxplot reflecting the distribution of the methylated *RASSF1A* in cases and controls. The two horizontal sides of the box identify the 25th and 75th centile, the horizontal line inside the box indicates the median and the limit of the two whiskers indicates the extreme measured values.

The AUC values (Table 2 and Figure 5) computed for each biomarker (univariate logistic model) indicated a weak/satisfactory level of predictive capability by ranging between 0.64 ($BRAF^{V600E}$) to 0.85 (cfDNA). Of note for all the considered biomarkers the 95% Confidence Interval (95%CI) of the AUC fails to include the 0.5 value (i.e. absence of predictive capability).

As reported in Table 3, cfDNA, integrity index 180/67 and methylated *RASSF1A* retained a statistically significant (p-value < 0.05) association with disease status also in the multivariate final logistic model. A good predictive capability was observed for the final logistic model with an AUC of 0.95 (95% CI: 0.91-0.98) (Table 3 and Figure 6).

Finally, the contribution of each variable to the predictive capability of the final model (AUC: 0.95, 95%CI: 0.91-0.98) was investigated by comparing the AUC value in the model with that of the same model without the variable itself: the highest predictive capability was given by cfDNA (AUC:0.86, 95%CI: 0.80-0.92) followed by integrity index 180/67 (AUC:0.90, 95%CI: 0.85-0.95) and methylated *RASSF1A* (AUC:0.89, 95%CI: 0.84-0.95).

Biomarker	OR[a]	OR 95%CI	p value[b]	AUC	AUC 95%CI	p value
cfDNA (ng/ml plasma)	5.621	3.102-10.185	<0.0001	0.853	0.788-0.918	<0.0001
Integrity Index 180/67	4.790	2.356-9.740	<0.0001	0.759	0.677-0.840	<0.0001
Methylated *RASSF1A* (GE/ml plasma)	1.413	1.112-1.795	0.005	0.688	0.621-0.754	<0.0001
BRAF[V600E] (ng/ml plasma)	6.061	1.650-22.263	0.007	0.635	0.540-0.730	0.005

Abbreviations: OR, Odds Ratio; CI, Confidence Interval; AUC, area under the ROC curve.
[a] Odds Ratio for any increase of one unit.
[b] p-value of the Wald statistic.

Table 2: Univariate logistic analysis.

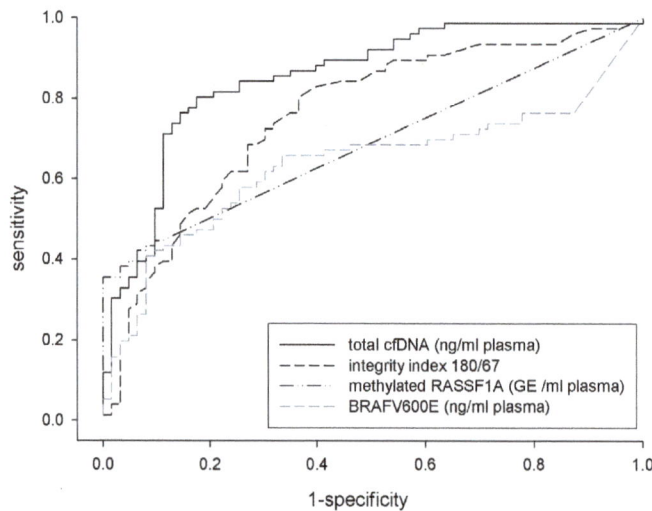

Figure 5: ROC Curves deriving from the univariate logistic analysis. ROC curves derived from the univariate logistic analysis corresponding to cfDNA (AUC = 0.85), integrity index 180/67 (AUC = 0.76), methylated *RASSF1A* (AUC = 0.69) and *BRAF[V600E]* (AUC = 0.64).

Biomarker	OR[a]	OR 95%CI	p value[b]	AUC	AUC 95%CI	p value
Total cfDNA (ng/ml plasma)	6.592	3.084-14.088	<0.0001	0.945	0.910-0.980	<0.0001
Integrity Index 180/67	7.783	2.944-20.579	<0.0001			
Methylated RASSF1A (GE/ml plasma	1.450	1.100-1.910	0.008			

Abbreviations: OR, Odds Ratio; CI, Confidence Interval; AUC, area under the ROC curve.
[a]Odds Ratio for any increase of one unit.
[b]p-value of the Wald statistic.

Table 3: Final multivariate logistic model.

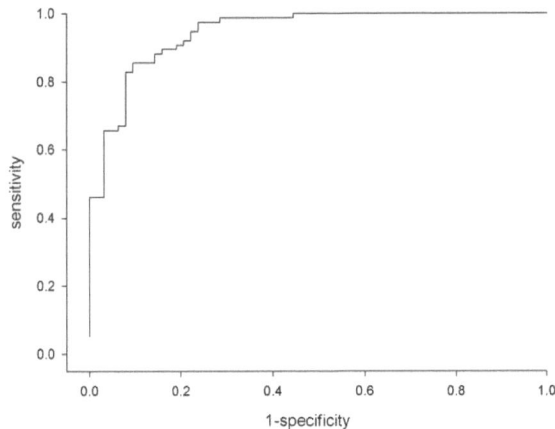

Figure 6 : ROC Curve deriving from the multivariate final logistic model. ROC curve derived from the final multivariate logistic model (AUC = 0.95).

4   Discussion

The analysis of cfDNA may have the potential to complement or replace the existing cancer tissue and blood biomarkers in the future (Schwarzenbach *et al.*, 2011). In order to reach this goal, specific and sensitive analytical procedures must be developed and optimized to compute proper circulating target molecules showing differences between patients and healthy subjects. It is now widely accepted that a single biomarker cannot fully discriminate between controls and patients and consequently an approach based on different markers is preferable in order to achieve a stronger predictive ability (Pinsky and Zhu, 2011). It has been demonstrated that in prenatal screening a combination of multiple markers, each of which by itself has limited sensitivity and/or specificity, can lead to a powerful screening test (Malone *et al.*, 2005). Analogously, Schneider and Mizejewski (2007) suggest to develop a multi-marker screening approach for cancer. The authors observed that so far the approach for cancer testing has been limited to the research of single biomarkers. Unfortunately this strategy has been proven unsuccessful, notwithstanding the high number of new biomarkers reported in the literature. There are already some examples on prostate and ovarian cancer clearly showing that multi-marker screening can have its place in early cancer detection (Schneider & Mizejewski 2007).

In this preliminary study the principal aim was to investigate the diagnostic performance of four markers associated to cfDNA in identifying melanoma patients. Particular efforts were dedicated to the technical aspects of the methods adopted for each single parameter allowing to reach accurate and reproducible measurements. Following the standard approach (Verderio *et al* 2010) for the clinical validation of biomarkers for early detection we are planning new studies focused on the assessment of the impact of these biomarkers on clinical practice including the identification of the most suitable thresholds to use for the early detection of melanoma by clinicians.

Here we considered total cfDNA concentration by a qPCR assay for the single copy gene *APP*, as well as its fragmentation expressed by the integrity index 180/67. On the other hand, tumour contribution to cfDNA was assessed by quantifying $BRAF^{V600E}$ mutated alleles and *RASSF1A* promoter methylation. These markers have been used in a panel in all patients, thus representing a simple model potentially adoptable by any laboratory. Our preliminary results show that by jointly considering the panel of biomarkers here investigated the highest predictive capability is given by cfDNA followed by integrity index 180/67 and methylated *RASSF1A*. According to these results, an approach based on the simultaneous determination of the three biomarkers (cfDNA, integrity index 180/67 and methylated *RASSF1A*) could be suggested to improve the diagnostic performance in melanoma (Salvianti *et al* 2012).

Even though each biomarker investigated in the present work is not exclusively associated with melanoma, their combination reveals a high specificity for melanoma detection.

Acknowledgement

This paper is dedicated to Prof. Claudio Orlando who initiated the research on cell-free DNA in our Laboratory.

References

Chan, K. C., Ding, C., Gerovassili, A., Yeung, S. W., Chiu, R. W., Leung, T. N., Lau, T. K., Chim, S. S., Chung, G. T., Nicolaides, K. H., & Lo, Y. M. (2006). Hypermethylated RASSF1A in maternal plasma: A universal fetal DNA marker that improves the reliability of noninvasive prenatal diagnosis. Clinical Chemistry, 52, 2211-2218.

Daniotti, M., Vallacchi, V., Rivoltini, L., Patuzzo, R., Santinami, M., Arienti, .F, Cutolo, G., Pierotti, M. A., Parmiani, G., & Rodolfo, M. (2007). Detection of mutated BRAFV600E variant in circulating DNA of stage III-IV melanoma patients. International Journal of Cancer, 120, 2439-2444.

Davies, H., Bignell, G. R., Cox, C., Stephens, P., Edkins, .S, Clegg, S., Teague, J., Woffendin, H., Garnett, M. J., Bottomley, W., Davis, N., Dicks, E., Ewing, R., Floyd, Y., Gray, K., Hall, S., Hawes, R., Hughes, J., Kosmidou, V., Menzies, A., Mould, C., Parker, A., Stevens, C., Watt, S., Hooper, S., Wilson, R., Jayatilake, H., Gusterson, B.A., Cooper, C., Shipley, J., Hargrave, D., Pritchard-Jones, K., Maitland, N., Chenevix-Trench, G., Riggins, G.J., Bigner, D. D., Palmieri, G., Cossu, A., Flanagan, A., Nicholson, A., Ho, J. W., Leung, S. Y., Yuen, S. T., Weber, B. L., Seigler, H. F., Darrow, T. L., Paterson, H., Marais, R., Marshall, C. J., Wooster, R., Stratton, M. R., & Futreal, P. A. (2002). Mutations of the BRAF gene in human cancer. Nature, 417, 949-954.

Dhomen, N. & Marais, R.(2007). New insight into BRAF mutations in cancer. Current Opinion in Genetics & Development, 17, 31-39.

Donninger, H., Vos, M. D., & Clark, G. J.(2007). The RASSF1A tumor suppressor. Journal of Cell Science, 120, 3163-3172.

Flaherty, K., Puzanov, I., & Sosman, J. (2009). Phase I study of PLX4032: proof of concept for V600E BRAF mutation as a therapeutic target in human cancer. Journal of Clinical Oncology, 27, 15s, abstr 9000.

Fleischhacker, M. & Schmidt, B. (2007). Circulating nucleic acids (CNAs) and cancer-a survey. Biochimica et Biophysica Acta, 1775, 181-232.

Gasparini, G., Bonoldi, E., Viale, G., Verderio, P., Boracchi, P., Panizzoni, G. A., Radaelli, U., Di Bacco, A., Guglielmi, R. B., & Bevilacqua, P. (1996). Prognostic and predictive value of tumour angiogenesis in ovarian carcinomas. International Journal of Cancer, 69, 205-211.

Hanley, J. A. & McNeil, B. J. (1982) The meaning and use of the area under a receiver operating characteristic (ROC) curve. Radiology, 143, 29-36.

Hanley, R., Rieger-Christ, K. M., Canes, D., Emara, N.R., Shuber, A.P., Boynton, K. A., Libertino, J.A., & Summerhayes, I.C. (2006). DNA integrity assay: a plasma-based screening tool for the detection of prostate cancer. Clinical Cancer Research, 12, 4569-4574.

Hauser, S., Zahalka, T., Ellinger, J., Fechner, G., Heukamp, L. C., VON Ruecker, A., Müller, S. C., & Bastian, P. J. (2010). Cell-free circulating DNA: Diagnostic value in patients with renal cell cancer. Anticancer Research, 30, 2785-2789.

Hodgson, D. R., Wellings, R., Orr, M. C., McCormack, R., Malone, M., Board, R. E., & Cantarini, M. V. (2010). Circulating tumour-derived predictive biomarkers in oncology. Drug Discovery Today, 15, 98-101.

Hollander, M. &Wolfe, D. A. (1999). Nonparametric Statistical Methods, Second ed. New York: John Wiley & Sons

Hoon, D.S., Bostick, P., Kuo, C., Okamoto, T., Wang, H.J., Elashoff, R., & Morton, D. L. (2000). Molecular markers in blood as surrogate prognostic indicators of melanoma recurrence. Cancer Research, 60, 2253-2257.

Hosmer, D. W. & Lemeshow, S. (1989). Applied Logistic Regression. New York: John Wiley & Sons.

Huang, P. H. & Marais, R. (2009). Cancer: Melanoma troops massed. Nature, 459, 336-337.

Jiang, W. W., Zahurak, M., Goldenberg, D., Milman, Y., Park, H.L., Westra, W. H., Koch, W., Sidransky, D., & Califano, J. (2006). Increased plasma DNA integrity index in head and neck cancer patients. International Journal of Cancer, 119, 2673-2676.

Jung, K., Fleischhacker, M., & Rabien, A. (2010). Cell-free DNA in the blood as a solid tumor biomarker--a critical appraisal of the literature. Clinica Chimica Acta, 411, 1611-1624.

Koyanagi, K., Mori, T., O'Day, S. J., Martinez, S. R., Wang, H. J., & Hoon, D. S. (2006). Association of circulating tumor cells with serum tumor-related methylated DNA in peripheral blood of melanoma patients. Cancer Research, 66, 6111-6117.

Lehmann, U., Glöckner, S., Kleeberger, W., vonWasielewski, H. F., & Kreipe, H. (2000). Detection of gene amplification in archival breast cancer specimens by laser-assisted microdissection and quantitative real-time polymerase chain reaction. The American Journal of Pathology, 156, 1855–1864.

Malone, F. D., Canick, J. A., Ball, R. H., Nyberg, D. A., Comstock, C. H., Bukowski, R., Berkowitz, R. L., Gross, S. J., Dugoff, L., Craigo, S. D., Timor-Tritsch, I. E., Carr, S. R., Wolfe, H. M., Dukes, K., Bianchi, D. W., Rudnicka, A. R., Hackshaw, A. K., Lambert-Messerlian, G., Wald, N. J., & D'Alton, M. E. (2005). First- and Second-Trimester Evaluation of Risk (FASTER) Research Consortium. First-trimester or second-trimester screening, or both, for Down's syndrome. The New England Journal of Medicine, 353, 2001-2011.

Marini, A., Mirmohammadsadegh, A., Nambiar, S., Gustrau, A., Ruzicka, T., & Hengge, U. R. (2006). Epigenetic inactivation of tumor suppressor genes in serum of patients with cutaneous melanoma. The Journal of Investigative Dermatology, 126, 422-431.

Mori, T., O'Day, S. J., Umetani, N., Martinez, S. R., Kitago, M., Koyanagi, K., Kuo, C., Takeshima, T. L., Milford, R., Wang, H. J., Vu, V. D., Nguyen, S. L., & Hoon, D. S. (2005). Predictive utility of circulating methylated DNA in serum of melanoma patients receiving biochemotherapy. Journal of Clinical Oncology, 23, 9351-9358.

Omholt, K., Platz, A., Kanter, L., Ringborg, U., & Hansson, J. (2003). NRAS and BRAF mutations arise early during melanoma pathogenesis and are preserved throughout tumor progression. Clinical Cancer Research, 9, 6483-6488.

Pinsky, P. F. & Zhu, C.S. (2011). Building Multi-Marker Algorithms for Disease Prediction-The Role of Correlations Among Markers. Biomarker Insights, 6, 83-93.

Pinzani, P., Salvianti, F., Cascella, R., Massi, D., De Giorgi, V., Pazzagli, M., & Orlando, C. (2010). Allele specific Taqman-based real-time PCR assay to quantify circulating BRAFV600E mutated DNA in plasma of melanoma patients. Clinica Chimica Acta, 411, 1319-1324.

Pinzani, P., Salvianti, F., Zaccara, S., Massi, D., De Giorgi, V., Pazzagli, M., & Orlando, C. (2011) .Circulating cell-free DNA in plasma of melanoma patients: qualitative and quantitative considerations. Clinica Chimica Acta 412, 2141-2145.

Pollock, P. M., Harper, U. L., Hansen, K. S., Yudt, L. M., Stark, M., Robbins, C. M., Moses, T. Y., Hostetter, G., Wagner, U., Kakareka, J., Salem, G., Pohida, T., Heenan, P., Duray, P., Kallioniemi, O., Hayward, N. K., Trent, J. M., & Meltzer, P. S.(2003). High frequency of BRAF mutations in nevi. Nature Genetics, 33, 19-20.

Salvianti, F., Pinzani, P., Verderio, P., Ciniselli, C. M., Massi, D., De Giorgi, V., Grazzini, M., Pazzagli, M., & Orlando, C. (2012). Multiparametric analysis of cell-free DNA in melanoma patients. PLoS One, 7, e49843.

Schneider, E. & Mizejewski, G.(2007). Multi-marker testing for cancer: what can we learn from modern prenatal testing for Trisomy-21. Cancer Informatics, 2, 44-47.

Schwarzenbach, H., Hoon, D. S., & Pantel, K. (2011) Cell-free nucleic acids as biomarkers in cancer patients. Nature Reviews. Cancer, 11, 426–437.

Spugnardi, M., Tommasi, S., Dammann, R., Pfeifer, G. P., Hoon, D. S. (2003). Epigenetic inactivation of RAS association domain family protein 1 (RASSF1A) in malignant cutaneous melanoma. Cancer Research, 63, 1639-1643.

Tanemura, A., Terando, A. M., Sim, M.S., van Hoesel, A. Q., de Maat, M. F., Morton, D. L., & Hoon, D. S. (2009). CpG island methylator phenotype predicts progression of malignant melanoma. Clinical Cancer Research, 15, 1801-1807.

Tomita, H., Ichikawa, D., Ikoma, D., Sai, S., Tani, N., Ikoma, H., Fujiwara, H., Kikuchi, S., Okamoto, K., Ochiai, T., & Otsuji, E. (2007). Quantification of circulating plasma DNA fragments as tumor markers in patients with esophageal cancer. Anticancer Research, 27, 2737-2741.

Umetani, N., Giuliano, A. E., Hiramatsu, S. H., Amersi, F., Nakagawa, T., Martino, S., & Hoon, D. S. (2006). Prediction of breast tumor progression by integrity of free circulating DNA in serum. Journal of Clinical Oncology, 24, 4270-4276.

Umetani, N., Kim, J., Hiramatsu, S., Reber, H. A., Hines, O. J., Bilchik, A. J., & Hoon, D. S.(2006). Increased integrity of free circulating DNA in sera of patients with colorectal or periampullary cancer: direct quantitative PCR for ALU repeats. Clinical Chemistry, 52, 1062-1069.

Verderio, P., Mangia, A., Ciniselli, C.M., Tagliabue, P., Paradiso, A.(2010) Biomarkers for Early Cancer Detection - Methodological Aspects. Breast Care; 5, 62-65.

Wang, B. G., Huang, H. Y., Chen, Y. C., Bristow, R. E., Kassauei, K., Cheng, C. C., Roden, R., Sokoll, L. J., Chan, D. W., & Shih, IeM. (2003). Increased plasma DNA integrity in cancer patients. Cancer Research, 63, 3966-3968.

Yancovitz, M., Yoon, J., Mikhail, M., Gai, W., Shapiro, R. L., Berman, R. S., Pavlick, A. C., Chapman, P. B., Osman, .I, & Polsky, D. (2007). Detection of mutant BRAF alleles in the plasma of patients with metastatic melanoma. The Journal of Molecular Diagnostics, 9, 178-183.

Role of the pRb-E2F Pathway in TGFβ-Mediated Tumour Suppression

Juliana Korah
Department of Surgical Research
Division of Medical Oncology, Faculty of Medicine
McGill University, Canada

Jean-Jacques Lebrun
Division of Medical Oncology
Faculty of Medicine
McGill University, Canada

1   Introduction

The transforming growth factor-β (TGFβ) superfamily comprises widespread and evolutionarily conserved polypeptide growth factors that are involved in the regulation of a multitude of diverse fundamental cellular processes, including the regulation of cell proliferation, differentiation, immortalization, and apoptosis (Massague, 1990; Siegel & Massague, 2003). TGFβ, the prototype of the family, is a vital factor in the maintenance of homeostasis between cell growth and apoptosis. TGFβ ligands signal through serine/threonine kinase receptors that, once activated by ligand binding, recruit and phosphorylate the canonical downstream mediators, Smad2 and Smad3. Once phosphorylated, Smad2 and Smad3 interact with their common partner Smad4 to then translocate to the nucleus where the Smad complex associates with diverse DNA binding factors to regulate expression of target genes in a cell- and tissue-specific manner (Massague, 1998). These partner proteins, which act as co-activators or co-repressors, are differentially expressed in different cell types and are thus thought to provide a basis for tissue and cell type-specific functions for TGFβ ligands (Feng & Derynck, 2005; Massague & Wotton, 2000).

Alternatively, TGFβ also activates other intracellular signalling pathways independently of the Smads. These non-canonical mediators of TGFβ signalling include the stress-activated kinases p38 and c-Jun N-terminal kinase (JNK), which are phosphorylated and activated by TGFβ, and can actually synergize with Smad signalling to induce apoptosis and epithelial-to-mesenchymal transition (EMT) (Bakin *et al.*, 2002; Cocolakis *et al.*, 2001; de Guise *et al.*, 2006; Hanafusa *et al.*, 1999; Yan *et al.*, 1994). TGFβ also signals through the mitogen-activated protein kinase (MAPK) pathway, by activating the extracellular signal-regulated kinases 1 and 2 (ERK1 and ERK2), leading to the induction of EMT (Davies *et al.*, 2005; M. K. Lee *et al.*, 2007; Yan *et al.*, 1994). Moreover, TGFβ activates the phosphoinositide 3-kinase (PI3K)/Akt pathway to regulate cell growth inhibition (R. H. Chen *et al.*, 1998) and induction of EMT (Lamouille & Derynck, 2007; Peron *et al.*, 2001). Finally, TGFβ has also been shown to signal through the Rho-like GTPase pathway, by activating RhoA, Cdc42, and Rac, leading to cytoskeleton reorganization, cell motility and invasion (Bhowmick *et al.*, 2001; Edlund *et al.*, 2002).

TGFβ and its receptors are widely expressed in virtually all tissues and TGFβ signal transduction pathways play a significant role in human diseases, particularly cancer. Intriguingly, while TGFβ acts as a tumour suppressor in normal cells and early carcinoma, its protective effects are often lost during cancer progression. Concurrently, its tumour promoting and pro-invasive responses prevail, leading to further tumour growth and metastasis (Lebrun, 2012). Loss or mutation of TGFβ signalling components is frequently observed in human cancer, thus defining a tumour suppressive role for this growth factor (Levy & Hill, 2006; Pardali & Moustakas, 2007). TGFβ exerts its tumour suppressive effects by inhibiting cell cycle progression, preventing immortalization through inhibition of telomerase activity, and inducing apoptosis. These are outlined in Figure 2.

1.1   Cell Cycle Inhibition

Cell cycle progression is tightly regulated by cyclin-dependent kinases (Cdks), which associate with their regulatory cyclins. These cyclin-Cdk complexes phosphorylate members of the retinoblastoma (Rb) protein family, which release E2F transcription factors that mediate the transcription of numerous cell cycle regulatory genes, allowing for cell cycle progression from G1 to S phase (Dyson, 1998; Massague, 2004). TGFβ induces cell cycle arrest in G1 through transcriptional induction of the Cdk inhibitors p15[INK4B] (J. M. Li *et al.*, 1995) and p21[CIP1] (Datto *et al.*, 1995). This regulation is Smad-dependent and requires Smad association with the transcription factors FoxO (Seoane *et al.*, 2004) and Sp1 (Ho *et al.*, 2004; Pardali *et al.*, 2000). p15[INK4B] binding to the Cdk4/6-cyclinD complexes also displaces p21[CIP1] or

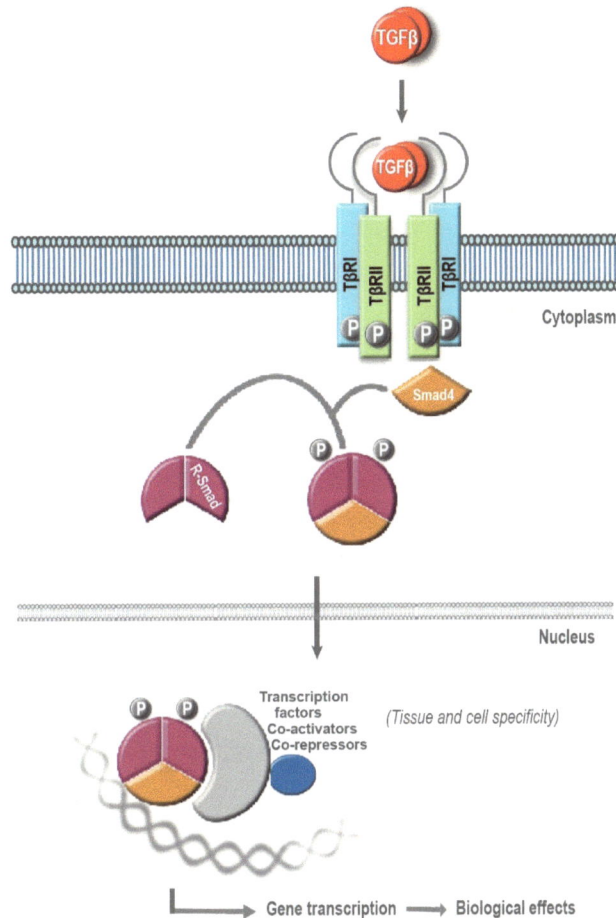

Figure 1: TGFβ Signalling Through the Canonical Smad Pathway. Signalling is initiated with TGFβ ligand binding to its type-II receptor (TβRII) that exhibits constitutive serine-threonine protein kinase activity. Upon ligand binding, TβRII recruits and transphosphorylates TβRI which in turn phosphorylates the canonical downstream mediators, the receptor-regulated Smads (R-Smads), Smad2 and Smad3. The phosphorylated R-Smads then detach from the receptor complex and associate with common partner Smad4 within the cytoplasm. The resulting activated Smad2/3/4 heterotrimeric complex translocates to the nucleus, where it interacts with various transcription factors, co-activators and/or co-repressors, to modulate target gene expression.

the related p27^{KIP1} from their pre-existing Cdk4/6 complexes, allowing them to bind and inactivate Cdk2-cyclinA/E complexes (Figure 2A, orange arrows) (Reynisdottir *et al.*, 1995; Sandhu *et al.*, 1997).

The antiproliferative effect of TGFβ also relies on transcriptional inhibition of growth-promoting factors, such as c-Myc (C. R. Chen *et al.*, 2002), Cdc25A (Iavarone & Massague, 1999), and Id transcription factors (Kang *et al.*, 2003; Kowanetz *et al.*, 2004; Lasorella *et al.*, 2000). While c-Myc is a well-established activator of cell growth and proliferation (Eisenman, 2001; Grandori *et al.*, 2000), it also directly inhibits p15^{INK4B} (Warner *et al.*, 1999) and p21$^{CIP1/WAF1}$ (Claassen & Hann, 2000). Thus, inhibition of c-Myc expression by TGFβ not only relieves its proliferative role but also further contributes to the induction of the Cdk inhibitors and cell cycle arrest (Seoane *et al.*, 2001). The Cdk tyrosine phosphatase

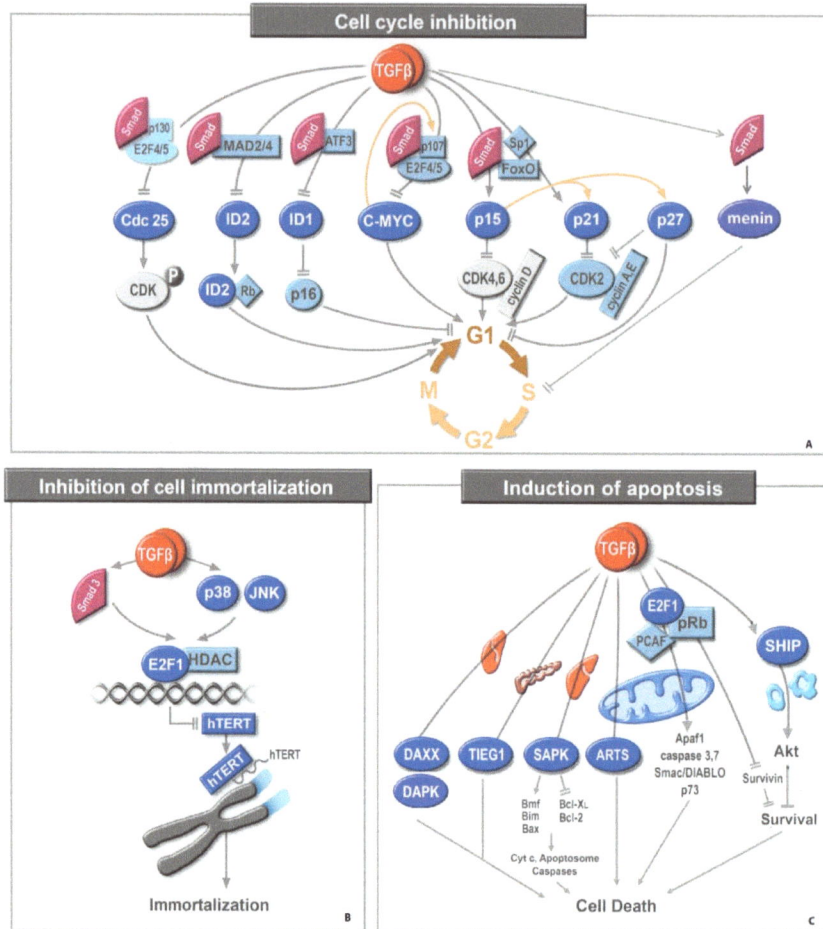

Figure 2: TGFβ Tumour Suppressive Pathways. In normal cells and early carcinoma, TGFβ exerts its tumour suppressive effects by inhibiting cell cycle progression, preventing immortalization through inhibition of telomerase activity, and inducing apoptosis. See text for details.

Cdc25A normally dephosphorylates inhibitory sites on Cdk4 and Cdk6, resulting in their activation. Transcriptional repression of Cdc25A by TGFβ allows for sustained phosphorylation and inactivation of these Cdks, thus preventing cell cycle progression (Iavarone & Massague, 1997). TGFβ inhibits both c-Myc and Cdc25A by recruiting Smad-E2F4/5-pRb family member repressor complexes to these gene promoters (C. R. Chen *et al.*, 2002; Iavarone & Massague, 1999). The Id (Inhibitor of Differentiation/DNA binding) family of transcription factors prevents differentiation, promote cell proliferation through interaction with pRb, and have been implicated in promoting tumourigenesis (Lasorella *et al.*, 2000; Norton, 2000). Id1 has also been shown to delay cellular senescence in primary mammalian cells through repression of the cell cycle regulatory protein p16^{INK4a} (Alani *et al.*, 2001). TGFβ transcriptionally induces activating transcription factor 3 (ATF3), which associates with Smad3 to inhibit Id1 expression (Kang *et al.*, 2003). Id2 overexpression results from transcriptional activation by c-Myc (Lasorella *et al.*, 2000), thus c-Myc down-regulation by TGFβ contributes to inhibition of Id2 expression. Repression of these transcription factors by TGFβ largely contributes to this growth factor's anti-proliferative effect.

Moreover, previous studies from our laboratory demonstrated that TGFβ induces expression of the tumour suppressor menin in pituitary adenoma cells, leading to G1 arrest. We further found that menin interacts with Smad3, and that inactivating menin expression blocks TGFβ signalling and antagonizes TGFβ-mediated cell growth inhibition (Hendy *et al.*, 2005; Kaji *et al.*, 2001; Lebrun, 2009).

1.2 Inhibition of Immortalization

TGFβ also exerts its tumour suppressive effects through inhibition of cell immortalization in both normal and cancer cells. Most normal human cells are only able to replicate a limited number of times due to the progressive shortening of the ends of the chromosomes (telomeres) with each cell division, as DNA polymerases fail to fully replicate the genetic material. Consequently, the length of the telomeres shortens to a critical point, triggering cell senescence or cell death to avoid genomic instability and loss of important chromosomal DNA (Cong *et al.*, 2002). Conversely, cancer cells are not limited by such a fixed number of replication cycles but instead achieve immortalization. This is due to the constitutive activity of telomerase, an enzyme that adds telomeric DNA repeats at the ends of newly duplicated telomeres, thereby preserving their length throughout successive replication cycles and protecting chromosomes from degradation (Blasco, 2005).

Human telomerase is a specialized reverse transcriptase complex composed of both an RNA component (hTR) that provides the template for the addition of new telomeric repeats, and a catalytic protein subunit known as human telomerase reverse transcriptase (hTERT). Although hTR is highly expressed in virtually all mammalian cells, the expression of hTERT is restricted to cells that exhibit telomerase activity, indicating that hTERT expression is the rate-limiting component of the telomerase enzyme (Cong *et al.*, 2002; Olaussen *et al.*, 2006). Most somatic cells have little or no telomerase activity due to a strong repression of hTERT. Exceptions include cells with high proliferative potential, such as basal cells of the epidermis, embryonic cells, germ cells, activated lymphocytes, intestinal crypt cells, and certain stem cells, which require telomerase activity for proliferation and long-term viability (Meyerson *et al.*, 1997). In contrast, the expression of hTERT is elevated in 85-90% of cancer cells (Blasco, 2005; Kim *et al.*, 1994; Neumann & Reddel, 2002). This is by far the most commonly observed abnormality acquired by tumour cells and is used as a diagnostic marker for cancer. Reactivation of telomerase activity is mainly due to the loss of repression of the hTERT gene in cancer cells. Though telomerase activity is regulated at various levels, such as mRNA splicing, hTR and hTERT modification, and accessibility of the telomeres, transcriptional control of the hTERT gene is considered the key event in the activation of telomerase activity observed in cancer cells (Cong & Bacchetti, 2000; Meyerson *et al.*, 1997).

TGFβ inhibits telomerase activity in various cell lines, however the precise mechanisms by which it represses hTERT expression remain unclear. Several factors have been implicated in the inhibition of telomerase by TGFβ. For instance, TGFβ has been shown to suppress human and rat TERT expression indirectly by inhibiting c-Myc expression (Hu *et al.*, 2006; H. Yang *et al.*, 2001). However, another study in MCF-7 breast cancer cells suggested that hTERT expression is not repressed by the inhibition of c-Myc but rather by direct action of Smad3 on the hTERT promoter in response to TGFβ (H. Li *et al.*, 2006). In this proposed pathway, TGFβ mediates Smad3 binding to c-Myc and inactivates its expression, while c-Myc recruits Smad3 to the hTERT promoter resulting in transcriptional repression of the hTERT gene (H. Li *et al.*, 2006). Another study revealed a role for the Smad interacting protein-1 (SIP1) in TGFβ-mediated hTERT repression (S. Y. Lin & Elledge, 2003). The different mechanisms observed in different cell systems may in fact reflect cell type-specific effects rather than a central mechanism.

Studies from our laboratory demonstrate that repression of telomerase by TGFβ is mediated not only through the Smad pathway but also requires the Erk1/2 and p38 kinase pathways, as well as histone deacetylase activity (Lacerte *et al.*, 2008). We also found that the inhibitory effect of TGFβ on hTERT expression is dependent on the transcription factor E2F1, highlighting E2F1 as an important mediator of TGFβ tumour suppressive effects. Results from this study will be discussed here in detail.

1.3   Induction of Apoptosis

Finally, TGFβ also prevents tumour growth and progression by inducing apoptosis. Programmed cell death by apoptosis is a fundamental mechanism for regulating cell number and tissue homeostasis (Meier *et al.*, 2000; Thompson, 1995). The apoptotic programme is tightly controlled through the action of numerous effectors, both pro- and anti-apoptotic factors.

TGFβ induces a number of apoptotic responses and its ability to do so varies greatly depending on the tissue or cell type (Siegel & Massague, 2003). Understanding the basis of this variability requires elucidating the molecular mechanisms involved in regulating TGFβ-mediated cell death. Several apoptotic regulators have been implicated in mediating TGFβ apoptotic responses. In hepatocarcinomas, TGFβ transcriptionally induces the death-associated protein kinase (DAPK), which promotes cell death in a Smad-dependent manner by modulating the activation potential of the mitochondrial membrane, potentially contributing to cytochrome *c* release and caspase activation(Jang *et al.*, 2002). In pancreatic epithelial cells, TGFβ induces the zinc finger transcription factor TGFβ-inducible early-response gene (TIEG1), leading to cell death (Tachibana *et al.,* 1997). Moreover, TGFβ promotes delocalization of the mitochondrial septin-like protein ARTS (apoptosis-related protein in TGFβ signalling pathway) from the mitochondrion to the nucleus where it binds to and inactivates inhibitors of apoptosis (IAPs), resulting in activation of caspases and the apoptotic programme (Larisch *et al.*, 2000). Previous work from our lab showed that TGFβ can also induce apoptosis by antagonizing PI3K/Akt signalling activity through Smad-mediated transcriptional induction of the lipid phosphatase SHIP (SH2-domain-containing inositol-5-phosphatase) in haematopoietic cells. Increased SHIP expression impedes the phosphorylation and activation of Akt, a major pro-survival kinase, resulting in cell death in both B and T lymphocytes (Valderrama-Carvajal *et al.*, 2002).

TGFβ also antagonizes survival signalling by inhibiting expression of survivin, a member of the mammalian IAPs, through the association of Smad3 with Akt, leading to programmed cell death in colon cancer (Conery *et al.*, 2004; Remy *et al.*, 2004; J. Wang *et al.*, 2008). In normal cells, survivin expression is confined to the G_2/M phase of the cell cycle and is required for regulating mitosis (Altieri, 2003b). Conversely, survivin expression is highly overexpressed in numerous cancers and has been associated with inhibition of various apoptotic pathways, thus contributing to tumour maintenance and progression (Ambrosini *et al.*, 1997; Hoffman *et al.*, 2002; Islam *et al.*, 2000; Mahotka *et al.*, 1999; Mirza *et al.*, 2002; A. Suzuki *et al.*, 2000; Tamm *et al.*, 1998). In fact, antagonizing survivin expression or activity induces spontaneous apoptosis, enhances apoptosis induced by chemotherapeutic agents, and/or inhibits tumour growth (Altieri, 2003a, 2003c). In prostate cancer, it has been proposed that de-regulated TGFβ-survivin signalling may contribute to tumour progression, as survivin expression positively correlates with tumour stage or loss of expression of the TGFβ receptors (Kishi *et al.*, 2004; Shariat *et al.*, 2004). In prostate epithelial cells, transcriptional repression of survivin by TGFβ is Smad2- and Smad3-dependent and involves recruitment of a pRb/E2F4 repressive complex to the survivin promoter (J. Yang *et al.*, 2008).

Moreover, the stress-activated protein kinase/c-Jun N-terminal kinase (SAPK/JNK) signalling pathway also plays a critical role in mediating TGFβ apoptotic responses, through Smad interaction with the activator protein 1 (AP1) (Atfi *et al.*, 1997; Yamamura *et al.*, 2000). TGFβ causes both Smad- and SAPK/p38-dependent transcriptional induction of the pro-apoptotic Bcl-2 family members Bmf and Bim, which in turn activate Bax, leading to mitochondrial release of cytochrome *c* and activation of the apoptosome, resulting in caspase-dependent apoptosis in hepatocytes and B-lymphocytes (Ohgushi *et al.*, 2005; Wildey *et al.*, 2003). Conversely, TGFβ inhibits expression of the anti-apoptotic factors Bcl-X$_L$ and Bcl-2 in various cell types (Chipuk *et al.*, 2001; Francis *et al.*, 2000; Kanamaru *et al.*, 2002; Saltzman *et al.*, 1998).

Each of these signalling events eventually couples the TGFβ signalling pathway to the apoptotic machinery, leading to changes in expression, localization, and activation of various apoptotic effectors (Schuster & Krieglstein, 2002). The TGFβ apoptotic response in normal and tumour cells is multifaceted, incorporating both pro-apoptotic and pro-survival pathways and an array of cytoplasmic and nuclear effectors. The net decision of whether TGFβ will promote apoptosis or favor survival likely depends on additional signalling inputs that the cell receives. Though numerous TGFβ apoptotic mediators and pathways have been defined, these regulatory mechanisms have been mostly cell type- and tissue-specific (Siegel & Massague, 2003). Recently, a more wide-ranging mechanism of TGFβ-mediated cell death was uncovered, based on a study from our laboratory which will be described herein.

1.4   Rationale

Our first study described here demonstrates that the TGFβ inhibitory effect on telomerase activity and cell immortalization is dependent on both Smad3 and the transcription factor E2F1, highlighting E2F1 as an important mediator of TGFβ tumour suppressive effects (Lacerte *et al.*, 2008).

The E2F family of transcription factors is a group of DNA-binding proteins that are central regulators of cell cycle progression. The transcriptional activity of E2F1 through 5 is regulated primarily via their association with members of the retinoblastoma family of pocket proteins, which include the retinoblastoma tumour suppressor protein, pRb/p105, and its homologs p107 and p130 (Dyson, 1998). E2F1, the founding member and best-characterized of the family, has a unique role compared to other E2Fs, showing characteristics of being both an oncogene and a tumour suppressor, as it is able to induce both cell cycle progression and apoptosis. Though an increase in E2F1 activity has been reported in several types of tumours (Eymin *et al.*, 2001; T. Suzuki *et al.*, 1999) supporting an oncogenic role for E2F1, transgenic mice overexpressing E2F1 display aberrant cell apoptosis (D. Wang *et al.*, 2000). Furthermore, E2F1 knockout mice develop highly malignant tumours and show defects in thymocyte apoptosis, highlighting E2F1 as a potent tumour suppressor (Yamasaki *et al.*, 1996). The nature of this dichotomy is proposed to be based on the degree to which E2F1 is expressed in the context of the cell cycle and/or following DNA damage, and the notion that different threshold levels of E2F1 are required for differential transactivation of its target gene promoters, which may favor either survival or apoptosis (Crosby & Almasan, 2004). Moreover, posttranslational modifications of E2F1 in response to DNA damage have been shown to direct E2F1 from cell cycle progression to apoptotic E2F target genes, resulting in apoptotic induction (Carnevale *et al.*, 2012; Pediconi *et al.*, 2003). Interestingly, E2F1 mutants that are unable to promote cell cycle progression retain their ability to induce programmed cell death, indicating that induction of the cell cycle and apoptosis are separable functions of E2F1 (Phillips *et al.*, 1997). Given our previous findings that E2F1 is required for TGFβ-mediated inhibition of hTERT (Lacerte *et al.*, 2008) and that TGFβ promotes increased E2F-DNA-binding activity in pre-apoptotic hepatoma cell nuclear extracts (Fan *et al.*, 2002), we investigated whether E2F1 could also mediate another arm of the TGFβ tumour suppressive response and regulate apoptosis. Indeed, we uncovered a central mechanism by which TGFβ induces apoptosis in both normal and cancer cells of various origins. We found TGFβ to increase E2F1 expression post-translationally, further leading to the formation and binding of a transcriptionally active E2F1-pRb-P/CAF complex on multiple TGFβ pro-apoptotic target gene promoters, thereby activating their transcription and highlighting E2F1 as a central mediator of the TGFβ apoptotic programme (Korah et al., 2012). Results of this study will also be discussed in this chapter.

2   Results

2.1   TGFβ Represses hTERT Gene Expression in a HDAC-Dependent Manner

To investigate the regulation of hTERT by TGFβ, we used human epithelial cancer cell lines originating from different tissues; immortalized human keratinocytes (HaCaT), human hepatocarcinoma cells (HuH7), and human breast adenocarcinoma cells (MCF-7), as well as Chinese hamster ovary (CHO) cells. We first analyzed the effect of TGFβ on hTERT gene promoter activity. To do so, a 2-kb region (−1978 to +73) of the hTERT promoter was cloned upstream of luciferase gene. The resulting hTERT-lux reporter construct was then transfected in the different cell lines, and the cells were stimulated or not with TGFβ. As shown in Figure 3a, TGFβ significantly decreased hTERT gene promoter activity in all cell lines tested. The TGFβ effect was strongest in HaCaT cells (76% ± 8% inhibition), while more modest in HuH7 cells (32% ± 13% inhibition) and CHO cells (46% ± 24% inhibition), and minor in MCF-7 cells (24% ± 4% inhibition). We then examined whether the repressed hTERT promoter activity translated into reduced hTERT mRNA and protein levels. As illustrated in Figure 3b, TGFβ treatment of HaCaT cells resulted in a strong and rapid decrease in hTERT mRNA expression levels (left panels) followed by a significant decrease in hTERT protein levels (right panels). Together, our results indicate that TGFβ acts as a potent inhibitor of hTERT expression in epithelial cancer cells.

Previous studies have reported that histone deacetylases (HDACs) are involved in repressing telomerase activity (Cong & Bacchetti, 2000). To assess whether inhibition of hTERT expression by TGFβ requires HDAC activity, we examined the effect of Trichostatin A (TSA), a class I and II HDAC inhibitor, on hTERT promoter activity. As shown in Figure 3c, increasing concentrations of TSA fully impeded the inhibitory effect of TGFβ on hTERT promoter activity and endogenous hTERT mRNA levels. To further elucidate whether both class I and II HDACs are involved in regulating hTERT, we overexpressed a class I histone deacetylase (HDAC1) or a class II histone deacetylase (HDAC4/5) in HaCaT cells and assessed their effect on hTERT gene promoter activity in the presence or the absence of TGFβ. Interestingly, while overexpression of HDAC1 did not demonstrate any significant effect on hTERT promoter activity (Figure 3d), overexpression of HDAC4 or HDAC5 significantly repressed hTERT gene promoter activity, indicating that specifically class II HDACs are required for this regulation.

2.2   The Smad, Erk, and p38 MAPK Pathways are Required for TGFβ-Mediated hTERT Inhibition

The receptor-regulated Smads, Smad2 and Smad3, are central to TGFβ signalling (Derynck & Zhang, 2003). Blocking TGFβ receptor signalling by overexpressing Smad7, a potent inhibitor that restrains Smad2/3 phosphorylation by the TGFβ type I receptor (Hayashi et al., 1997) and further targets the receptor complex to degradation (Ebisawa et al., 2001; Kavsak et al., 2000), completely blocked the TGFβ inhibition of hTERT (Figure 4a).

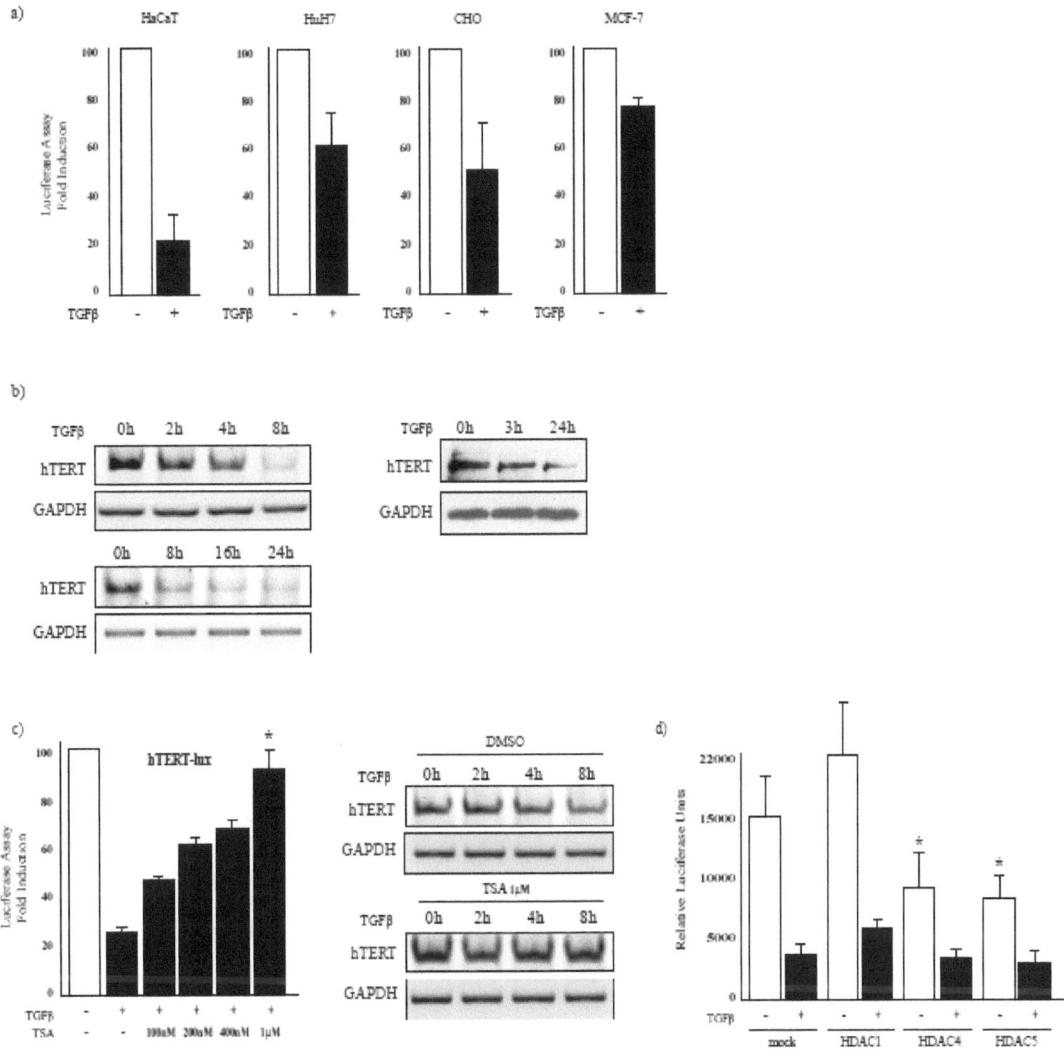

Figure 3: TGFβ Represses hTERT Gene Expression in a HDAC-Dependent Manner. a) The specified cell lines were transfected with the hTERT(−1934)-lux reporter, untreated or treated with TGFβ for 16h, and assessed for luciferase. b) RT-PCR (left) and Western blot (right) analysis of hTERT mRNA and protein levels, respectively, in HaCaT cells stimulated with TGFβ for the indicated times. c) hTERT-lux transfected HaCaT cells were pre-treated with the indicated concentrations of Trichostatin A (TSA) and stimulated with TGFβ before being assessed for luciferase (left) and hTERT mRNA levels by RT-PCR (right). d) HaCaT cells were transfected with the hTERT-lux and HDAC1, HDAC4, and HDAC5 expression vectors, as indicated, and untreated or treated with TGFβ, before being assessed for luciferase.

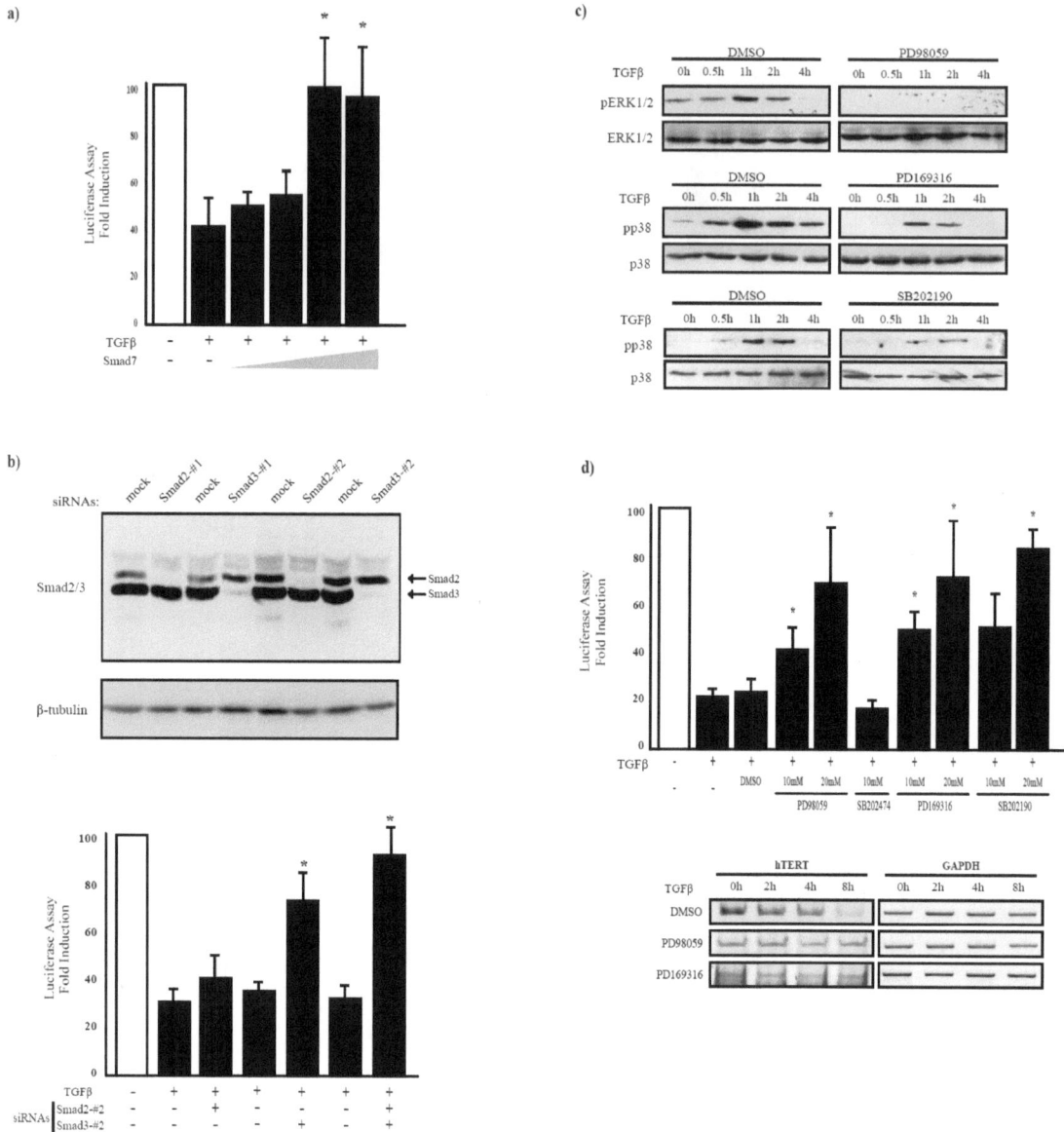

Figure 4: The Smad, Erk, and p38 MAPK Pathways are Required for TGFβ-Mediated hTERT Inhibition. a) HaCaT cells transfected with hTERT-lux and increasing amounts of Smad7 cDNA (0.1 to 0.8 μg) were stimulated or not with TGFβ before being assessed for luciferase. b) HaCaT cells were transfected with two different sets of siR-NAs against human Smad2 or Smad3 and the efficiency of Smad knockdown was verified by immunoblotting with a Smad2/3-specific antibody (upper panel). HaCaT cells were then transfected with hTERT-lux and Smad2/3 siRNAs, as indicated, stimulated with TGFβ and assessed for luciferase (lower panel). c) HaCaT cells were pre-treated for 30 min with the Erk1/2 inhibitor PD98059, or p38 kinase inhibitors, PD169316 or SB202190, as indicated, stimulated with TGFβ and protein phosphorylation levels were monitored by Western blot using phospho-specific antibodies. d) HaCaT cells were transfected with hTERT-lux, then pre-treated with or without the different MAPK inhibitors at the indicated concentrations, stimulated or not with TGFβ and assessed for luciferase (upper panel). Following treatment of HaCaT cells with MAPK inhibitors, hTERT and GAPDH mRNA levels were measured by RT-PCR (lower panel).

This demonstrated that functional TGFβ receptors and proper Smad2/3 signalling are required for inhibition of hTERT expression. To further address the relative contribution of Smad2 and Smad3, we used specific siRNAs to selectively block their expression. As shown in Figure 4b (upper panel), transfection of these siRNAs led to potent inhibition of their relative expression. Importantly, the siRNAs were highly specific since the siRNAs targeting Smad2 not affect expression of Smad3 and vice versa. Interestingly, we found that the TGFβ inhibitory effect on hTERT promoter activity is specifically mediated through Smad3 and is independent of Smad2 (Figure 4b, lower panel). This is in fact consistent with a recent study showing that TGFβ-mediated inhibition of hTERT is Smad3-dependent (H. Li *et al.*, 2006). However, since the Smad3 knockdown only partially impeded the TGFβ effect, this suggested that the Smad pathway is indeed required but perhaps not sufficient for TGFβ to inhibit hTERT expression and raised the question as to whether additional pathways might be involved. TGFβ has been reported to use other intracellular signalling cascades such as the p38 and Erk MAP kinases (Derynck & Zhang, 2003). To determine whether these pathways were activated by TGFβ, HaCaT cells were stimulated with TGFβ for different periods of time and the levels of Erk1/2 and p38 phosphorylation were examined. As shown in Figure 4c, both Erk1/2 and p38 kinases were strongly activated in response to TGFβ and these effects were specifically blocked when cells were treated with either a specific Erk1/2 inhibitor (PD98059) or two different specific p38 kinase inhibitors (PD169316 and SB202190). To address the contribution of these two pathways in TGFβ-mediated regulation of the hTERT promoter, HaCaT cells were transfected with hTERT-lux and stimulated or not with TGFβ in the presence or absence of increasing concentrations of the specific inhibitors. As shown in Figure 4d (upper panel), TGFβ-mediated inhibition of the hTERT promoter was significantly blocked when cells were pre-treated with the different kinase inhibitors, while not affected in cells treated with a non-functional analog of the PD169316 inhibitor (SB202474). Moreover, the TGFβ effect on hTERT mRNA repression was also impeded in cells pre-treated with PD169316 or PD98059 (Figure 4d, lower panel), further suggesting a role for Erk and p38 kinases in regulating hTERT inhibition by TGFβ.

2.3   The hTERT Core Promoter Region Comprises E2F DNA Binding Elements Required for TGFβ-Mediated Transcriptional Repression of hTERT

To further identify the hTERT gene promoter elements which confer the TGFβ response, progressive deletion mutants of the hTERT promoter were generated and assessed for their TGFβ responsiveness by luciferase assays. As shown in Fig. 5a, the results clearly indicated that the critical regulatory region for TGFβ-mediated inhibition of hTERT promoter activity was located between nucleotides −252 and +3. Interestingly, this 255-bp sequence of the hTERT promoter corresponds to the previously reported minimal promoter sequence necessary for its activity (Cong & Bacchetti, 2000).

The −252 to +3 hTERT promoter region contains two E-box DNA binding sites and five GC-boxes (Kyo *et al.*, 2008). E-box DNA binding elements of the hTERT promoter are recognized by the Myc/Mad/Max transcription factor family. In many cases, c-Myc expression parallels hTERT expression, in that both are increased in highly dividing cells and down regulated during differentiation. On the other hand, Mad overexpression results in decreased hTERT promoter activity (Gunes *et al.*, 2000; Oh *et al.*, 2000). Both c-Myc and Mad protein expression levels are known to be controlled by TGFβ signalling (Siegel *et al.*, 2003; Waddell *et al.*, 2004; Yagi *et al.*, 2002). For this reason, and as it was previously suggested that TGFβ inhibits hTERT through the repression of c-Myc (H. Yang *et al.*, 2001), we evaluated the potential contribution of each E-box to TGFβ-mediated inhibition of hTERT promoter activity by specific point mutations which would disrupt DNA binding (Kyo *et al.*, 2000). Mutation of the E-box sites, either individually or combined, did not affect TGFβ-mediated inhibition of the promoter activity (Figure 5b). The GC-boxes are DNA binding elements for the Sp1 transcription factor family. Sp1 transcription factors have been shown to cooperate with Smad proteins to regulate expression of several target genes (Feng *et al.*, 2000). Similarly, mutational analysis of the GC-box sites within the hTERT promoter did not affect hTERT inhibition by TGFβ signalling (data not shown), suggesting that neither of these regulatory binding sites are involved in the TGFβ response.

The −252 to +3 core hTERT promoter region also contains four E2F DNA binding elements and the dynamic assembly of an E2F/pocket protein/HDAC complex has been shown to play a role in hTERT regulation (Won *et al.*, 2004). We therefore evaluated the potential role of these E2F DNA binding sites in TGFβ-induced hTERT repression by mutational analysis. Interestingly, while single, double and triple mutations of the E2F binding sites had little or no effect, mutating all four E2F DNA sites (4XE2F mutant) abolished the TGFβ inhibitory response (Figure 5c), suggesting that the transcriptional repression of hTERT by TGFβ is mediated through several E2F binding sites located throughout the 255-bp core promoter region.

To further investigate whether E2F transcription factors are required for TGFβ to inhibit hTERT expression, we used two dominant negative forms of E2F. We first used E2F1 (1–374), a truncated E2F1 mutant, that contains the DNA binding domain but lacks the transactivation domain as well as the pocket protein-binding site. Overexpression of this mutant was previously shown to act as a dominant negative by displacing endogenous E2F-complexes from E2F DNA binding sites (Lukas *et al.*, 1996). Transcriptional activity of E2F family members is regulated by interactions with pocket proteins (pRb, p107, p130) that recruit HDACs to repress target genes (Classon & Dyson, 2001; Dyson, 1998). Thus, we also used a mutated form of E2F1 (Y411C) which is unable to bind pocket proteins (Lukas *et al.*, 1996). Interestingly, overexpression of increasing amounts of either mutant significantly impeded TGFβ-mediated inhibition of the hTERT promoter (Figure 5d and 5e). Altogether, these results suggest that TGFβ inhibits telomerase activity through binding of an E2F/repressor complex, within the proximal region of the hTERT promoter.

2.4   TGFβ-Mediated Repression of hTERT is Lost in Embryonic Fibroblasts from E2F1-Null Mutant Mice

To further define the role and contribution of E2F1 downstream of TGFβ in normal cells, we used mouse embryonic fibroblasts (MEFs) isolated from E2F1 knockout mice (Yamasaki *et al.*, 1996). Importantly, both wild-type (E2F1$^{+/+}$) and E2F1-null (E2F1$^{-/-}$) MEFs responded equally to TGFβ stimulation, as assessed by the induction of Smad phosphorylation (Figure 6a). To then investigate the contribution of E2F1 to TGFβ-mediated inhibition of mTERT, wild-type and E2F1$^{-/-}$ MEFs were stimulated with TGFβ for different periods of time and mTERT mRNA and protein levels were analyzed. While TGFβ potently inhibited both mTERT mRNA and protein levels in wild-type cells, this effect was lost in the E2F1 knockout cells (Figure 6b and 6c), further highlighting the critical role of E2F1 in TGFβ-mediated TERT repression.

Given these findings and that TGFβ has also been shown to promote increased E2F-DNA-binding activity in pre-apoptotic hepatoma cell nuclear extracts (Fan *et al.*, 2002), we investigated whether E2F1 could also mediate another arm of the TGFβ tumour suppressive response and regulate apoptosis.

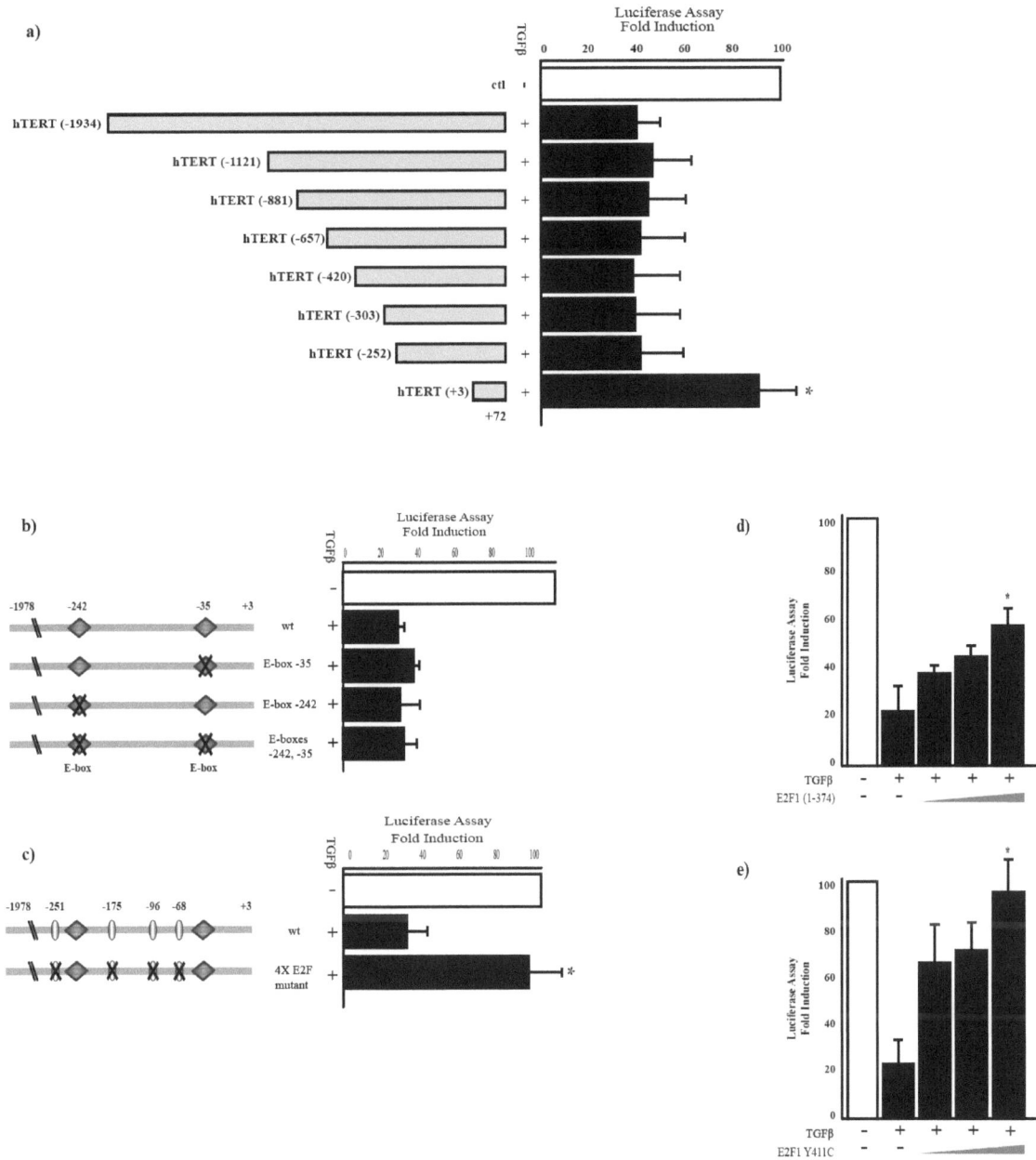

Figure 5: The hTERT Core Promoter Region Comprises E2F DNA Binding Elements Required for TGFβ-Mediated Repression of hTERT. a) Progressive deletion mutants of the hTERT gene promoter were transfected in HaCaT cells and assessed for luciferase in response to TGFβ. E-box mutants (b) and quadruple E2F binding site mutants (c) of hTERT-lux were transfected in HaCaT cells as indicated and assessed for luciferase in response to TGFβ. d, e) Dominant negative forms of E2F, E2F1 (1–374) and E2F1 Y411C were transfected in HaCaT cells as indicated and luciferase activity assessed in response to TGFβ.

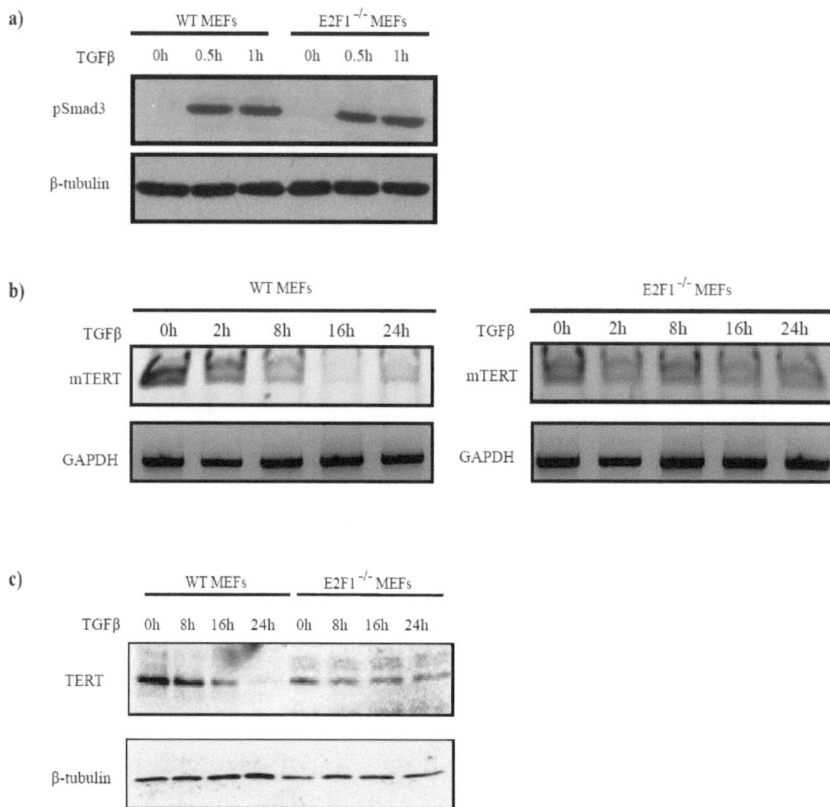

Figure 6: TGFβ-Mediated Repression of hTERT is Lost in Embryonic Fibroblasts from E2F1-Null Mutant Mice. a) Wild-type (WT) and E2F1$^{-/-}$ mouse embryonic fibroblasts (MEFs) were untreated or treated with TGFβ for the indicated times and phospho-Smad3 levels of total cell lysates were analyzed by Western blotting. b, c) Following TGFβ treatment, TERT mRNA (b) and TERT protein (c) levels were assessed by Western blotting and RT-PCR, respectively.

2.5   TGFβ-Mediated Apoptosis is E2F1-Dependent

We first examined the apoptotic effect of TGFβ in various model cells systems, including two human hepatoma cell lines (HuH7 and HepG2), a human melanoma cell line (WM278), and a human keratino-cyte cell line (HaCaT). Cells were treated with TGFβ and the apoptotic response was assessed by cell viability assay (MTT) as well as calcein-AM assay, which has been defined as a more sensitive assay for early apoptosis detection (Gatti *et al.*, 1998). All cell lines tested were strongly growth-inhibited by TGFβ treatment in a time-dependent manner (Figure 7a and b). To address the contribution of E2F1 in mediating this TGFβ response, we used RNA interference to reduce the expression of endogenous E2F1. Interestingly, we found that the effect of TGFβ on cell viability (Figure 7c) and early apoptosis (Figure 7d) in all cell lines tested was almost completely abolished when E2F1 expression was silenced, indicat-ing that E2F1 is indeed required for mediating the TGFβ pro-apoptotic response in multiple cell lines of various origin.

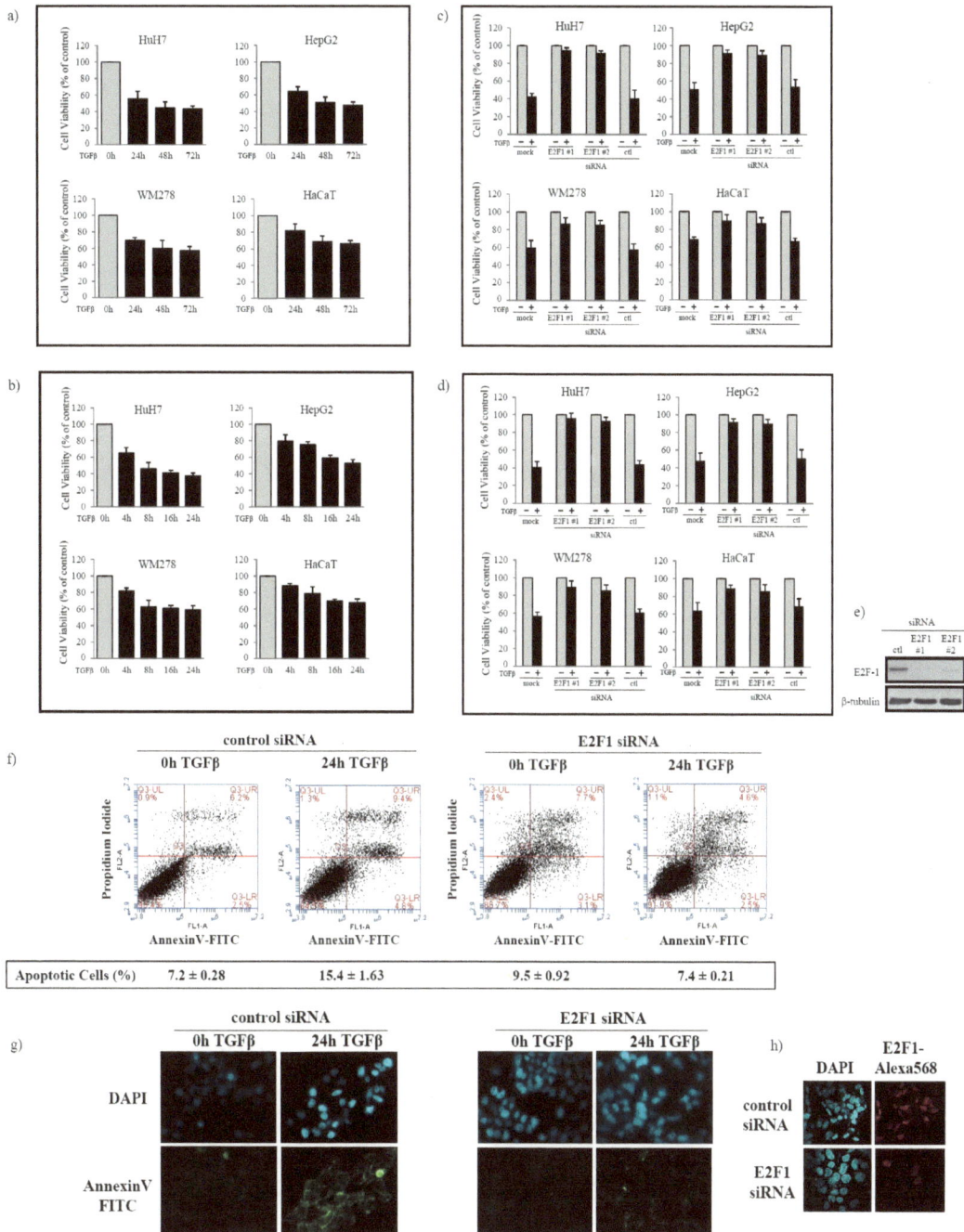

Figure 7: TGFβ-Mediated Apoptosis is E2F1-Dependent. The specified cell lines were untreated or treated with TGFβ for the indicated times and assessed for cell viability by MTT (a) and Calcein-AM (b) assays. Data are represented as mean ± SD. c, d) Cells were transiently transfected with two different siRNAs against human E2F1 or a control non-silencing siRNA and assessed by MTT (c) and Calcein-AM assays (d). e) The efficiency of E2F1 knockdown was verified by immunoblotting with an E2F1-specific antibody. Activation of the apoptotic program by TGFβ was assessed by AnnexinV staining followed by FACS (f) or fluorescence microscopy (g), in HuH7 cells transiently transfected with a control, non-targeting siRNA or E2F1 siRNA. In (f), values represent the percentage of early and late apoptotic cells and represent the mean ± SD. (h) Expression of endogenous E2F1 in these cells was assessed by immunofluorescence.

To further investigate the role of E2F1 in TGFβ-mediated apoptosis we performed fluorescence-activated cell sorting (FACS) following AnnexinV and PI staining. While TGFβ treatment markedly increased the number of apoptotic cells in control (non-targeting) siRNA-transfected HuH7 cells (Figure 7f, left panels), E2F1 knockdown completely impeded this effect (Figure 7f, right panels), consistent with cell viability and calcein-AM results. Fluorescence imaging following AnnexinV staining further confirmed these findings (Figure 7g). Taken together, these results indicate that TGFβ has a potent pro-apoptotic function in various cell lines and that these effects require the transcription factor E2F1.

2.6   E2F1 is Required for TGFβ-Mediated Transcriptional Induction of Pro-Apoptotic Target Genes

TGFβ signalling activates multiple pro-apoptotic genes and pathways in a cell- and tissue-specific manner (Siegel & Massague, 2003). Independently of TGFβ, the E2F pathway has also been implicated in multiple distinct cell death mechanisms. E2F1 alone has been shown to activate numerous pro-apoptotic genes, including *Apaf-1*(apoptotic protease activating factor 1), *p14ARF*, *p73*, *Caspase 3*, *Caspase 7*, *Caspase 8*, *Chk2* (checkpoint kinase 2), *Ask*-1 (apoptosis signal-regulating kinase 1), and *Smac/DIABLO* (second mitochondrial-derived activator of caspase/direct IAP-binding protein with low pI) in various cell types and tissues (Elliott *et al.*, 2001; Furukawa *et al.*, 2002; M. Irwin *et al.*, 2000; Kherrouche *et al.*, 2006; Rogoff *et al.*, 2004; Xie *et al.*, 2006; H. L. Yang *et al.*, 2000).

To determine whether TGFβ and E2F1 share any common downstream apoptotic targets, we examined the regulation of representative E2F1-responsive apoptotic genes in TGFβ-treated HuH7 cells, which express both functional p53 and pRb. As shown in Figure 8a, TGFβ transcriptionally induced *Apaf1*, *Caspase 3*, *Caspase 7*, *p73*, and *Smac/DIABLO* expression, suggesting that TGFβ induces apoptosis in HuH7 cells by the intrinsic mitochondrial pathway. Importantly, this analysis also revealed *Smac/DIABLO* as a novel TGFβ target. Moreover, E2F1 knockdown markedly impaired the TGFβ-mediated induction of each of these target genes (Figure 8b), indicating that TGFβ-mediated regulation of multiple pro-apoptotic downstream target genes is E2F1-dependent. These data provide a novel pathway by which TGFβ regulates these genes and reveals E2F1 as a widespread co-transducer of TGFβ-induced activation of the intrinsic mitochondrial pathway. It would be interesting in future to assess the contribution of E2F1 to TGFβ-mediated mitochondrial outer membrane permeabilization (MOMP) and cytochrome *c* release. We then examined whether these pro-apoptotic genes were direct or indirect targets of TGFβ signalling. To do so, cells were treated or not with the translational inhibitor cycloheximide (CHX) and stimulated with TGFβ as indicated. Interestingly, CHX treatment completely impaired the induction of these genes by TGFβ (Figure 8c), suggesting that TGFβ indirectly regulates the expression of its downstream pro-apoptotic target genes and that this regulation requires the induction of a TGFβ-responsive transcriptional activator. As a control, we also examined the mRNA expression levels of Smad7, which is known to be a direct TGFβ target gene and, as expected, transcriptional induction of Smad7 by TGFβ was not affected by CHX treatment.

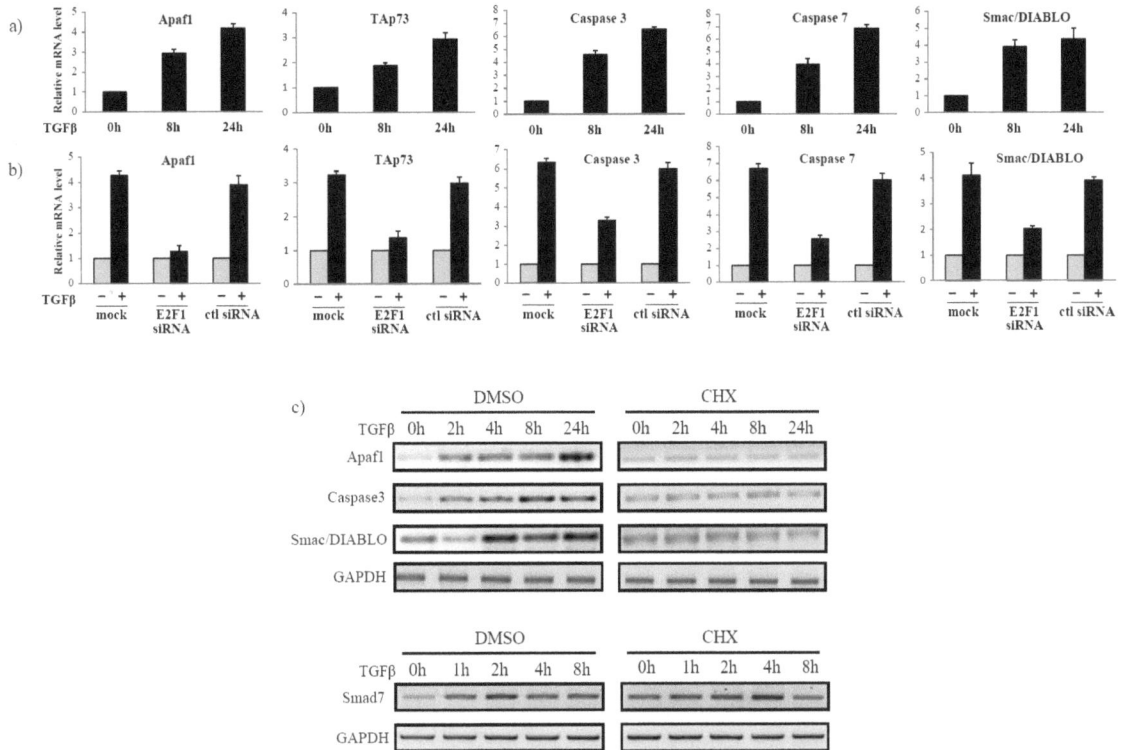

Figure 8: E2F1 is required for TGFβ-Mediated Transcriptional Induction of Pro-Apoptotic Target Genes. a) HuH7 cells were stimulated with TGFβ and mRNA levels for the indicated genes were measured by real-time qPCR. Results are normalized to GAPDH and shown relative to levels observed in untreated cells (set to 1). Data are represented as mean ± SD. b) HuH7 cells were transiently transfected with siRNA against E2F1 or a control non-silencing siRNA and stimulated with TGFβ for 24h. The mRNA levels for the indicated genes were measured as in (a). c) HuH7 cells were pre-treated for 30 min with cycloheximide (10 μM) or vehicle and then stimulated with TGFβ for the indicated times. The mRNA levels for the indicated genes were analyzed by RT-PCR and amplified products were analyzed by DNA gel electrophoresis.

2.7   TGFβ Rapidly and Transiently Increases E2F1 Protein Expression Levels

Having shown that TGFβ indirectly induces the expression of these pro-apoptotic target genes and that E2F1 is required for this process, we next sought to determine whether E2F1 expression itself was regulated by TGFβ. We found that TGFβ induced a time-dependent decrease in E2F1 mRNA levels in HaCaT cells (Figure 9a), which corresponds with previous studies (J. M. Li *et al.*, 1997; Spender & Inman, 2009). Surprisingly, however, we also found TGFβ to rapidly and transiently induce E2F1 protein expression levels in these cells (Figure 9b). Moreover, as shown in Figure 9c, this effect was observed in various human epithelial cancer cell lines (melanoma, hepatocarcinoma, and colon carcinoma). The induction of E2F1 was transient, however, as longer exposure to TGFβ resulted in a return to basal E2F1 protein levels in all cell lines. Interestingly, in all cases the increase in E2F1 expression in response to TGFβ was rapid (within 30 minutes of TGFβ treatment), suggesting that TGFβ potentially induces post-translational stabilization of the E2F1 protein. To address this, we performed a cycloheximide chase in HaCaT cells treated or not with TGFβ (Figure 9d). In the presence of cycloheximide, untreated cells demonstrated

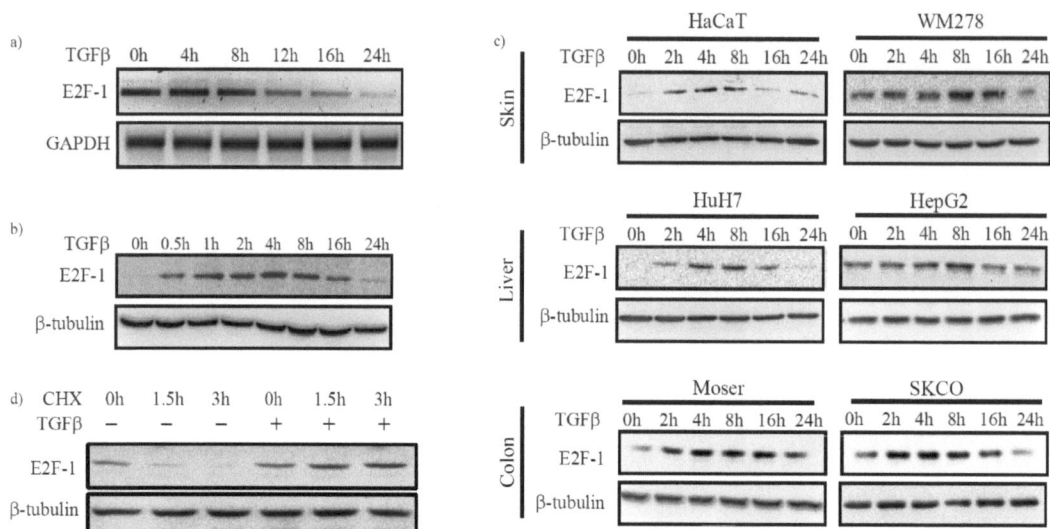

Figure 9: TGFβ Rapidly and Transiently Increases E2F1 Protein Expression Levels. HaCaT cells were stimulated with TGFβ for the indicated times and subjected to RT-PCR (a) and Western blotting (b) to measure E2F1 RNA and protein levels, respectively. c) Western blot analysis of total E2F1 protein levels in TGFβ-treated cells of various origins, as indicated. d) Cycloheximide (CHX) chase analysis in HaCaT cells to address the potential contribution of TGFβ in E2F1 post-translational stabilization. Cells were incubated with CHX (50 µg/mL) and treated or not with TGFβ for the indicated times. Total cell lysates were analyzed for E2F1 protein levels by Western blotting.

progressively diminished levels of E2F1 over time. Conversely, TGFβ treatment maintained E2F1 levels throughout the chase, indicating that TGFβ is indeed able to prolong E2F1 half-life, by stabilizing E2F1 protein levels post-translationally.

2.8   TGFβ Pro-Apoptotic Effects are Impaired in E2F1-Null Embryonic Fibroblasts

Having determined that TGFβ-induced apoptosis in various epithelial cancer cell lines is E2F1-dependent, we then investigated whether E2F1 contributes to TGFβ-mediated cell death in normal cells as well. To do so, we used mouse embryonic fibroblasts (MEFs) isolated from wild-type and E2F1-deficient mice. Interestingly, the TGFβ-mediated apoptotic response greatly differed in these two cell types. While cell viability of the wild-type E2F1$^{+/+}$ MEFs was potently decreased in response to TGFβ, this effect was severely impaired in the E2F1$^{-/-}$ MEFs (Figure 10a). Correspondingly, the TGFβ-mediated transcriptional induction *Caspase 7* and *Smac/DIABLO* was significantly reduced in the E2F1$^{-/-}$ MEFs (Figure 10b). These findings highlight a prominent role for E2F1 downstream of TGFβ signalling in regulating cell death in a normal cell setting in addition to multiple cell lines of various cancer origins.

2.9   E2F1 DNA-Binding, Transactivation, and pRb-Interaction are Required for TGFβ-Mediated Apoptosis

To further elucidate the molecular mechanisms by which E2F1 plays a role in TGFβ-mediated programmed cell death, we examined the contribution of the retinoblastoma tumour suppressor protein, pRb,

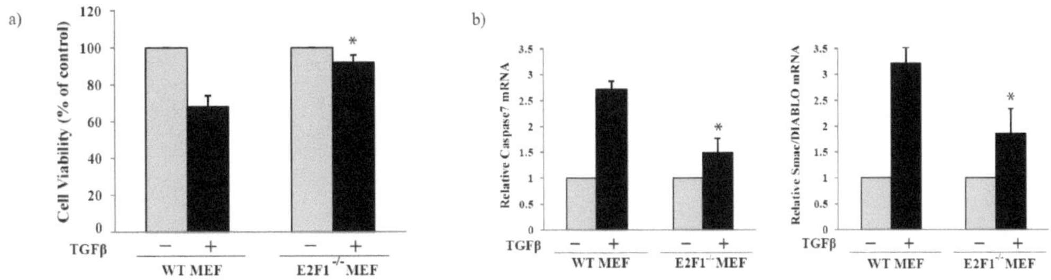

Figure 10: TGFβ Pro-Apoptotic Effects are Impaired in E2F1-Null Embryonic Fibroblasts.
a) WT and E2F1[-/-] MEFs were stimulated or not with TGFβ for 24h and cell viability assessed by calcein-AM assay. b) Caspase 7 and Smac/DIABLO mRNA levels in TGFβ-treated WT and E2F1[-/-] MEFs were measured by real-time qPCR analysis. Results are normalized to GAPDH and shown relative to levels observed in untreated cells (set to 1). Data are represented as mean ± SD, (* $p < 0.05$).

which is the principal regulator of E2F1 activity. For this, we used dominant negative E2F1 mutant forms to alter E2F1 function and/or binding to pRb. Importantly, the DNA-binding deficient mutant, E2F1 (E132), and the transactivation-defective mutant, E2F1 (1-374), are both reportedly unable to activate transcription, whereas the E2F1 Y411C mutant, which has lost its ability to interact with pRb, retains similar transcriptional activating potential as its wild-type E2F1 (Lukas *et al.*, 1996). Interestingly, ectopic expression of each of these mutants remarkably impaired the TGFβ effect on cell viability in HuH7 cells (Figure 11a). The antagonistic effect of these E2F1 mutants was further established at the transcriptional level, as their overexpression greatly impeded the transcriptional induction of *Caspase 7* and *Smac/DIABLO* in response to TGFβ (Figure 11b). These data indicate that TGFβ requires not only proper E2F1 function (DNA binding and transactivation), but additionally the ability of E2F1 to interact with pRb in order to successfully induce apoptosis. To further address this, we examined whether TGFβ could induce association between pRb and E2F1 using co-immunoprecipitation studies. As shown in Figure 11c, TGFβ treatment indeed promotes endogenous pRb-E2F1 association. These results indicate that pRb-E2F binding is required for TGFβ to induce apoptotic gene expression and cell death. Moreover, this association is induced by TGFβ itself, strongly supporting that the pRb-E2F1 complex plays a role downstream of TGFβ-mediated cell signalling, leading to apoptosis.

2.10 TGFβ Induces Formation of a Transcriptionally Active Complex Comprising pRb, E2F1, and P/CAF, onto Pro-Apoptotic Gene Promoters

Given the classical model of E2F regulation, which implies that E2F1 must be released from its regulatory pRb in order to activate transcription, this raised the question as to how E2F1 activates these pro-apoptotic genes in response to TGFβ while remaining in its seemingly transcriptionally repressive pRb-E2F complex. We therefore examined whether TGFβ could in fact recruit positive regulators of transcription to the pRb-E2F1 complex. As TGFβ has been shown to activate gene transcription through histone acetyltransferases (HATs), including p300/CBP (CREB-binding protein) and p300/CBP-associated factor (P/CAF) (Itoh *et al.*, 2000), we screened for the presence of these HATs in E2F1 and pRb immunoprecipitates in untreated versus TGFβ-treated cells. Interestingly, we found that TGFβ strongly promotes the association of both E2F1 and pRb to the acetyltransferase P/CAF (Figure 12a). Moreover, these complexes were P/CAF-specific, as no association was observed between pRb-E2F1 and p300/CBP.

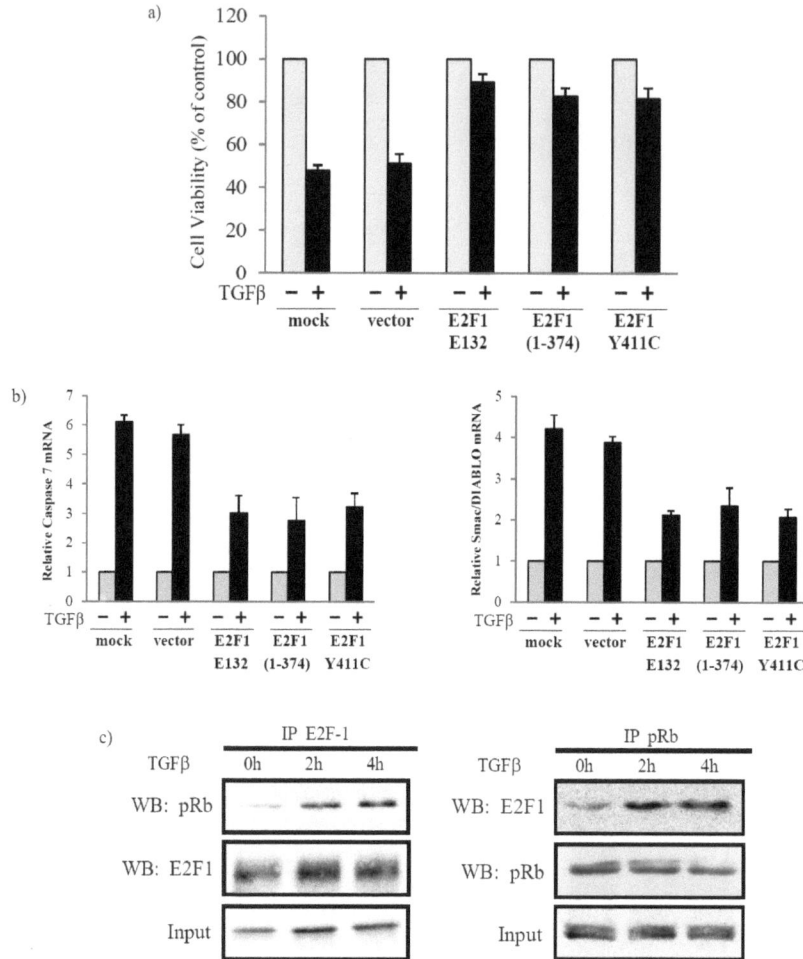

Figure 11: E2F1 DNA-Binding, Transactivation, and pRb-Interaction are required for TGFβ-Mediated Apoptosis. HuH7 cells transiently transfected with empty vector or mutant E2F1 expression constructs as indicated were untreated or treated with TGFβ for 24h. a) Cell viability was assessed by calcein-AM assay, with bars representing means ± SD. b) Caspase 7 and Smac/DIABLO mRNA levels were measured by real-time qPCR analysis. Results are normalized to GAPDH and show the mean ± SD, expressed as relative to levels observed in untreated cells (set to 1). c) HuH7 cells untreated or treated with TGFβ were subjected to immunoprecipitation (IP) with the specified antibodies followed by Western blotting (WB) to assess levels of associated E2F1 and pRb.

We subsequently addressed the contribution of P/CAF to TGFβ-mediated activation of E2F1-responsive pro-apoptotic genes and induction of apoptosis. As seen in Figure 12b, knockdown of P/CAF expression by RNA interference markedly reduced the TGFβ pro-apoptotic effect in these cells. Moreover, the transcriptional induction of *Caspase 7* and *Smac/DIABLO* in response TGFβ was also significantly impaired when P/CAF expression was silenced (Figure 12c). Since caspases require post-translational activation to become catalytically active and mediate cell death (Nahle *et al.*, 2002), we then investigated whether the loss of TGFβ-induced caspase expression due to P/CAF knockdown also resulted in a de-

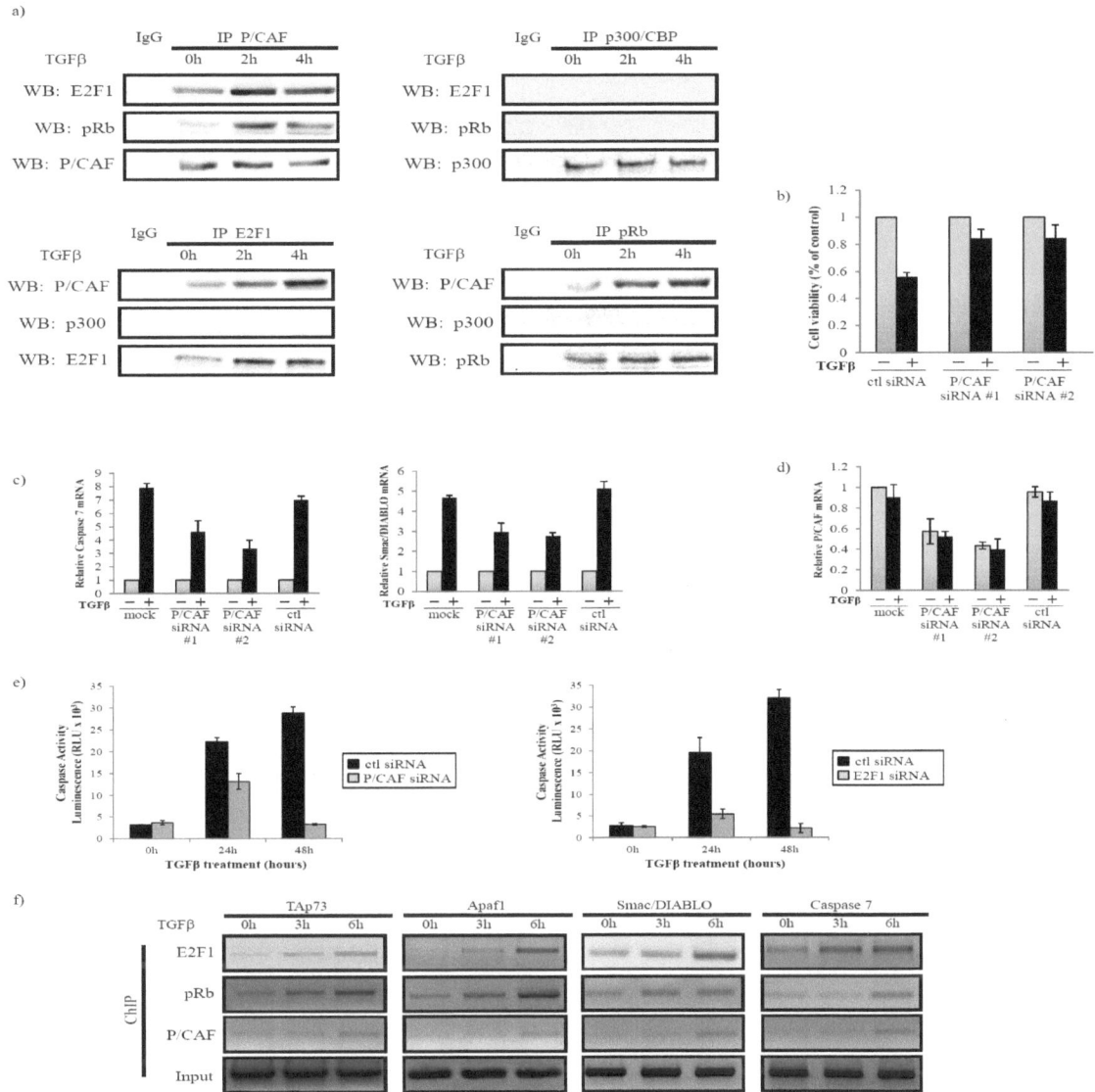

Figure 12: TGFβ Induces Formation of a Transcriptionally Active Complex Comprising pRb, E2F1, and P/CAF, onto Pro-Apoptotic Gene Promoters. a) Untreated and TGFβ-treated HuH7 cells were subjected to immunoprecipitation (IP) with the specified antibodies followed by Western blotting (WB) to assess levels of P/CAF or CBP/p300 and associated E2F1 and pRb. b, c) HuH7 cells were transiently transfected with siRNA against P/CAF or a control non-silencing siRNA and treated with TGFβ for 24h. Cell viability was assessed by calcein-AM assay (b), and Caspase 7 and Smac/DIABLO mRNA levels were measured by real-time qPCR analysis (c). Results are normalized to GAPDH and shown relative to levels observed in untreated cells (set to 1). Data are represented as mean ± SD. d) The efficiency of P/CAF knockdown by siRNA was verified by real-time qPCR. e) HuH7 cells were transiently transfected with a control siRNA or siRNA again P/CAF (left panel) or E2F1 (right panel) and treated with TGFβ as indicated. Activation of Caspase 3/7 was measured by Caspase-Glo® 3/7 Assay (Promega). Data are represented as mean ± SD. f) HuH7 cells were untreated or treated with TGFβ for the indicated times, and the binding of E2F1, pRb, and p/CAF to the p73, Apaf1, Smac/DIABLO, and Caspase7 gene promoters was determined by chromatin immunoprecipitation (ChIP).

crease in caspase activity. Indeed, as shown in Figure 12e (left panel), silencing P/CAF expression severely suppressed TGFβ-mediated Caspase 3/7 activation. Similarly, silencing E2F1 expression also suppressed caspase activation by TGFβ (Figure 6E, right panel). Following 48 hours of TGFβ treatment, loss of either P/CAF or E2F1 expression nearly completely abolished TGFβ-induced caspase activation. Collectively, these findings support a critical role for P/CAF downstream of TGFβ in the E2F1-dependent activation of pro-apoptotic genes and the mediation of programmed cell death.

Finally, to investigate the functional relevance of the TGFβ-induced pRb-E2F1-P/CAF complex in regulating TGFβ transcriptional responses, we performed chromatin immunoprecipitation (ChIP) assays to determine whether this complex is recruited to pro-apoptotic target gene promoters in response to TGFβ. To do so, we examined the promoters of the TGFβ- and E2F1-responsive pro-apoptotic genes identified above. Interestingly, we found that TGFβ treatment markedly induced recruitment of all three partners (E2F1, pRb and P/CAF) to the *p73*, *Apaf1*, *Caspase 7*, and *Smac/DIABLO* gene promoters (Figure 12f), which concurs with the transcriptional induction of these pro-apoptotic genes and activation of the apoptotic programme that we observed in response to TGFβ. These results highlight the E2F1-pRb-P/CAF pathway as a major signalling axis leading to apoptosis downstream of TGFβ in normal and cancer cells.

3   Discussion

Replicative senescence is a telomere-dependent mechanism that defines a limited number of successive cell divisions in somatic cells (Shay & Wright, 2005). It has been proposed that cellular senescence may have evolved, in part, to protect long-lived organisms such as humans against the early development of cancer (Bodnar *et al.*, 1998). Consequently, upregulation of telomerase in order to bypass senescence may be critical for continuous tumour cell growth. Contrary to normal cells, tumour cells exhibit no net loss of average telomere length with cell division, strongly suggesting that telomere stability may be required for cells to escape replicative senescence and proliferate indefinitely (Kim *et al.*, 1994). Cell immortalization may occur through gene mutation(s) in the telomerase repression pathway. Reactivation of telomerase activity may therefore be a rate-limiting step required for the continuing proliferation of advanced cancers.

There is mounting evidence that telomere-associated events are relevant to carcinogenesis. Numerous studies have demonstrated that ectopic expression of telomerase in telomerase-null, mortal human cells stabilizes telomeres and promotes immortalization, which is crucial for cell transformation (Bodnar *et al.*, 1998; Counter *et al.*, 1998; Halvorsen *et al.*, 1999). Others have shown that the conversion of human fibroblasts or epithelial cells to transformed cancer cells by an activated oncogene such as Ras is facilitated by hTERT expression and requires immortalization (Hahn *et al.*, 1999). Furthermore, inhibition of telomerase in immortal human cancer cell lines leads to apoptosis or senescence (Herbert *et al.*, 1999; Zhang *et al.*, 1999).

Our results indicate that TGFβ signalling plays a major role in suppressing hTERT expression and, as most normal human cell types respond to TGFβ, this suggests that this growth factor provides a protective barrier against abnormal hTERT expression, thereby contributing to replicative senescence in normal somatic cells. Our data indicate that specifically Smad3 is important for hTERT repression by TGFβ. This concurs with previous observations by Li *et al.*, highlighting hTERT as a Smad3-specific target gene (H. Li *et al.*, 2006). We found that Smad3 is indeed essential but not sufficient for TGFβ to regulate hTERT expression, which also requires both the Erk and p38 kinase pathways. Such crosstalk between these three pathways has previously been described to be important for the activation of the aggrecan gene (Watanabe *et al.*, 2001) and the collagenase-3 gene (Selvamurugan *et al.*, 2004), downstream of TGFβ in other cell systems. These results further strengthen the current paradigm that, in addition to the canonical Smad pathway, TGFβ signals through different cascades in a cell-type dependent manner (Selvamurugan *et al.*, 2004).

We also found that E2F and HDAC activity are necessary for the mediation of the TGFβ inhibitory effect on hTERT expression. We further identified four critical E2F binding sites, within the proximal region of the core hTERT promoter, that confer the TGFβ response. Moreover, using the E2F1 knockout MEFs, we showed that the loss of E2F1 abolishes the TGFβ inhibitory effect on TERT expression in normal mouse embryonic fibroblasts. Previous studies investigating the role of E2F1 in hTERT regulation have generated some contradictory results. While some studies suggested that E2F1 was required for telomerase activity in mouse and human cancer cells (Crowe & Nguyen, 2001), others showed that E2F1 induced repression of the hTERT gene (Crowe *et al.*, 2001; Shats *et al.*, 2004; Won *et al.*, 2004). Moreover, it has been proposed that E2F1 exerts opposing regulatory roles on hTERT gene expression, by repressing hTERT in cancer cells, while activating hTERT in normal somatic cells (Won *et al.*, 2002). Our results indicate that E2F1 plays a central role in regulating telomerase activity and that E2F1 effects, at least downstream of TGFβ signalling, lead to hTERT repression in both normal and cancer cells.

Histone deacetylases have also previously been implicated in hTERT gene repression in normal cells, as treatment with HDAC inhibitors results in increased telomerase activity (Cong & Bacchetti, 2000; Crowe *et al.*, 2001; Shats *et al.*, 2004; S. Wang & Zhu, 2003) and HDAC complexes are shown to be recruited to the hTERT promoter via uncharacterized factors, Sp1 and/or pRb/E2F being potential candidates. Additionally, an assembly of complexes made up of E2F pocket proteins and HDACs has been demonstrated to regulate hTERT gene expression in normal human fibroblasts (Won *et al.*, 2004). A role for E2F1 in regulating hTERT activity has previously been suggested, as E2F1 overexpression in human cells leads to telomerase repression (Crowe *et al.*, 2001). Moreover, another study demonstrated that endogenous p53 represses hTERT expression through a p21- and pRb/E2F-dependent pathway (Shats *et al.*, 2004). They found that p53-induced p21 expression leads to decreased pRb phosphorylation and induces the recruitment of E2F family members and histone deacetylases to form complexes that inhibit transcription (Shats *et al.*, 2004). These data are complementary to our results and, combined, these studies highlight E2F and HDAC proteins as critical mediators of TGFβ-induced telomerase repression.

TGFβ-mediated inhibition of telomerase activity is of profound impact for this growth factor's tumour suppressive role. While hTERT involvement in cell immortalization is well-characterized, recent studies indicate that telomerase has additional functions not related to net telomere length that enhance cell survival and proliferation. Studies in mice provide for a good model to examine the impact of telomerase activation on cell proliferation since mice naturally have very long telomeres (25-40 kb) and so the role of telomerase in lengthening shortened telomeres is less critical. In fact, during tumourigenesis in mice, telomerase activity increases even in the presence of long telomeres (Artandi *et al.*, 2002; Blasco *et al.*, 1996; Broccoli *et al.*, 1996; Gonzalez-Suarez *et al.*, 2001). First generation telomerase knockout mice develop 33% less skin tumours than wild-type mice when induced with chemical carcinogens. In contrast, transgenic mice overexpressing mTERT are twice as likely to develop epidermal tumours when exposed to carcinogens (Gonzalez-Suarez *et al.*, 2001). Moreover, mice with constitutive mTERT expression are more susceptible to developing both induced and spontaneous tumours as they age, compared to wild-type controls (Artandi *et al.*, 2002; Gonzalez-Suarez *et al.*, 2001). These studies strongly suggest that telomerase expression may cooperate with oncogenic factors (and more frequently with age) to promote tumourigenesis in mice. This is supported by the observation that these transgenic mice, when young, display normal phenotype in terms of viability and development.

In human epithelial or neural cultured cells, overexpression of hTERT induces resistance to pro-apoptotic or anti-proliferative signals, including TGFβ (Stampfer *et al.*, 2001). In fibroblast cells, overexpression of hTERT with H-Ras produced tumours in nude mice, while a defective form of hTERT, which is unable to lengthen telomeres, was still able to cooperate with H-Ras to induce tumour formation. This further suggests that the hTERT effect on tumour progression includes a non-telomere function (Stewart *et al.*, 2002). Moreover, telomerase is able to stimulate proliferation of epithelial cells by controlling expression of genes involved in cell proliferation (Smith *et al.*, 2003). Telomerase activation therefore promotes tumour formation in two ways: by rescuing tumour cells with critically short telomeres and by inducing proliferation independently of telomere length during tumourigenesis. Thus, the TGFβ inhibitory effect on hTERT activity not only leads to repression of immortalization, but might also represent an important component of the cytostatic programme induced by this growth factor to inhibit cell proliferation.

Results from our hTERT study prompted us to investigate whether E2F1 could also be involved in mediating another arm of the TGFβ tumour suppressive response and regulate programmed cell death. While various apoptotic mediators and signalling pathways have been implicated in TGFβ-mediated apoptosis, these defined regulatory mechanisms have been largely cell type- and tissue-specific (Siegel & Massague, 2003). A better understanding of the specific regulatory mechanisms responsible for TGFβ-mediated apoptosis would provide clearer insight into the basis of this variability and, potentially, allow for the eventual integration of these various observations into a comprehensive pathway or global TGFβ apoptotic programme. Our second study described here defines a novel process of gene activation by the TGFβ-E2F1 signalling axis and highlights the pRb-E2F1-P/CAF pathway as a wide-ranging and critical mediator of the TGFβ apoptotic programme in multiple target tissues and cell types.

We identified a number of key pro-apoptotic TGFβ target genes that trigger the intrinsic apoptosis pathway through the induction of E2F1, as loss or mutation of E2F1 expression abrogates regulation of these genes by TGFβ. Notably, we highlighted Smac/DIABLO, a critical mediator of the mitochondrial apoptotic pathway, as a novel TGFβ target, and determined that it is also regulated in an E2F1-dependent manner. While these genes are functionally interrelated, our results imply that TGFβ regulates the intrinsic apoptosis pathway at multiple levels, consistent with the potent pro-apoptotic effect played by this growth factor in its target tissues. However, we do not exclude the possibility that other genes or pathways might also contribute to E2F1-dependent TGFβ-mediated cell death. Importantly, these results are corroborated using the E2F1 knockout mouse model, in which the TGFβ pro-apoptotic effects observed in wild-type MEFs were strikingly impaired in E2F1-null MEFs. In addition to supporting that E2F1 indeed plays a prominent role in TGFβ-induced cell death, this demonstrates that the TGFβ-E2F1 signalling pathway mediates this process not only in a diseased state, but in a normal cell setting as well. As TGFβ has also been implicated in both positively and negatively regulating numerous anti-apoptotic factors, such as members of the Bcl-2 family, in a cell type-specific manner (Francis *et al.*, 2000; Hague *et al.*, 1998; Lafon *et al.*, 1996; J. H. Lee *et al.*, 2002; Prehn *et al.*, 1994; Tobin *et al.*, 2001), it would be interesting to investigate whether the pRb/E2F1 pathway also mediates expression of these genes downstream of TGFβ.

While it is well-established that E2F1 activity is intimately controlled through association with pRb, the precise mechanisms of this regulation are somewhat contradictory. The prevailing view holds that the pRb-E2F1 complex acts as a repressor of E2F target genes (Dyson, 1998). Accordingly, disruption of this pRb-E2F1 complex is required to release free E2F1 in order to induce transcription of its target genes. Paradoxically, pRb-E2F1 complexes were recently shown to transcriptionally activate pro-apoptotic genes in response to DNA damage, through recruitment of a histone acetyltransferase to the pRb-E2F1 complex (Ianari *et al.*, 2009). Interestingly, our results also challenge this dogma, and support a non-classic transcriptionally active pRb-E2F1 regulatory complex, as we show here that the pRb-E2F1 complex can also recruit an actyltransferase (P/CAF) to activate transcription of pro-apotic genes in response to TGFβ. Indeed, analysis with dominant negative E2F1 mutants revealed that, in fact, pRb binding to E2F1 is required for TGFβ-mediated apoptosis.

Another intriguing finding in this study is that TGFβ upregulates E2F1 protein levels, albeit transiently, acting at the post-translational level in a several cell lines of varying cancer origins. Interestingly, numerous studies have demonstrated that the E2Fs are often regulated by post-translational modifications such as phosphorylation (W. C. Lin *et al.*, 2001), acetylation (Martinez-Balbas *et al.*, 2000), and by the ubiquitin-proteasome pathways (B. Wang *et al.*, 2004). Moreover, the pRb binding to E2F1 protects E2F1 from ubiquitination and proteolytic degradation (Hofmann *et al.*, 1996), thereby increasing its stability. As TGFβ maintains pRb in a hypophosphorylated form, causing it to remain bound to E2F1 and suppressing activation of E2F1-responsive cell cycle regulatory genes (Laiho *et al.*, 1990), it is likely that the TGFβ effect on E2F1 protein levels is mediated through induction of pRb-E2F1 association, revealing a new level of E2F1 regulation. The association of P/CAF to E2F1 may also potentially contribute to the increased E2F1 protein stability observed in response to TGFβ, as P/CAF also binds and acetylates E2F1, prolonging its half-life. In fact, E2F1 acetylation by P/CAF has three functional effects on E2F1 activity: increased protein-half life, DNA-binding ability, and activation potential (Martinez-Balbas *et al.*, 2000). Accordingly, P/CAF binding to E2F1 in response to TGFβ may in fact have multiple functional consequences, affecting not only E2F1 stability but also its transcriptional activating capability. In future, it would be interesting to identify the factors involved in E2F1 stabilization in response to TGFβ. In addition to pRb and P/CAF, potential candidates include the Smads and various kinases (such as MAPK, p38, and JNK) that act downstream of TGFβ signalling, promoting its tumour suppressive effects.

Moreover, additional post-translational modifications of E2F1 and/or pRb may also influence the formation of the pro-apoptotic complex on target gene promoters. Notably, pRb holds an alternate E2F1-specific binding site that does not interfere with the E2F1 transactivation domain (Dick & Dyson, 2003). It is interesting to consider, then, whether TGFβ could somehow induce pRb and E2F1 to assume this alternate conformation. If so, this conformation should also allow for recruitment of P/CAF, which we have established is necessary for TGFβ-mediated activation of E2F1-dependent pro-apoptotic target genes. The coordinated recruitment of E2F1, pRb, and P/CAF to these pro-apoptotic gene promoters suggests the potential formation of a transcriptionally active pRb-E2F1 complex, which mediates the regulation of TGFβ pro-apoptotic targets. Collectively, these results strongly support a pro-apoptotic role for the pRb/E2F1 pathway downstream of TGFβ signalling and provide a potential mechanism for the transcriptional activation of E2F1-responsive pro-apoptotic genes in response to TGFβ.

It is interesting to consider that TGFβ tumour suppressive effects might utilize the functional interplay among the E2F family members, which plays a role in affecting E2F activity. It is well-established that TGFβ prevents cell cycle progression by inducing Cdk inhibitors (Datto *et al.*, 1995; J. M. Li *et al.*, 1995) and by inhibiting both Cdc25a (Iavarone & Massague, 1999) and c-Myc (C. R. Chen *et al.*, 2002) through Smad-E2F4/5-pocket protein repressor complexes. Thus, the rapid surge in E2F1 that we observe in response to TGFβ may effectively initiate the TGFβ apoptotic programme without affecting cell cycle, since TGFβ maintains transcriptional repression of factors required for S phase entry through other E2F family members. Indeed, this notion is supported by a previous study that demonstrated that TGFβ greatly increased E2F1-DNA-binding activity and that this increase led to apoptosis and not cell cycle progression (Fan *et al.*, 2002). Additionally, E2F4 (in complex with pRb or p107) is capable of binding to E2F binding sites on the E2F1 promoter leading to its repression after 4 hours of TGFβ treatment (J. M. Li *et al.*, 1997). Hence, it is plausible that TGFβ treatment leads to increased levels of E2F1, triggering the activation of pro-apoptotic genes. Subsequently, in addition to directly inhibiting cell-cycle regulatory genes, E2F4 may repress E2F1 levels following longer stimulation with TGFβ, further preventing cell cycle progression.

This study defines a novel process of gene activation by the TGFβ-E2F1 signalling axis and supports a role for the E2F family as potent co-transducers of TGFβ signals. Combined with previous studies from our lab and others, these findings highlight the prominent role for the E2F family in regulating TGFβ tumour suppressive effects. We propose the following model of E2F tumour suppressive action downstream of TGFβ (Figure 13):

1. TGFβ induces E2F4/5 recruitment into classical repressive pRb-E2F-HDAC complexes which target key cell-cycle regulators, such as *Cdc25a* (Iavarone & Massague, 1999) and *c-Myc* (C. R. Chen *et al.*, 2002; Frederick *et al.*, 2004), preventing cell cycle entry.

2. TGFβ also induces E2F1 recruitment into repressive E2F-HDAC complexes, inhibiting hTERT expression (Lacerte et al., 2008) and suppressing immortalization. Moreover, the assembly of complexes formed of E2F, pocket proteins (potentially pRb) and HDACs have been shown to repress hTERT gene expression (Won et al., 2004), indicating that each of these is a key regulator of telomerase activity in human cells.

3. TGFβ can also recruit E2F1 into transcriptionally active pRb-E2F1-P/CAF complexes, increasing the expression of multiple pro-apoptotic target genes and inducing programmed cell death (Korah et al., 2012).

4. In certain cancer cell types, TGFβ also transcriptionally suppresses the inhibitor of apoptosis survivin through Smad signalling and recruitment of a pRb-E2F4 repressive complex to the survivin promoter (J. Yang et al., 2008), thus promoting apoptosis.

Interestingly, the E2F family acts via distinct pathways to regulate specific genes, yet all toward a global action of tumour suppression. We can thus consider E2F family members as "super-mediators" of TGFβ tumour suppressive effects. A better understanding of the mechanisms by which both TGFβ and pRb/E2F signalling mediate their tumour suppressive roles may prove useful for the development of novel therapeutic strategies aimed at restoring tumour suppressive response of the E2Fs in human cancer.

In fact, many of the E2F-dependent TGFβ tumour suppressive target genes described here have previously been investigated for their potential diagnostic and therapeutic value in cancer. For instance, both hTERT and survivin are highly expressed in tumours but not in normal tissue, rendering them attractive candidates for targeted cancer therapy. Numerous studies have shown promising potential therapeutic effects using various telomerase inhibitors. For instance, the very potent hTR antagonist GRN163L has been demonstrated to inhibit telomerase activity and trigger senescence and widespread apoptosis after progressive telomere shortening in various cell lines, including human multiple myeloma and non-Hodgkin lymphoma cell lines (E. S. Wang *et al.*, 2004). Moreover, many studies have successfully used the hTERT promoter to drive proapoptotic genes *in vitro*, including *Bax* (Gu *et al.*, 2002), *caspases 6-8* (Koga *et al.*, 2001; Komata *et al.,* 2001), and *TRAIL* (Jacob *et al.*, 2005).

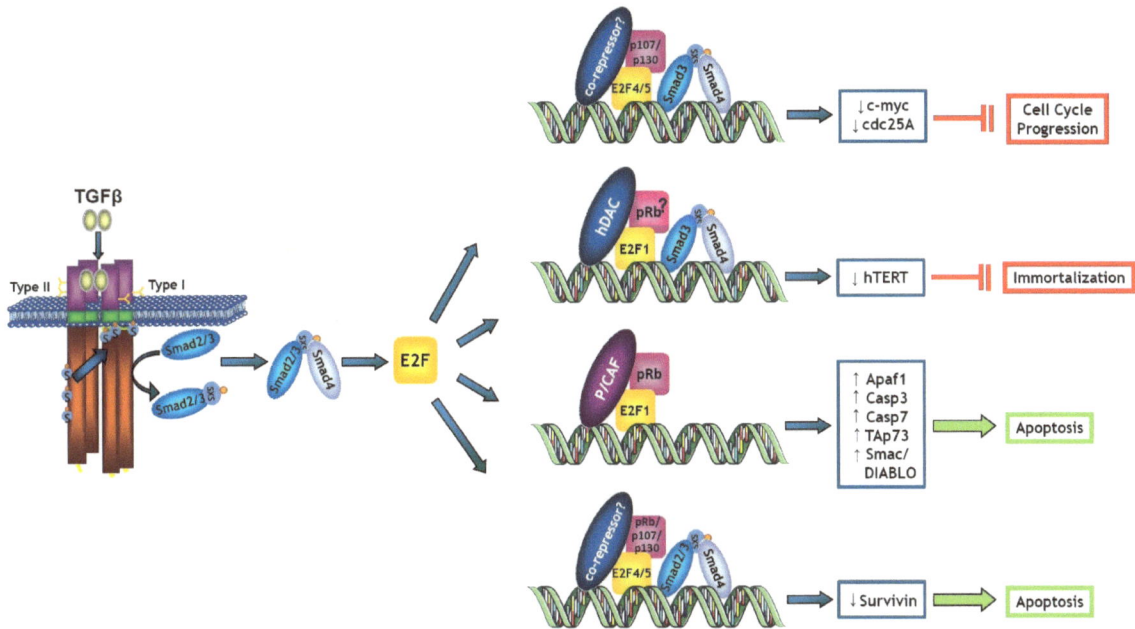

Figure 13: Model for the Role of the pRb/E2F Pathway in TGFβ-Mediated Tumour Suppression. The pRb/E2F signalling pathway mediates multiple distinct arms of TGFβ-mediated tumour suppressive effects.

This strategy selectively affects cells that are telomerase-positive, while sparing telomerase-negative cells. In contrast, survivin contributes to tumour maintenance and progression primarily by conferring apoptotic resistance. Antagonizing survivin expression or function has been shown to induce spontaneous apoptosis, sensitize tumour cells to chemotherapeutic agents, and reduce tumour growth potential (Altieri, 2003a, 2003c). Notably, Pennati *et al.* demonstrated that inhibiting survivin expression in human prostate cancer cells enhanced their susceptibility to cisplatin-induced apoptosis and prevented tumour formation when cells were xenografted in athymic nude mice (Pennati, Binda, Colella, *et al.*, 2004). They further showed that survivin suppression in human melanoma cells increased sensitivity to gamma-irradiation (Pennati, Binda, De Cesare, *et al.*, 2004). A better understanding of the role of both hTERT and survivin in tumour versus normal cells would be instrumental for the design of optimal strategies to selectively target these genes in cancer.

In recent years, a number of pre-clinical studies have also investigated whether E2F1 may be utilized as an anti-cancer therapeutic. The frequent deregulation of E2F1 in human cancer, along with its apoptotic potential and its stabilization following DNA damage, suggest that E2F1 may in fact contribute to the enhanced sensitivity of tumour cells to DNA damage-induced cell death (Putzer, 2007). Numerous *in vitro* and *in vivo* studies have evaluated the effect of E2F1 overexpression on tumour growth in several types of human cancer including glioma (Fueyo *et al.*, 1998), melanoma (Dong *et al.*, 1999), breast and ovarian carcinoma (Hunt *et al.*, 1997), head and neck squamous cell carcinoma (Liu *et al.*, 1999), gastric carcinoma (Atienza *et al.*, 2000), pancreatic carcinoma (Rodicker *et al.*, 2001), and nonsmall-cell lung carcinoma (Kuhn *et al.*, 2002). Remarkably, these studies clearly demonstrated that apoptosis induction by adenoviral-expressed E2F1 results in growth suppression of tumour cells without significantly affecting normal tissues. Moreover, increased E2F1 expression enhanced tumour cell chemosensitivity.

Additionally, the downstream TGFβ- and E2F1-proapoptotic target p73 was established as a promising candidate for targeted cancer therapy. In a similar manner, p73 overexpression induced apoptosis and increased the tumour cell sensitivity to chemotherapy, thus providing a basis for selective killing of cancer cells, including p53-defective tumour cells, by DNA-damaging agents (M. S. Irwin *et al.*, 2003; Tuve *et al.*, 2006). Since manipulating apoptotic signalling can produce abundant changes in cell death, the genes and proteins involved in controlling the apoptotic programme are thus potential therapeutic drug targets.

Though there is much evidence to support that various effectors of TGFβ and pRb/E2F1 tumour suppressive signalling can significantly and specifically kill cancer cells, their role as targets for cancer therapeutics depends on further elucidation of their precise regulatory mechanisms. The potential exploitation of these pRb/E2F and TGFβ signalling tumour suppressive pathways may provide new avenues for the development of novel cancer therapies and management of human cancers.

4   Materials and Methods

4.1   Cell Culture and Transfections

HuH7, MCF-7, CHO, HepG2, Moser and SKCO cell lines, as well as mouse embryonic fibroblasts (MEFs) were cultured in DMEM (HyClone), and WM278 cells in RPMI-1640 (HyClone). Medium for all cells was supplemented with 10% fetal bovine serum (FBS) (HyClone) and 2mM L-glutamine (GIBCO) and cells were grown at 37°C in 5% CO_2 conditions. Prior to treatment, cells were serum-starved for 24 hours and all stimulations were done in serum-free medium containing 100pM TGFβ1 (Peprotech). Cells were transiently transfected with different siRNAs against Smad 2, Smad 3, E2F1 (Ambion) or P/CAF (Sigma-Aldrich), or with wild-type and mutant E2F1 expression vectors using Lipofectamine[TM] 2000 reagent (Invitrogen), according to the manufacturer's instructions.

4.2   Plasmid Constructions

The hTERT-2k GFP reporter construct was digested with BamHI and KpnI to separate the hTERT promoter insert (−1934 to +78, ATG as +1, GenBank sequence gi: 4210970) from the pGFP vector. This hTERT promoter insert was ligated into pGL3-basic vector digested with BglII and KpnI. The resulting hTERT (−1934)-lux reporter construct was confirmed by sequencing. Sequential deletion mutants of the hTERT promoter reporter were done using Erase-a-Base System (Promega) according to the manufacturer's instructions. All constructs were confirmed by sequencing.

4.3   Luciferase Assays

HaCaT cells were transfected using Lipofectamine[TM] 2000 reagent (Invitrogen) with 0.5 µg of luciferase reporter construct, 0.5 µg of β-galactosidase (pCMV-lacZ) expression vector. The next day, cells were stimulated or not with TGFβ in starvation media. When inhibitors were used, they were added 30 min prior to TGFβ treatment. Luminescence of each sample was measured using an EG & G Berthold luminometer. All experiments were repeated independently six times and the luciferase activity normalized to β-galactosidase values.

4.4   RNA Isolation, RT-PCR, and Real-Time Quantitative PCR

Total RNA was isolated from cell lines using TRIzol reagent (Invitrogen) and reverse transcribed using random hexamers and M-MLV Reverse Transcriptase (Invitrogen), as per the manufacturer's instructions. For RT-PCR, densitometry analysis following DNA gel electrophoresis was performed using Alpha Innotech Fluorochem Imaging software. The linear amplification range of each PCR was tested on the adjusted cDNA. The conditions were chosen so that none of the RNA analyzed reached a plateau at the end of the amplification protocol, (i.e. they were in the exponential phase of amplification.) Real-time qPCR was carried out using SsoFast™ EvaGreen® Supermix (BioRad) in a RotorGene 6000 PCR detection system (Corbett Life Science). Conditions for qPCR were as follows: 95°C for 30sec, 40 cycles of 95°C for 5sec and 60°C for 20sec. Primer sequences are listed in Table 1 of the Appendix.

4.5   Immunoblotting and Immunoprecipitation

Cells were lysed in cold RIPA buffer (50mM Tris-HCl pH 7.4, 150 mM NaCl, 1% Triton X-100, 0.1% SDS, 1 mM EDTA), containing 1 mM sodium orthovanadate, 1mM phenylmethylsulphonyl fluoride, 5 µg/ml aprotinin, 2 µg/ml leupeptin, and 1 µg/ml pepstatin. Lysates were separated by SDS-PAGE, transferred to nitrocellulose, and incubated with the specified antibodies overnight at 4°C: anti-hTERT (Calbiochem), anti-phospho-Erk, anti-Erk, anti-phospho-p38, anti-p38 (Cell Signaling Technology), anti-phospho-Smad3 (BioSource), anti-Smad2/3 (Santa Cruz Biotechnology), anti-E2F1 (KH95, Santa Cruz Biotechnology), anti-β-tubulin (Sigma). Following primary antibody incubation, membranes were washed twice in TBST (50mM Tris-HCl at pH 7.6, 200mM NaCl, 0.05% Tween20), and incubated with secondary antibody coupled to horseradish peroxidase (Sigma) at 1:10,000 dilution for 1h at room temperature. Membranes were then washed in TBST four times for 15 min. Immunoreactivity was revealed by chemiluminescence and detected using an Alpha Innotech Fluorochem Imaging system (Packard Canberra). Immunoprecipitations were performed overnight at 4°C using antibodies against E2F1 (C-20, Santa Cruz Biotechnology), pRb (Cell Signaling), P/CAF (Abcam) and CBP/p300 (Santa Cruz Biotechnology). Protein A-sepharose (Amersham Biosciences) was added for 2 hours at 4°C and beads were then washed four times with cold lysis buffer. The immunoprecipitates were eluted with 2xSDS Laemmli sample buffer, boiled for 5 min, and subjected to immunoblotting.

4.6   Viability Assays

Cells were seeded in triplicate in 96-well plates, at 10,000 cells/100 µl in medium supplemented with 2% FBS and in the presence or absence of 100pM TGFβ. Mitochondrial viability was determined by 3-(4,5-Dimethylthiazol-2-yl)-2,5-diphenyltetrazolium bromide (MTT) colorimetric assay. Briefly, following 24 to 72 hours of TGFβ treatment, cells were incubated with 1 mg/ml MTT solution (Sigma) in the culture media for 2 hours. Formazan crystals were solubilized overnight in 50% dimethyl formamide, 20% SDS, pH 4.7, and the absorbance of each well was measured at 570 nm using a Bio-Tek microplate reader. Alternatively, cell viability was determined by the fluorescent calcein acetoxymethyl ester (calcein-AM) method. Briefly, following 4 to 24 hours of TGFβ treatment, original culture medium was replaced with serum-free medium containing 2 ug/ml calcein-AM (BD Biosciences) for 60 min at 37°C. Cells were then washed twice with PBS and the fluorescence of each well was monitored from the bottom of the wells at excitation and emission wavelengths of 485 and 520 nm, respectively, using a FLUOstar Optima microplate reader.

4.7   AnnexinV Apoptotic Assays

Apoptotic cells were analyzed using an AnnexinV apoptosis detection kit (Santa Cruz Biotechnology). Following TGFβ treatment, cells were collected by trypsinization, pelleted by centrifugation, washed with PBS and each sample was incubated with 0.5 µg AnnexinV-FITC and 10 µl Propidium Iodide (50 µg/ml) in the supplied incubation buffer for 15 min. Cells were then analyzed using FACS in an Accuri C6 flow cytometer (BD Biosciences). For fluorescence microscopy, cells were plated on glass coverslips at 80% confluence. Following TGFβ treatment, cells were washed with PBS and subjected to AnnexinV-FITC staining for 15 minutes as described above. Stained coverslips were mounted onto slides with SlowFade® Gold Antifade with DAPI (Invitrogen), and immediately examined.

4.8   Immunofluorescence

Cells plated on glass coverslips were fixed with 4% paraformaldehyde, permeabilized in PBS containing 0.1% Triton X-100 for 3 min, washed with PBS, and blocked with 2% bovine serum albumin (BSA) for 30 min. Cells were then incubated with anti-E2F1 antibody (Santa Cruz Biotechnology) for 1 hour, washed with PBS, and incubated with AlexaFluor568 goat anti-mouse IgG secondary antibody (Invitrogen) for 1 hour. After a final wash, stained coverslips were mounted with SlowFade® Gold Antifade with DAPI (Invitrogen) and examined using a Zeiss LSM-510 Meta Axiovert confocal microscope.

4.9   Caspase Activity Assay

Cells were plated in triplicate in 96-well dishes, at 10,000 cells/100 µl in medium supplemented with 2% FBS and in the presence or absence of 100pM TGFβ. Caspase 3/7 activity was measured using the Caspase-Glo® 3/7 Assay (Promega) according to the manufacturer's instructions. Briefly, following TGFβ treatment, cells were incubated with Caspase-Glo® reagent for 1.5 hours at room temperature, and the luminescence of each sample was measured using an EG & G Berthold luminometer.

4.10   Cycloheximide Chase

Cells were seeded in 60-mm^2 plates and grown to 85% confluence. Following overnight serum-starvation, the cells were incubated, in the presence or absence of 100pM TGFβ, with 50 µg/ml cyclo-heximide (Sigma) for the indicated times, and analyzed by immunoblotting.

4.11   Chromatin Immunoprecipitation

Protein complexes were cross-linked to DNA by adding formaldehyde directly to tissue culture medium to a final concentration of 1%. Crosslinking was allowed to proceed for 10 min at room temperature and was then stopped by the addition of glycine to a final concentration of 0.125 M. Cross-linked cells were harvested, washed with PBS, pelleted by centrifugation at 2000 rpm for 5 min at 4°C, and lysed in nucle-ar lysis buffer (1% SDS, 10 mM EDTA, 50 mM Tris-HCl (pH 8.1), supplemented with 1 mM PMSF, 10 µg/ml aprotinin, 10 µg/ml leupeptin, and 2 µg/ml pepstatin, for 10 min on ice. The resulting chromatin solution was sonicated for five pulses of 20 seconds to generate 300–2000 bp DNA fragments. After cen-trifugation at 14,000 rpm for 10min at 4°C, the supernatant was immunocleared by incubation with pro-tein A-sepharose beads for 2 hours at 4°C. Immunocleared chromatin was immunoprecipitated overnight with 5 µg of the indicated antibodies. Antibody-protein-DNA complexes were then isolated by immuno-precipitation with 40 µl protein A-sepharose beads (Amersham) for 2 hours with rotation at 4°C. Beads were washed consecutively for 10 min each with low salt wash buffer (0.1% SDS, 1% Triton X-100, 2 mM EDTA, 150 mM NaCl, 20 mM Tris-HCl, pH 8.1), high salt wash buffer (0.1% SDS, 1% Triton X-100, 2 mM EDTA, 500 mM NaCl, 20 mM Tris-HCl, pH 8.1), and LiCl wash buffer (0.25 M LiCl, 1% NP-40, 1% Na-deoxycholate, 1mM EDTA, 10mM Tris-HCl, pH 8.1), and twice in TE buffer. Complexes were then eluted twice in 150 µl of freshly made elution buffer (1% SDS, 0.1 M NaHCO3), by incubating at 65°C for 10 min. To reverse cross-linking, 0.2 M NaCl and 1µl of 10 mg/ml RNaseA was added each sample, and they were incubated at 65°C overnight. Following this, 5mM EDTA and 2 µl of 10 mg/ml proteinase K was added, and samples were incubated for at 45°C for 2h. DNA was recovered using the QIAquick spin columns (Qiagen, Maryland, USA) as per the manufacturer's protocol and PCR analysis was performed using primers specific for the indicated promoters, as listed in Table 2 of the Appendix.

4.12 Statistical Analysis

Results are expressed as mean ± standard deviation of at least 3 independent experiments. Statistical differences were determined by one-way ANOVA or two-tailed unpaired t-test, where appropriate. $p < 0.05$ was considered statistically significant.

Acknowledgements

We thank Dr. Shiaw-Yih Lin for kindly providing the hTERT-2k GFP reporter construct and Dr. Kristian Helin for generously providing the mutant E2F1 expression vectors. We are also greatly thankful to Dr. Lili Yamasaki for providing the wild-type and E2F1 knockout MEFs. This work was supported by grants from the NCIC (015257 to JJL) and the Canadian Institutes for Health Research (CIHR, MOP-114904 to JJL). JJL is the recipient of the McGill Sir William Dawson Research Chair and JK holds a CIHR Frederick Banting and Charles Best Doctoral Research Award.

Appendix

To whom correspondence should be addressed: Jean-Jacques Lebrun, Department of Medicine, Royal Victoria Hospital, 687 Pine Avenue West, Montreal, Quebec H3A 1A1, Canada. Tel: +1 514 843 1553; Fax: +1 514 982 0893; E-mail address: JJ.Lebrun@mcgill.ca

Primer Name	Sequence
hTERT forward	5'-CGGAAGAGTGTCTGGAGCAA-3'
hTERT reverse	5'-GGATGAAGCGGAGTCTGGA-3'
E2F1 forward	5'-TGCAGAGCAGATGGTTATGG-3'
E2F1 reverse	5'-ATCTGTGGTGAGGGATGAGG-3'
Apaf1 forward	5'-CTCTCATTTGCTGATGTCGC-3'
Apaf1 reverse	5'-TCGAAATACCATGTTTGGTCA-3'
TAp73 forward	5'-CATGGAGACGAGGACACGTA-3'
TAp73 reverse	5'-CTGTAACCCTTGGGAGGTGA-3'
Caspase3 forward	5'-AGCGAATCAATGGACTCTGG-3'
Caspase3 reverse	5'-CGGCCTCCACTGGTATTTTA-3'
Caspase7 forward	5'-GCAGTGGGATTTGTGCTTCT-3'
Caspase7 reverse	5'-CCCTAAAGTGGGCTGTCAAA-3'

Smac/DIABLO forward	5'-AATGTGATTCCTGGCGGTTA-3'
Smac/DIABLO reverse	5'-AGCTGGAAACCACTTGGATG-3'
GAPDH forward	5'-GCCTCAAGATCATCAGCAATGCCT-3'
GAPDH reverse	5'-TGTGGTCATGAGTCCTTCCACGAT-3'
Smad7 forward	5'-TCCTGCTGTGCAAAGTGTTC-3'
Smad7 reverse	5'-CAGGCTCCAGAAGAAGTTGG-3'

Table 1: PCR primer sequences

Primer Name	Sequence
Apaf1 forward	5'-GCCCCGACTTCTTCCGGCTCTTCA-3'
Apaf1 reverse	5'-GAGCTGGCAGCTGAAAGACTC-3'
TAp73 forward	5'-TGAGCCATGAAGATGTGCGAG-3'
TAp73 reverse	5'-GCTGCTTATGGTCTGATGCTTATGG-3'
Caspase7 forward	5'-TTTGGGCACTTGGAGCGCG-3'
Caspase7 reverse	5'-AAGAGCCCAAAGCGACCCGT-3'
Smac/DIABLO forward	5'-TTCCCTTCAAGCCCTGGCCCGAAC-3'
Smac/DIABLO reverse	5'-ACGCCCCCACCCAAGGAAGCAGTC-3'

Table 2: ChIP primer sequences

References

Alani, R. M., Young, A. Z., & Shifflett, C. B. (2001). Id1 regulation of cellular senescence through transcriptional repression of p16/Ink4a. Proc Natl Acad Sci U S A, 98(14), 7812-7816.

Altieri, D. C. (2003a). Blocking survivin to kill cancer cells. Methods Mol Biol, 223, 533-542.

Altieri, D. C. (2003b). Survivin, versatile modulation of cell division and apoptosis in cancer. Oncogene, 22(53), 8581-8589.

Altieri, D. C. (2003c). Validating survivin as a cancer therapeutic target. Nat Rev Cancer, 3(1), 46-54.

Ambrosini, G., Adida, C., & Altieri, D. C. (1997). A novel anti-apoptosis gene, survivin, expressed in cancer and lymphoma. Nat Med, 3(8), 917-921.

Artandi, S. E., Alson, S., Tietze, M. K., Sharpless, N. E., Ye, S., Greenberg, R. A., et al. (2002). Constitutive telomerase expression promotes mammary carcinomas in aging mice. Proc Natl Acad Sci U S A, 99(12), 8191-8196.

Atfi, A., Buisine, M., Mazars, A., & Gespach, C. (1997). Induction of apoptosis by DPC4, a transcriptional factor regulated by transforming growth factor-beta through stress-activated protein kinase/c-Jun N-terminal kinase (SAPK/JNK) signaling pathway. J Biol Chem, 272(40), 24731-24734.

Atienza, C., Jr., Elliott, M. J., Dong, Y. B., Yang, H. L., Stilwell, A., Liu, T. J., et al. (2000). Adenovirus-mediated E2F-1 gene transfer induces an apoptotic response in human gastric carcinoma cells that is enhanced by cyclin dependent kinase inhibitors. Int J Mol Med, 6(1), 55-63.

Bakin, A. V., Rinehart, C., Tomlinson, A. K., & Arteaga, C. L. (2002). p38 mitogen-activated protein kinase is required for TGFbeta-mediated fibroblastic transdifferentiation and cell migration. J Cell Sci, 115(Pt 15), 3193-3206.

Bhowmick, N. A., Ghiassi, M., Bakin, A., Aakre, M., Lundquist, C. A., Engel, M. E., et al. (2001). Transforming growth factor-beta1 mediates epithelial to mesenchymal transdifferentiation through a RhoA-dependent mechanism. Mol Biol Cell, 12(1), 27-36.

Blasco, M. A. (2005). Telomeres and human disease: ageing, cancer and beyond. Nat Rev Genet, 6(8), 611-622.

Blasco, M. A., Rizen, M., Greider, C. W., & Hanahan, D. (1996). Differential regulation of telomerase activity and telomerase RNA during multi-stage tumorigenesis. Nat Genet, 12(2), 200-204.

Bodnar, A. G., Ouellette, M., Frolkis, M., Holt, S. E., Chiu, C. P., Morin, G. B., et al. (1998). Extension of life-span by introduction of telomerase into normal human cells. Science, 279(5349), 349-352.

Broccoli, D., Godley, L. A., Donehower, L. A., Varmus, H. E., & de Lange, T. (1996). Telomerase activation in mouse mammary tumors: lack of detectable telomere shortening and evidence for regulation of telomerase RNA with cell proliferation. Mol Cell Biol, 16(7), 3765-3772.

Carnevale, J., Palander, O., Seifried, L. A., & Dick, F. A. (2012). DNA damage signals through differentially modified E2F1 molecules to induce apoptosis. Mol Cell Biol, 32(5), 900-912.

Chen, C. R., Kang, Y., Siegel, P. M., & Massague, J. (2002). E2F4/5 and p107 as Smad cofactors linking the TGFbeta receptor to c-myc repression. Cell, 110(1), 19-32.

Chen, R. H., Su, Y. H., Chuang, R. L., & Chang, T. Y. (1998). Suppression of transforming growth factor-beta-induced apoptosis through a phosphatidylinositol 3-kinase/Akt-dependent pathway. Oncogene, 17(15), 1959-1968.

Chipuk, J. E., Bhat, M., Hsing, A. Y., Ma, J., & Danielpour, D. (2001). Bcl-xL blocks transforming growth factor-beta 1-induced apoptosis by inhibiting cytochrome c release and not by directly antagonizing Apaf-1-dependent caspase activation in prostate epithelial cells. J Biol Chem, 276(28), 26614-26621.

Claassen, G. F., & Hann, S. R. (2000). A role for transcriptional repression of p21CIP1 by c-Myc in overcoming transforming growth factor beta -induced cell-cycle arrest. Proc Natl Acad Sci U S A, 97(17), 9498-9503.

Classon, M., & Dyson, N. (2001). p107 and p130: versatile proteins with interesting pockets. Exp Cell Res, 264(1), 135-147.

Cocolakis, E., Lemay, S., Ali, S., & Lebrun, J. J. (2001). The p38 MAPK pathway is required for cell growth inhibition of human breast cancer cells in response to activin. J Biol Chem, 276(21), 18430-18436.

Conery, A. R., Cao, Y., Thompson, E. A., Townsend, C. M., Jr., Ko, T. C., & Luo, K. (2004). Akt interacts directly with Smad3 to regulate the sensitivity to TGF-beta induced apoptosis. Nat Cell Biol, 6(4), 366-372.

Cong, Y. S., & Bacchetti, S. (2000). Histone deacetylation is involved in the transcriptional repression of hTERT in normal human cells. J Biol Chem, 275(46), 35665-35668.

Cong, Y. S., Wright, W. E., & Shay, J. W. (2002). Human telomerase and its regulation. Microbiol Mol Biol Rev, 66(3), 407-425, table of contents.

Counter, C. M., Hahn, W. C., Wei, W., Caddle, S. D., Beijersbergen, R. L., Lansdorp, P. M., et al. (1998). Dissociation among in vitro telomerase activity, telomere maintenance, and cellular immortalization. Proc Natl Acad Sci U S A, 95(25), 14723-14728.

Crosby, M. E., & Almasan, A. (2004). Opposing roles of E2Fs in cell proliferation and death. Cancer Biol Ther, 3(12), 1208-1211.

Crowe, D. L., & Nguyen, D. C. (2001). Rb and E2F-1 regulate telomerase activity in human cancer cells. Biochim Biophys Acta, 1518(1-2), 1-6.

Crowe, D. L., Nguyen, D. C., Tsang, K. J., & Kyo, S. (2001). E2F-1 represses transcription of the human telomerase reverse transcriptase gene. Nucleic Acids Res, 29(13), 2789-2794.

Datto, M. B., Li, Y., Panus, J. F., Howe, D. J., Xiong, Y., & Wang, X. F. (1995). Transforming growth factor beta induces the cyclin-dependent kinase inhibitor p21 through a p53-independent mechanism. Proc Natl Acad Sci U S A, 92(12), 5545-5549.

Davies, M., Robinson, M., Smith, E., Huntley, S., Prime, S., & Paterson, I. (2005). Induction of an epithelial to mesenchymal transition in human immortal and malignant keratinocytes by TGF-beta1 involves MAPK, Smad and AP-1 signalling pathways. J Cell Biochem, 95(5), 918-931.

de Guise, C., Lacerte, A., Rafiei, S., Reynaud, R., Roy, M., Brue, T., et al. (2006). *Activin inhibits the human Pit-1 gene promoter through the p38 kinase pathway in a Smad-independent manner. Endocrinology, 147(9), 4351-4362.*

Derynck, R., & Zhang, Y. E. (2003). *Smad-dependent and Smad-independent pathways in TGF-beta family signalling. Nature, 425(6958), 577-584.*

Dick, F. A., & Dyson, N. (2003). *pRB contains an E2F1-specific binding domain that allows E2F1-induced apoptosis to be regulated separately from other E2F activities. Mol Cell, 12(3), 639-649.*

Dong, Y. B., Yang, H. L., Elliott, M. J., Liu, T. J., Stilwell, A., Atienza, C., Jr., et al. (1999). *Adenovirus-mediated E2F-1 gene transfer efficiently induces apoptosis in melanoma cells. Cancer, 86(10), 2021-2033.*

Dyson, N. (1998). *The regulation of E2F by pRB-family proteins. Genes Dev, 12(15), 2245-2262.*

Ebisawa, T., Fukuchi, M., Murakami, G., Chiba, T., Tanaka, K., Imamura, T., et al. (2001). *Smurf1 interacts with transforming growth factor-beta type I receptor through Smad7 and induces receptor degradation. J Biol Chem, 276(16), 12477-12480.*

Edlund, S., Landstrom, M., Heldin, C. H., & Aspenstrom, P. (2002). *Transforming growth factor-beta-induced mobilization of actin cytoskeleton requires signaling by small GTPases Cdc42 and RhoA. Mol Biol Cell, 13(3), 902-914.*

Eisenman, R. N. (2001). *Deconstructing myc. Genes Dev, 15(16), 2023-2030.*

Elliott, M. J., Dong, Y. B., Yang, H., & McMasters, K. M. (2001). *E2F-1 up-regulates c-Myc and p14(ARF) and induces apoptosis in colon cancer cells. Clin Cancer Res, 7(11), 3590-3597.*

Eymin, B., Gazzeri, S., Brambilla, C., & Brambilla, E. (2001). *Distinct pattern of E2F1 expression in human lung tumours: E2F1 is upregulated in small cell lung carcinoma. Oncogene, 20(14), 1678-1687.*

Fan, G., Ma, X., Kren, B. T., & Steer, C. J. (2002). *Unbound E2F modulates TGF-beta1-induced apoptosis in HuH-7 cells. J Cell Sci, 115(Pt 15), 3181-3191.*

Feng, X. H., & Derynck, R. (2005). *Specificity and versatility in tgf-beta signaling through Smads. Annu Rev Cell Dev Biol, 21, 659-693.*

Feng, X. H., Lin, X., & Derynck, R. (2000). *Smad2, Smad3 and Smad4 cooperate with Sp1 to induce p15(Ink4B) transcription in response to TGF-beta. EMBO J, 19(19), 5178-5193.*

Francis, J. M., Heyworth, C. M., Spooncer, E., Pierce, A., Dexter, T. M., & Whetton, A. D. (2000). *Transforming growth factor-beta 1 induces apoptosis independently of p53 and selectively reduces expression of Bcl-2 in multipotent hematopoietic cells. J Biol Chem, 275(50), 39137-39145.*

Frederick, J. P., Liberati, N. T., Waddell, D. S., Shi, Y., & Wang, X. F. (2004). *Transforming growth factor beta-mediated transcriptional repression of c-myc is dependent on direct binding of Smad3 to a novel repressive Smad binding element. Mol Cell Biol, 24(6), 2546-2559.*

Fueyo, J., Gomez-Manzano, C., Yung, W. K., Liu, T. J., Alemany, R., McDonnell, T. J., et al. (1998). *Overexpression of E2F-1 in glioma triggers apoptosis and suppresses tumor growth in vitro and in vivo. Nat Med, 4(6), 685-690.*

Furukawa, Y., Nishimura, N., Satoh, M., Endo, H., Iwase, S., Yamada, H., et al. (2002). *Apaf-1 is a mediator of E2F-1-induced apoptosis. J Biol Chem, 277(42), 39760-39768.*

Gatti, R., Belletti, S., Orlandini, G., Bussolati, O., Dall'Asta, V., & Gazzola, G. C. (1998). *Comparison of annexin V and calcein-AM as early vital markers of apoptosis in adherent cells by confocal laser microscopy. J Histochem Cytochem, 46(8), 895-900.*

Gonzalez-Suarez, E., Samper, E., Ramirez, A., Flores, J. M., Martin-Caballero, J., Jorcano, J. L., et al. (2001). *Increased epidermal tumors and increased skin wound healing in transgenic mice overexpressing the catalytic subunit of telomerase, mTERT, in basal keratinocytes. EMBO J, 20(11), 2619-2630.*

Grandori, C., Cowley, S. M., James, L. P., & Eisenman, R. N. (2000). *The Myc/Max/Mad network and the transcriptional control of cell behavior. Annu Rev Cell Dev Biol, 16, 653-699.*

Gu, J., Andreeff, M., Roth, J. A., & Fang, B. (2002). hTERT promoter induces tumor-specific Bax gene expression and cell killing in syngenic mouse tumor model and prevents systemic toxicity. Gene Ther, 9(1), 30-37.

Gunes, C., Lichtsteiner, S., Vasserot, A. P., & Englert, C. (2000). Expression of the hTERT gene is regulated at the level of transcriptional initiation and repressed by Mad1. Cancer Res, 60(8), 2116-2121.

Hague, A., Bracey, T. S., Hicks, D. J., Reed, J. C., & Paraskeva, C. (1998). Decreased levels of p26-Bcl-2, but not p30 phosphorylated Bcl-2, precede TGFbeta1-induced apoptosis in colorectal adenoma cells. Carcinogenesis, 19(9), 1691-1695.

Hahn, W. C., Counter, C. M., Lundberg, A. S., Beijersbergen, R. L., Brooks, M. W., & Weinberg, R. A. (1999). Creation of human tumour cells with defined genetic elements. Nature, 400(6743), 464-468.

Halvorsen, T. L., Leibowitz, G., & Levine, F. (1999). Telomerase activity is sufficient to allow transformed cells to escape from crisis. Mol Cell Biol, 19(3), 1864-1870.

Hanafusa, H., Ninomiya-Tsuji, J., Masuyama, N., Nishita, M., Fujisawa, J., Shibuya, H., et al. (1999). Involvement of the p38 mitogen-activated protein kinase pathway in transforming growth factor-beta-induced gene expression. J Biol Chem, 274(38), 27161-27167.

Hayashi, H., Abdollah, S., Qiu, Y., Cai, J., Xu, Y. Y., Grinnell, B. W., et al. (1997). The MAD-related protein Smad7 associates with the TGFbeta receptor and functions as an antagonist of TGFbeta signaling. Cell, 89(7), 1165-1173.

Hendy, G. N., Kaji, H., Sowa, H., Lebrun, J. J., & Canaff, L. (2005). Menin and TGF-beta superfamily member signaling via the Smad pathway in pituitary, parathyroid and osteoblast. Horm Metab Res, 37(6), 375-379.

Herbert, B., Pitts, A. E., Baker, S. I., Hamilton, S. E., Wright, W. E., Shay, J. W., et al. (1999). Inhibition of human telomerase in immortal human cells leads to progressive telomere shortening and cell death. Proc Natl Acad Sci U S A, 96(25), 14276-14281.

Ho, J., de Guise, C., Kim, C., Lemay, S., Wang, X. F., & Lebrun, J. J. (2004). Activin induces hepatocyte cell growth arrest through induction of the cyclin-dependent kinase inhibitor p15INK4B and Sp1. Cell Signal, 16(6), 693-701.

Hoffman, W. H., Biade, S., Zilfou, J. T., Chen, J., & Murphy, M. (2002). Transcriptional repression of the anti-apoptotic survivin gene by wild type p53. J Biol Chem, 277(5), 3247-3257.

Hofmann, F., Martelli, F., Livingston, D. M., & Wang, Z. (1996). The retinoblastoma gene product protects E2F-1 from degradation by the ubiquitin-proteasome pathway. Genes Dev, 10(23), 2949-2959.

Hu, B., Tack, D. C., Liu, T., Wu, Z., Ullenbruch, M. R., & Phan, S. H. (2006). Role of Smad3 in the regulation of rat telomerase reverse transcriptase by TGFbeta. Oncogene, 25(7), 1030-1041.

Hunt, K. K., Deng, J., Liu, T. J., Wilson-Heiner, M., Swisher, S. G., Clayman, G., et al. (1997). Adenovirus-mediated overexpression of the transcription factor E2F-1 induces apoptosis in human breast and ovarian carcinoma cell lines and does not require p53. Cancer Res, 57(21), 4722-4726.

Ianari, A., Natale, T., Calo, E., Ferretti, E., Alesse, E., Screpanti, I., et al. (2009). Proapoptotic function of the retinoblastoma tumor suppressor protein. Cancer Cell, 15(3), 184-194.

Iavarone, A., & Massague, J. (1997). Repression of the CDK activator Cdc25A and cell-cycle arrest by cytokine TGF-beta in cells lacking the CDK inhibitor p15. Nature, 387(6631), 417-422.

Iavarone, A., & Massague, J. (1999). E2F and histone deacetylase mediate transforming growth factor beta repression of cdc25A during keratinocyte cell cycle arrest. Mol Cell Biol, 19(1), 916-922.

Irwin, M., Marin, M. C., Phillips, A. C., Seelan, R. S., Smith, D. I., Liu, W., et al. (2000). Role for the p53 homologue p73 in E2F-1-induced apoptosis. Nature, 407(6804), 645-648.

Irwin, M. S., Kondo, K., Marin, M. C., Cheng, L. S., Hahn, W. C., & Kaelin, W. G., Jr. (2003). Chemosensitivity linked to p73 function. Cancer Cell, 3(4), 403-410.

Islam, A., Kageyama, H., Takada, N., Kawamoto, T., Takayasu, H., Isogai, E., et al. (2000). High expression of Survivin, mapped to 17q25, is significantly associated with poor prognostic factors and promotes cell survival in human neuroblastoma. Oncogene, 19(5), 617-623.

Itoh, S., Ericsson, J., Nishikawa, J., Heldin, C. H., & ten Dijke, P. (2000). The transcriptional co-activator P/CAF potentiates TGF-beta/Smad signaling. Nucleic Acids Res, 28(21), 4291-4298.

Jacob, D., Davis, J. J., Zhang, L., Zhu, H., Teraishi, F., & Fang, B. (2005). Suppression of pancreatic tumor growth in the liver by systemic administration of the TRAIL gene driven by the hTERT promoter. Cancer Gene Ther, 12(2), 109-115.

Jang, C. W., Chen, C. H., Chen, C. C., Chen, J. Y., Su, Y. H., & Chen, R. H. (2002). TGF-beta induces apoptosis through Smad-mediated expression of DAP-kinase. Nat Cell Biol, 4(1), 51-58.

Kaji, H., Canaff, L., Lebrun, J. J., Goltzman, D., & Hendy, G. N. (2001). Inactivation of menin, a Smad3-interacting protein, blocks transforming growth factor type beta signaling. Proc Natl Acad Sci U S A, 98(7), 3837-3842.

Kanamaru, C., Yasuda, H., & Fujita, T. (2002). Involvement of Smad proteins in TGF-beta and activin A-induced apoptosis and growth inhibition of liver cells. Hepatol Res, 23(3), 211-219.

Kang, Y., Chen, C. R., & Massague, J. (2003). A self-enabling TGFbeta response coupled to stress signaling: Smad engages stress response factor ATF3 for Id1 repression in epithelial cells. Mol Cell, 11(4), 915-926.

Kavsak, P., Rasmussen, R. K., Causing, C. G., Bonni, S., Zhu, H., Thomsen, G. H., et al. (2000). Smad7 binds to Smurf2 to form an E3 ubiquitin ligase that targets the TGF beta receptor for degradation. Mol Cell, 6(6), 1365-1375.

Kherrouche, Z., Blais, A., Ferreira, E., De Launoit, Y., & Monte, D. (2006). ASK-1 (apoptosis signal-regulating kinase 1) is a direct E2F target gene. Biochem J, 396(3), 547-556.

Kim, N. W., Piatyszek, M. A., Prowse, K. R., Harley, C. B., West, M. D., Ho, P. L., et al. (1994). Specific association of human telomerase activity with immortal cells and cancer. Science, 266(5193), 2011-2015.

Kishi, H., Igawa, M., Kikuno, N., Yoshino, T., Urakami, S., & Shiina, H. (2004). Expression of the survivin gene in prostate cancer: correlation with clinicopathological characteristics, proliferative activity and apoptosis. J Urol, 171(5), 1855-1860.

Koga, S., Hirohata, S., Kondo, Y., Komata, T., Takakura, M., Inoue, M., et al. (2001). FADD gene therapy using the human telomerase catalytic subunit (hTERT) gene promoter to restrict induction of apoptosis to tumors in vitro and in vivo. Anticancer Res, 21(3B), 1937-1943.

Komata, T., Kondo, Y., Kanzawa, T., Hirohata, S., Koga, S., Sumiyoshi, H., et al. (2001). Treatment of malignant glioma cells with the transfer of constitutively active caspase-6 using the human telomerase catalytic subunit (human telomerase reverse transcriptase) gene promoter. Cancer Res, 61(15), 5796-5802.

Korah, J., Falah, N., Lacerte, A., & Lebrun, J. J. (2012). A transcriptionally active pRb-E2F1-P/CAF signaling pathway is central to TGFβ-mediated apoptosis. Cell Death and Disease, in press.

Kowanetz, M., Valcourt, U., Bergstrom, R., Heldin, C. H., & Moustakas, A. (2004). Id2 and Id3 define the potency of cell proliferation and differentiation responses to transforming growth factor beta and bone morphogenetic protein. Mol Cell Biol, 24(10), 4241-4254.

Kuhn, H., Liebers, U., Gessner, C., Schumacher, A., Witt, C., Schauer, J., et al. (2002). Adenovirus-mediated E2F-1 gene transfer in nonsmall-cell lung cancer induces cell growth arrest and apoptosis. Eur Respir J, 20(3), 703-709.

Kyo, S., Takakura, M., Fujiwara, T., & Inoue, M. (2008). Understanding and exploiting hTERT promoter regulation for diagnosis and treatment of human cancers. Cancer Sci, 99(8), 1528-1538.

Kyo, S., Takakura, M., Taira, T., Kanaya, T., Itoh, H., Yutsudo, M., et al. (2000). Sp1 cooperates with c-Myc to activate transcription of the human telomerase reverse transcriptase gene (hTERT). Nucleic Acids Res, 28(3), 669-677.

Lacerte, A., Korah, J., Roy, M., Yang, X. J., Lemay, S., & Lebrun, J. J. (2008). Transforming growth factor-beta inhibits telomerase through SMAD3 and E2F transcription factors. Cell Signal, 20(1), 50-59.

Lafon, C., Mathieu, C., Guerrin, M., Pierre, O., Vidal, S., & Valette, A. (1996). Transforming growth factor beta 1-induced apoptosis in human ovarian carcinoma cells: protection by the antioxidant N-acetylcysteine and bcl-2. Cell Growth Differ, 7(8), 1095-1104.

Laiho, M., DeCaprio, J. A., Ludlow, J. W., Livingston, D. M., & Massague, J. (1990). Growth inhibition by TGF-beta linked to suppression of retinoblastoma protein phosphorylation. Cell, 62(1), 175-185.

Lamouille, S., & Derynck, R. (2007). Cell size and invasion in TGF-beta-induced epithelial to mesenchymal transition is regulated by activation of the mTOR pathway. J Cell Biol, 178(3), 437-451.

Larisch, S., Yi, Y., Lotan, R., Kerner, H., Eimerl, S., Tony Parks, W., et al. (2000). A novel mitochondrial septin-like protein, ARTS, mediates apoptosis dependent on its P-loop motif. Nat Cell Biol, 2(12), 915-921.

Lasorella, A., Noseda, M., Beyna, M., Yokota, Y., & Iavarone, A. (2000). Id2 is a retinoblastoma protein target and mediates signalling by Myc oncoproteins. Nature, 407(6804), 592-598.

Lebrun, J. J. (2009). Activin, TGF-beta and menin in pituitary tumorigenesis. Adv Exp Med Biol, 668, 69-78.

Lebrun, J. J. (2012). The Dual Role of TGFβ in Human Cancer: From Tumor Suppression to Cancer Metastasis. ISRN Molecular Biology, 2012, 1-28.

Lee, J. H., Wan, X. H., Song, J., Kang, J. J., Chung, W. S., Lee, E. H., et al. (2002). TGF-beta-induced apoptosis and reduction of Bcl-2 in human lens epithelial cells in vitro. Curr Eye Res, 25(3), 147-153.

Lee, M. K., Pardoux, C., Hall, M. C., Lee, P. S., Warburton, D., Qing, J., et al. (2007). TGF-beta activates Erk MAP kinase signalling through direct phosphorylation of ShcA. The EMBO journal, 26(17), 3957-3967.

Levy, L., & Hill, C. S. (2006). Alterations in components of the TGF-beta superfamily signaling pathways in human cancer. Cytokine Growth Factor Rev, 17(1-2), 41-58.

Li, H., Xu, D., Li, J., Berndt, M. C., & Liu, J. P. (2006). Transforming growth factor beta suppresses human telomerase reverse transcriptase (hTERT) by Smad3 interactions with c-Myc and the hTERT gene. J Biol Chem, 281(35), 25588-25600.

Li, J. M., Hu, P. P., Shen, X., Yu, Y., & Wang, X. F. (1997). E2F4-RB and E2F4-p107 complexes suppress gene expression by transforming growth factor beta through E2F binding sites. Proc Natl Acad Sci U S A, 94(10), 4948-4953.

Li, J. M., Nichols, M. A., Chandrasekharan, S., Xiong, Y., & Wang, X. F. (1995). Transforming growth factor beta activates the promoter of cyclin-dependent kinase inhibitor p15INK4B through an Sp1 consensus site. J Biol Chem, 270(45), 26750-26753.

Lin, S. Y., & Elledge, S. J. (2003). Multiple tumor suppressor pathways negatively regulate telomerase. Cell, 113(7), 881-889.

Lin, W. C., Lin, F. T., & Nevins, J. R. (2001). Selective induction of E2F1 in response to DNA damage, mediated by ATM-dependent phosphorylation. Genes Dev, 15(14), 1833-1844.

Liu, T. J., Wang, M., Breau, R. L., Henderson, Y., El-Naggar, A. K., Steck, K. D., et al. (1999). Apoptosis induction by E2F-1 via adenoviral-mediated gene transfer results in growth suppression of head and neck squamous cell carcinoma cell lines. Cancer Gene Ther, 6(2), 163-171.

Lukas, J., Petersen, B. O., Holm, K., Bartek, J., & Helin, K. (1996). Deregulated expression of E2F family members induces S-phase entry and overcomes p16INK4A-mediated growth suppression. Mol Cell Biol, 16(3), 1047-1057.

Mahotka, C., Wenzel, M., Springer, E., Gabbert, H. E., & Gerharz, C. D. (1999). Survivin-deltaEx3 and survivin-2B: two novel splice variants of the apoptosis inhibitor survivin with different antiapoptotic properties. Cancer Res, 59(24), 6097-6102.

Martinez-Balbas, M. A., Bauer, U. M., Nielsen, S. J., Brehm, A., & Kouzarides, T. (2000). Regulation of E2F1 activity by acetylation. EMBO J, 19(4), 662-671.

Massague, J. (1990). The transforming growth factor-beta family. Annu Rev Cell Biol, 6, 597-641.

Massague, J. (1998). TGF-beta signal transduction. Annu Rev Biochem, 67, 753-791.

Massague, J. (2004). G1 cell-cycle control and cancer. Nature, 432(7015), 298-306.

Massague, J., & Wotton, D. (2000). Transcriptional control by the TGF-beta/Smad signaling system. Embo J, 19(8), 1745-1754.

Meier, P., Finch, A., & Evan, G. (2000). Apoptosis in development. Nature, 407(6805), 796-801.

Meyerson, M., Counter, C. M., Eaton, E. N., Ellisen, L. W., Steiner, P., Caddle, S. D., et al. (1997). hEST2, the putative human telomerase catalytic subunit gene, is up-regulated in tumor cells and during immortalization. Cell, 90(4), 785-795.

Mirza, A., McGuirk, M., Hockenberry, T. N., Wu, Q., Ashar, H., Black, S., et al. (2002). Human survivin is negatively regulated by wild-type p53 and participates in p53-dependent apoptotic pathway. Oncogene, 21(17), 2613-2622.

Nahle, Z., Polakoff, J., Davuluri, R. V., McCurrach, M. E., Jacobson, M. D., Narita, M., et al. (2002). Direct coupling of the cell cycle and cell death machinery by E2F. Nat Cell Biol, 4(11), 859-864.

Neumann, A. A., & Reddel, R. R. (2002). Telomere maintenance and cancer -- look, no telomerase. Nat Rev Cancer, 2(11), 879-884.

Norton, J. D. (2000). ID helix-loop-helix proteins in cell growth, differentiation and tumorigenesis. J Cell Sci, 113 (Pt 22), 3897-3905.

Oh, S., Song, Y. H., Yim, J., & Kim, T. K. (2000). Identification of Mad as a repressor of the human telomerase (hTERT) gene. Oncogene, 19(11), 1485-1490.

Ohgushi, M., Kuroki, S., Fukamachi, H., O'Reilly, L. A., Kuida, K., Strasser, A., et al. (2005). Transforming growth factor beta-dependent sequential activation of Smad, Bim, and caspase-9 mediates physiological apoptosis in gastric epithelial cells. Mol Cell Biol, 25(22), 10017-10028.

Olaussen, K. A., Dubrana, K., Domont, J., Spano, J. P., Sabatier, L., & Soria, J. C. (2006). Telomeres and telomerase as targets for anticancer drug development. Crit Rev Oncol Hematol, 57(3), 191-214.

Pardali, K., Kurisaki, A., Moren, A., ten Dijke, P., Kardassis, D., & Moustakas, A. (2000). Role of Smad proteins and transcription factor Sp1 in p21(Waf1/Cip1) regulation by transforming growth factor-beta. J Biol Chem, 275(38), 29244-29256.

Pardali, K., & Moustakas, A. (2007). Actions of TGF-beta as tumor suppressor and pro-metastatic factor in human cancer. Biochim Biophys Acta, 1775(1), 21-62.

Pediconi, N., Ianari, A., Costanzo, A., Belloni, L., Gallo, R., Cimino, L., et al. (2003). Differential regulation of E2F1 apoptotic target genes in response to DNA damage. Nat Cell Biol, 5(6), 552-558.

Pennati, M., Binda, M., Colella, G., Zoppe, M., Folini, M., Vignati, S., et al. (2004). Ribozyme-mediated inhibition of survivin expression increases spontaneous and drug-induced apoptosis and decreases the tumorigenic potential of human prostate cancer cells. Oncogene, 23(2), 386-394.

Pennati, M., Binda, M., De Cesare, M., Pratesi, G., Folini, M., Citti, L., et al. (2004). Ribozyme-mediated down-regulation of survivin expression sensitizes human melanoma cells to topotecan in vitro and in vivo. Carcinogenesis, 25(7), 1129-1136.

Peron, P., Rahmani, M., Zagar, Y., Durand-Schneider, A. M., Lardeux, B., & Bernuau, D. (2001). Potentiation of Smad transactivation by Jun proteins during a combined treatment with epidermal growth factor and transforming growth factor-beta in rat hepatocytes. role of phosphatidylinositol 3-kinase-induced AP-1 activation. J Biol Chem, 276(13), 10524-10531.

Phillips, A. C., Bates, S., Ryan, K. M., Helin, K., & Vousden, K. H. (1997). Induction of DNA synthesis and apoptosis are separable functions of E2F-1. Genes Dev, 11(14), 1853-1863.

Prehn, J. H., Bindokas, V. P., Marcuccilli, C. J., Krajewski, S., Reed, J. C., & Miller, R. J. (1994). Regulation of neuronal Bcl2 protein expression and calcium homeostasis by transforming growth factor type beta confers wide-ranging protection on rat hippocampal neurons. Proc Natl Acad Sci U S A, 91(26), 12599-12603.

Putzer, B. M. (2007). E2F1 death pathways as targets for cancer therapy. J Cell Mol Med, 11(2), 239-251.

Remy, I., Montmarquette, A., & Michnick, S. W. (2004). PKB/Akt modulates TGF-beta signalling through a direct interaction with Smad3. Nat Cell Biol, 6(4), 358-365.

Reynisdottir, I., Polyak, K., Iavarone, A., & Massague, J. (1995). Kip/Cip and Ink4 Cdk inhibitors cooperate to induce cell cycle arrest in response to TGF-beta. Genes Dev, 9(15), 1831-1845.

Rodicker, F., Stiewe, T., Zimmermann, S., & Putzer, B. M. (2001). Therapeutic efficacy of E2F1 in pancreatic cancer correlates with TP73 induction. Cancer Res, 61(19), 7052-7055.

Rogoff, H. A., Pickering, M. T., Frame, F. M., Debatis, M. E., Sanchez, Y., Jones, S., et al. (2004). Apoptosis associated with deregulated E2F activity is dependent on E2F1 and Atm/Nbs1/Chk2. Mol Cell Biol, 24(7), 2968-2977.

Saltzman, A., Munro, R., Searfoss, G., Franks, C., Jaye, M., & Ivashchenko, Y. (1998). Transforming growth factor-beta-mediated apoptosis in the Ramos B-lymphoma cell line is accompanied by caspase activation and Bcl-XL downregulation. Exp Cell Res, 242(1), 244-254.

Sandhu, C., Garbe, J., Bhattacharya, N., Daksis, J., Pan, C. H., Yaswen, P., et al. (1997). Transforming growth factor beta stabilizes p15INK4B protein, increases p15INK4B-cdk4 complexes, and inhibits cyclin D1-cdk4 association in human mammary epithelial cells. Mol Cell Biol, 17(5), 2458-2467.

Schuster, N., & Krieglstein, K. (2002). Mechanisms of TGF-beta-mediated apoptosis. Cell Tissue Res, 307(1), 1-14.

Selvamurugan, N., Kwok, S., Alliston, T., Reiss, M., & Partridge, N. C. (2004). Transforming growth factor-beta 1 regulation of collagenase-3 expression in osteoblastic cells by cross-talk between the Smad and MAPK signaling pathways and their components, Smad2 and Runx2. J Biol Chem, 279(18), 19327-19334.

Seoane, J., Le, H. V., Shen, L., Anderson, S. A., & Massague, J. (2004). Integration of Smad and forkhead pathways in the control of neuroepithelial and glioblastoma cell proliferation. Cell, 117(2), 211-223.

Seoane, J., Pouponnot, C., Staller, P., Schader, M., Eilers, M., & Massague, J. (2001). TGFbeta influences Myc, Miz-1 and Smad to control the CDK inhibitor p15INK4b. Nat Cell Biol, 3(4), 400-408.

Shariat, S. F., Lotan, Y., Saboorian, H., Khoddami, S. M., Roehrborn, C. G., Slawin, K. M., et al. (2004). Survivin expression is associated with features of biologically aggressive prostate carcinoma. Cancer, 100(4), 751-757.

Shats, I., Milyavsky, M., Tang, X., Stambolsky, P., Erez, N., Brosh, R., et al. (2004). p53-dependent down-regulation of telomerase is mediated by p21waf1. J Biol Chem, 279(49), 50976-50985.

Shay, J. W., & Wright, W. E. (2005). Senescence and immortalization: role of telomeres and telomerase. Carcinogenesis, 26(5), 867-874.

Siegel, P. M., & Massague, J. (2003). Cytostatic and apoptotic actions of TGF-beta in homeostasis and cancer. Nat Rev Cancer, 3(11), 807-821.

Siegel, P. M., Shu, W., & Massague, J. (2003). Mad upregulation and Id2 repression accompany transforming growth factor (TGF)-beta-mediated epithelial cell growth suppression. J Biol Chem, 278(37), 35444-35450.

Smith, L. L., Coller, H. A., & Roberts, J. M. (2003). Telomerase modulates expression of growth-controlling genes and enhances cell proliferation. Nat Cell Biol, 5(5), 474-479.

Spender, L. C., & Inman, G. J. (2009). TGF-beta induces growth arrest in Burkitt lymphoma cells via transcriptional repression of E2F-1. J Biol Chem, 284(3), 1435-1442.

Stampfer, M. R., Garbe, J., Levine, G., Lichtsteiner, S., Vasserot, A. P., & Yaswen, P. (2001). Expression of the telomerase catalytic subunit, hTERT, induces resistance to transforming growth factor beta growth inhibition in p16INK4A(-) human mammary epithelial cells. Proc Natl Acad Sci U S A, 98(8), 4498-4503.

Stewart, S. A., Hahn, W. C., O'Connor, B. F., Banner, E. N., Lundberg, A. S., Modha, P., et al. (2002). Telomerase contributes to tumorigenesis by a telomere length-independent mechanism. Proc Natl Acad Sci U S A, 99(20), 12606-12611.

Suzuki, A., Ito, T., Kawano, H., Hayashida, M., Hayasaki, Y., Tsutomi, Y., et al. (2000). Survivin initiates procaspase 3/p21 complex formation as a result of interaction with Cdk4 to resist Fas-mediated cell death. Oncogene, 19(10), 1346-1353.

Suzuki, T., Yasui, W., Yokozaki, H., Naka, K., Ishikawa, T., & Tahara, E. (1999). Expression of the E2F family in human gastrointestinal carcinomas. Int J Cancer, 81(4), 535-538.

Tachibana, I., Imoto, M., Adjei, P. N., Gores, G. J., Subramaniam, M., Spelsberg, T. C., et al. (1997). Overexpression of the TGFbeta-regulated zinc finger encoding gene, TIEG, induces apoptosis in pancreatic epithelial cells. J Clin Invest, 99(10), 2365-2374.

Tamm, I., Wang, Y., Sausville, E., Scudiero, D. A., Vigna, N., Oltersdorf, T., et al. (1998). IAP-family protein survivin inhibits caspase activity and apoptosis induced by Fas (CD95), Bax, caspases, and anticancer drugs. Cancer Res, 58(23), 5315-5320.

Thompson, C. B. (1995). Apoptosis in the pathogenesis and treatment of disease. Science, 267(5203), 1456-1462.

Tobin, S. W., Brown, M. K., Douville, K., Payne, D. C., Eastman, A., & Arrick, B. A. (2001). Inhibition of transforming growth factor beta signaling in MCF-7 cells results in resistance to tumor necrosis factor alpha: a role for Bcl-2. Cell Growth Differ, 12(2), 109-117.

Tuve, S., Racek, T., Niemetz, A., Schultz, J., Soengas, M. S., & Putzer, B. M. (2006). Adenovirus-mediated TA-p73beta gene transfer increases chemosensitivity of human malignant melanomas. Apoptosis, 11(2), 235-243.

Valderrama-Carvajal, H., Cocolakis, E., Lacerte, A., Lee, E. H., Krystal, G., Ali, S., et al. (2002). Activin/TGF-beta induce apoptosis through Smad-dependent expression of the lipid phosphatase SHIP. Nat Cell Biol, 4(12), 963-969.

Waddell, D. S., Liberati, N. T., Guo, X., Frederick, J. P., & Wang, X. F. (2004). Casein kinase Iepsilon plays a functional role in the transforming growth factor-beta signaling pathway. J Biol Chem, 279(28), 29236-29246.

Wang, B., Liu, K., Lin, F. T., & Lin, W. C. (2004). A role for 14-3-3 tau in E2F1 stabilization and DNA damage-induced apoptosis. J Biol Chem, 279(52), 54140-54152.

Wang, D., Russell, J. L., & Johnson, D. G. (2000). E2F4 and E2F1 have similar proliferative properties but different apoptotic and oncogenic properties in vivo. Mol Cell Biol, 20(10), 3417-3424.

Wang, E. S., Wu, K., Chin, A. C., Chen-Kiang, S., Pongracz, K., Gryaznov, S., et al. (2004). Telomerase inhibition with an oligonucleotide telomerase template antagonist: in vitro and in vivo studies in multiple myeloma and lymphoma. Blood, 103(1), 258-266.

Wang, J., Yang, L., Yang, J., Kuropatwinski, K., Wang, W., Liu, X. Q., et al. (2008). Transforming growth factor beta induces apoptosis through repressing the phosphoinositide 3-kinase/AKT/survivin pathway in colon cancer cells. Cancer Res, 68(9), 3152-3160.

Wang, S., & Zhu, J. (2003). Evidence for a relief of repression mechanism for activation of the human telomerase reverse transcriptase promoter. J Biol Chem, 278(21), 18842-18850.

Warner, B. J., Blain, S. W., Seoane, J., & Massague, J. (1999). Myc downregulation by transforming growth factor beta required for activation of the p15(Ink4b) G(1) arrest pathway. Mol Cell Biol, 19(9), 5913-5922.

Watanabe, H., de Caestecker, M. P., & Yamada, Y. (2001). Transcriptional cross-talk between Smad, ERK1/2, and p38 mitogen-activated protein kinase pathways regulates transforming growth factor-beta-induced aggrecan gene expression in chondrogenic ATDC5 cells. J Biol Chem, 276(17), 14466-14473.

Wildey, G. M., Patil, S., & Howe, P. H. (2003). Smad3 potentiates transforming growth factor beta (TGFbeta)-induced apoptosis and expression of the BH3-only protein Bim in WEHI 231 B lymphocytes. J Biol Chem, 278(20), 18069-18077.

Won, J., Chang, S., Oh, S., & Kim, T. K. (2004). Small-molecule-based identification of dynamic assembly of E2F-pocket protein-histone deacetylase complex for telomerase regulation in human cells. Proc Natl Acad Sci U S A, 101(31), 11328-11333.

Won, J., Yim, J., & Kim, T. K. (2002). *Opposing regulatory roles of E2F in human telomerase reverse transcriptase (hTERT) gene expression in human tumor and normal somatic cells.* FASEB J, 16(14), 1943-1945.

Xie, W., Jiang, P., Miao, L., Zhao, Y., Zhimin, Z., Qing, L., et al. (2006). *Novel link between E2F1 and Smac/DIABLO: proapoptotic Smac/DIABLO is transcriptionally upregulated by E2F1.* Nucleic Acids Res, 34(7), 2046-2055.

Yagi, K., Furuhashi, M., Aoki, H., Goto, D., Kuwano, H., Sugamura, K., et al. (2002). *c-myc is a downstream target of the Smad pathway.* J Biol Chem, 277(1), 854-861.

Yamamura, Y., Hua, X., Bergelson, S., & Lodish, H. F. (2000). *Critical role of Smads and AP-1 complex in transforming growth factor-beta -dependent apoptosis.* J Biol Chem, 275(46), 36295-36302.

Yamasaki, L., Jacks, T., Bronson, R., Goillot, E., Harlow, E., & Dyson, N. J. (1996). *Tumor induction and tissue atrophy in mice lacking E2F-1.* Cell, 85(4), 537-548.

Yan, Z., Winawer, S., & Friedman, E. (1994). *Two different signal transduction pathways can be activated by transforming growth factor beta 1 in epithelial cells.* J Biol Chem, 269(18), 13231-13237.

Yang, H., Kyo, S., Takatura, M., & Sun, L. (2001). *Autocrine transforming growth factor beta suppresses telomerase activity and transcription of human telomerase reverse transcriptase in human cancer cells.* Cell Growth Differ, 12(2), 119-127.

Yang, H. L., Dong, Y. B., Elliott, M. J., Liu, T. J., & McMasters, K. M. (2000). *Caspase activation and changes in Bcl-2 family member protein expression associated with E2F-1-mediated apoptosis in human esophageal cancer cells.* Clin Cancer Res, 6(4), 1579-1589.

Yang, J., Song, K., Krebs, T. L., Jackson, M. W., & Danielpour, D. (2008). *Rb/E2F4 and Smad2/3 link survivin to TGF-beta-induced apoptosis and tumor progression.* Oncogene, 27(40), 5326-5338.

Zhang, X., Mar, V., Zhou, W., Harrington, L., & Robinson, M. O. (1999). *Telomere shortening and apoptosis in telomerase-inhibited human tumor cells.* Genes Dev, 13(18), 2388-2399.

Urokinase-Type Plasminogen Activator System in Breast Cancer

Ahmed H. Mekkawy
Department of Surgery, St George Hospital
University of New South Wales, Australia

Krishna Pillai
Department of Surgery, St George Hospital
University of New South Wales, Australia

David L. Morris
Department of Surgery, St George Hospital
University of New South Wales, Australia

1   Introduction

It has been widely reported that breast cancer is the most common cancer in women worldwide (Jemal *et al.*, 2011). In 2013, in the US only, more than 230,000 cases were diagnosed with breast cancer that leads to nearly 40,000 deaths. Therefore, breast cancer has been designated as the second most common cancer causing deaths in women (Siegel *et al.*, 2013). Over the last two decades, mortality rate due to breast cancer has declined by about 30% (Siegel *et al.*, 2013). Although a dramatic improvement in early detection, treatment and management of patients has taken place; these approaches are still costly and not achievable in developing countries (Anderson *et al.*, 2006).

Breast cancers have been sorted into six groups based on molecular expression prefilling. These groups are luminal subtype A, luminal subtype B, HER2 subtype, normal breast subtype, basal subtype and claudian-low subtype. A fraction of basal and claudian-low breast cancers that do not express estrogen receptor, progesterone receptor and the human epidermal growth factor receptor 2 (HER2) is known as triple negative breast cancers (TNBC) (Duffy *et al.*, 2012). As in many cancers, the main hurdle that has been affecting the development and treatment of breast cancer is the incomplete understanding of the molecular biology of the disease. Hence, currently rigorous research is underway examining the molecular biology that may contribute to the disease, and with time better prognosis and therapies will be forthcoming.

One of the molecular biology systems that has been well investigated is the urokinase plasminogen activator (uPA) system. Preclinical investigation indicates that uPA system plays a vital role in remodeling the surrounding tissues such as cleavage of basement membranes (BM) and extracellular matrix (ECM) along with the activation of latent growth factors. In addition, uPA system activates several signaling pathways involved in cell proliferation, migration, invasion, metastasis and angiogenesis (Figure 1 & 2) (Mekkawy *et al.*, 2009). In several malignancies, including breast cancer, increased expression of the uPA system results in tumor promotion. Recent studies seem to indicate that there is a strong correlation between the expression of uPA components and clinical outcome in breast cancer (Jelisavac-Cosic *et al.*, 2011; Harbeck *et al.*, 2013); hence it is currently an active area of research.

2   The structure of uPA system

The uPA system is made up of uPA enzyme, plasminogen substrate, the uPA receptors (uPAR) and three plasminogen inhibitors [PAI-1, PAI-2 and proteinas nexin 1 (PN-1)] (Mekkawy *et al.*, 2009).

2.1   Plasminogen and uPA

Although uPA is translated as a 48.5 kDa protein molecule, its weight normally increases to about 52 kDa with modification, post-transitionally (Petersen *et al.*, 1988). The gene coding for uPA is 6.4 kb long with 11 exons (Riccio *et al.*, 1985), and the transcribed uPA mRNA is 2.4 kb (Verde *et al.*, 1984). At a structural level, uPA is divided into three sections: the first being the inactive N-terminal fragment (uPA-ATF) that contains "the growth factor-like domain (GFD)" (residues 1-46) which is homologous to the epidermal growth factor (EGF), and is responsible for interaction with uPAR. The second section is a kringle domain with an unknown function. the third section is the carboxyl terminal sequence that contains the catalytically active motif (Stepanova & Tkachuk, 2002). The mature uPA presents itself as a two chain protein linked by a disulphide bond at cysteine 148 and 279. Similar to most mammalian proteases,

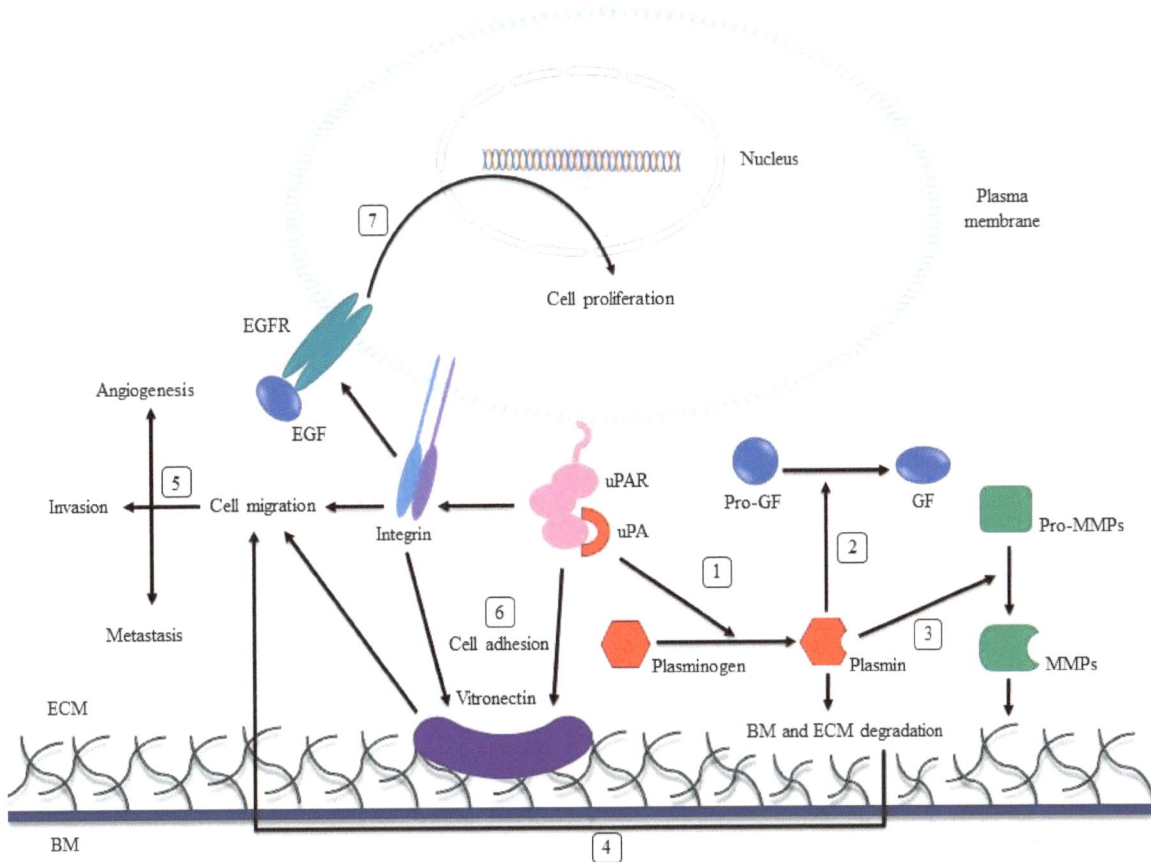

Figure 1: The urokinase-type plasminogen activator (uPA) system. The membrane anchored receptor (uPAR) binds its extracellular ligand (pro-uPA), causing activation of pro-uPA to uPA which then activates plasminogen to plasmin [1]. Plasmin afterward activates latent growth factors (GF) [2], Matrix metalloproteases (MMPs) [3]. Plasmin and activated MMPs breaks up the basement membranes (BM) and extracellular matrix (ECM) which allows endothelial cells to migrate [4] and to form new vasculature (angiogenesis). In addition, breaking up of ECM allows migration, invasion and metastasis of tumor cells [5]. uPAR also regulates cellular adhesion and migration via interaction with integrins and vitronectin [6]. Interaction between uPAR and integrins has been linked to EGFR-dependent cell proliferation [7].

it is synthesized as an inactive single chain polypeptide consisting of 411 amino acid residues, referred to as pro-uPA. Remarkably, pro-uPA acts on plasminogen (a zymogen), and converts it to plasmin that in turn converts the pro-uPA into the active two-chain high molecular weight uPA (HMW- uPA) (Stepanova & Tkachuk, 2002).

The N-terminal sequencing examination of uPA cleavage by plasmin revealed the formation of the two chain uPA by the cleavage of Lys158-Ile159. This cleavage is followed by the cleavage of Lys46-Ser47 in the region between GFD and the kringle domains. Hence, the removal of GFD resulted in the formation of two chain uPA with a molecular weight of 36-40 kDa. Further exposure to plasmin produces a lower molecular weight uPA (LMW-uPA) of 32 kDa without the kringle domain. Such findings suggest

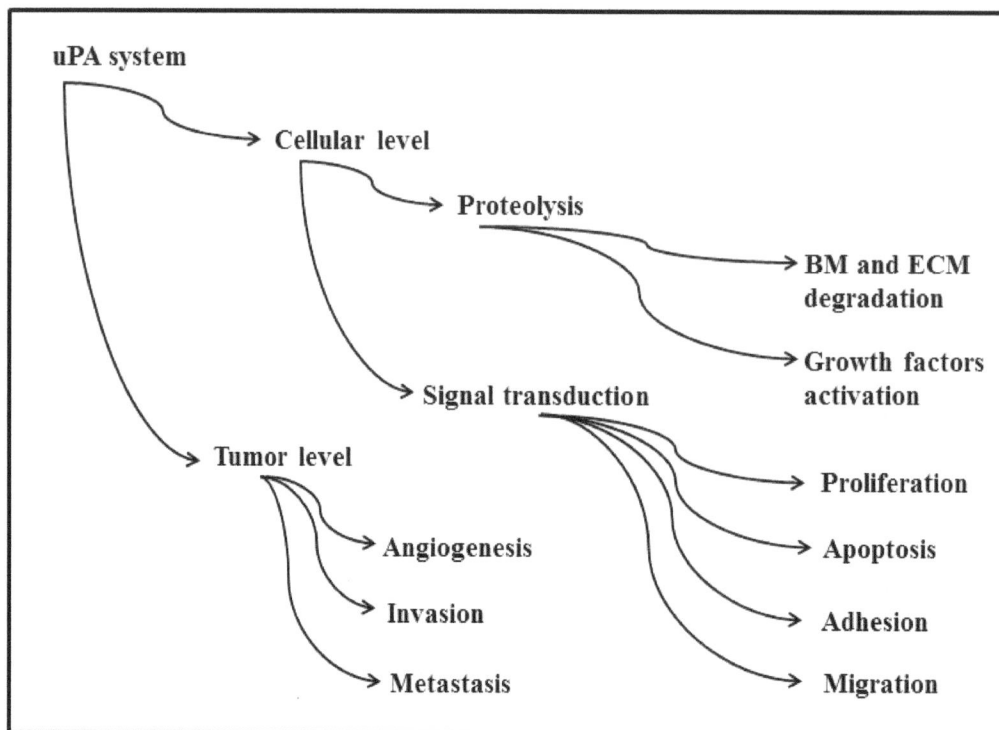

Figure 2: Tumor processes associated with urokinase-type plasminogen activator (uPA) system.

that besides proteolytic activation, plasmin can also sequentially split off the N-terminal domain of uPA with the production several proteolytically active forms. The uPA form lacking GFD is also generated on the cell surface through the action of plasmin (Poliakov *et al.*, 2001). Further, the full length, single and two-chain forms of uPA and its ATF can interact with uPAR on the cell surface whilst uPA lacking the GFD is unable to interact with uPAR. Thus, uPA can only bind uPAR on smooth muscle cells (SMC) and other cells either through the kringle domains or through the protease domain. This finding suggests that other uPAR may present on the plasma membrane. Additionally, there are indications that uPA fragments generated by extracellular proteases can affect cellular function independently or cross talk with uPAR (Stepanova & Tkachuk, 2002).Moreover, the interaction between uPA and uPAR can provoke signal transduction independent of the catalytic activity of uPA, as it can be induced by proteolytically inactive ATF of uPA (Stahl & Mueller, 1994; Resnati *et al.*, 1996; Rabbani *et al.*, 1997). uPA has also been found to mediate cell survival by stimulating the X-linked inhibitor of apoptosis protein and the PI3K/AKT pathway (Gondi *et al.*, 2007; Prager *et al.*, 2009).

Plasminogen is normally bound to cell membranes, and is activated to a serine protease known as plasmin by uPA (Collen & Lijnen, 1991). Plasminogen consists of 791 amino acid residues that are organized into seven structural domains, comprising of "a pre-activation peptide" (residues 1-77), 5 sequential homologous kringle domains which are triple-disulphide linked peptides (approximately 80 residues each), and the protease domain (residues 562-791) (Collen, 2001). The kringle domain contains lysine binding sites, and plays a vital role in specific binding to fibrin, cell surfaces and α2-anti-plasmin (main inhibitor of plasmin) (Collen, 2001). uPA bound to uPAR activates plasminogen to plasmin at the cell surface (Stefansson *et al.*, 2003). Although plasmin is well known for its anti-coagulant properties that degrade fibrin, it has ancillary role in remodeling surrounding tissues by facilitating the degradation of BM and ECM (Bergmann *et al.*, 2005). This property of plasmin enhances cell migration through tissue barriers under normal and pathological conditions such as embryogenesis, wound healing as well as angiogenesis (Castellino & Ploplis, 2005). Like uPA, plasmin is a serine protease but it acts on several ECM components including fibrin, laminin and fibronectin (Fn) (del Zoppo, 2010). Further, plasmin also assists the progress of ECM degradation by activating latent matrix metalloproteinases (MMPs) such as MMP-3, MMP-9, MMP-12, MMP-13 and growth factors (Fukao *et al.*, 1997; Lijnen, 2001). Moreover, both plasmin and MMPs activate growth factors (GFs) including vascular endothelial growth factor (VEGF) in ECM (Shevde & Welch, 2003; Steeg, 2003). VEGF is an important angiogenic factor which has also been implicated in vascular permeability that is mediated via activation of the uPA system (Behzadian *et al.*, 2003).

2.2 uPAR

uPAR is the cellular receptor for uPA (Vassalli *et al.*, 1985), and belongs to the Lys-6/uPAR/α-neurotoxin family of proteins (Ploug, 2003). Whilst the uPAR gene is 21.67 Kb long and located on chromosome 19q13, the complementary deoxyribonucleic acid (cDNA) for uPAR is 1.4 kDa encoding a 313 amino acid polypeptide (Roldan *et al.*, 1990). uPAR in its fully functional and mature form (CD87) is a single chain (45-65 kDa) glycoprotein with three domains and linked to cellular surface by a glycosyl phosphatidylinositol (GPI) anchor (Vassalli *et al.*, 1985). The three domains (DI, DII and DIII) are approximately 90 amino acid residue long, with DI carrying the primary ligand-binding region that is involved in high-affinity binding to the N-terminal of uPA (Behrendt *et al.*, 1991). However, DII and DIII host binding sites for other proteins such as kininogen and integrins (Behrendt *et al.*, 1996; Colman *et al.*, 1997; Ploug, 1998; Gardsvoll *et al.*, 1999).

The three domains of uPAR are connected together by short linker regions (Andreasen *et al.*, 2000), with the linker region between DI and II containing several cleavage sites that can react with trypsin, chemotrypsin, elastase, cathepsin G, MMPs, plasmin and uPA (Montuori *et al.*, 1999; Andolfo *et al.*, 2002; Beaufort *et al.*, 2004; Beaufort *et al.*, 2004). Once cleaved, uPAR lacking the N-terminal DI as well as the full length uPAR can exist as membrane bound or as soluble form (suPAR) (Montuori *et al.*, 2005). uPAR soluble forms have been found in the plasma of cancer patients, and is thought to be released from tumor cell surface (Riisbro *et al.*, 2001; Lomholt *et al.*, 2009).

The uPAR molecules were found to exist on cell surface predominantly in a monomeric form, and 10-30% in dimeric forms (Cunningham *et al.*, 2003). The binding sites of uPAR-uPAR interactions are completely different from that of uPA-binding sites on the uPAR molecule (Liang *et al.*, 2003).

2.3   Serine protease inhibitors

The PA system also has three major protease inhibitors that belong to the Serpins family. The inhibitors are PAI-1, PAI-2 and PN-1. The first two are uPA inhibitors whilst the third inhibits plasmin. Serpins belong to a super family of inhibitors that has 400 residues ranging from 38-70 kDa, depending on degree of glysoylation (Travis & Salvesen, 1983). Serpins are characterized by their highly conserved tertiary structure and unique substrate-inhibition mechanism. All the members of this family consist of three sheets (A, B and C), nine helices (A - I) and a surface-exposed loop near the C-terminal end that contains the active center peptide bond (Carrell & Boswell, 1986; Huber & Carrell, 1989). This bond performs as a pseudo-substrate by mimicking the interaction of the substrate with its target proteases (Laskowski &

Kato, 1980). As an alternative to cleaving the bond, the proteases are trapped in a stable inactive complex of 1:1 stoichiometry (Potempa *et al.*, 1994; Stein & Carrell, 1995).

PAI-1 (43 kDa) is a single-chain glycoprotein, and consists of 379 or 381 amino acid residues. PAI-1 is the main physiological inhibitor of uPA and has been shown to play a key role in cell migration and tissue remodeling (Durand *et al.*, 2004). In addition, PAI-1 has been found to bind to vitronectin (Vn), and this binding boosts the inhibition rates for thrombin by PAI-1 (Ehrlich *et al.*, 1990). PAI-1 has been also found to mediates apoptotic pathways (Soeda *et al.*, 2001; Horowitz *et al.*, 2008). PAI-2 has been found to repress invasion of human cancer cells *in vitro* (Laug *et al.*, 1993; Stahl & Mueller, 1994), and to inhibit pulmonary metastases of cancer cells in vivo (Mueller *et al.*, 1995). Unlike PAI-1, PAI-2 expression has been associated with good prognosis and prolonged survival in breast cancer patients (Croucher *et al.*, 2008). In addition, elevated level of PAI-1 has been correlated to poor prognosis even more than uPA itself (Grondahl-Hansen *et al.*, 1993; Foekens *et al.*, 1994; Foekens *et al.*, 2000). However, breast cancer patients with high PAI-2 levels showed a longer response to tamoxifen (Meijer-van Gelder *et al.*, 2004). Differential interaction with Vn might clarify the discrepancy between PAI-1 and PAI-2 in breast cancer prognosis. It has been found that $\alpha5\beta3$ integrin binding site on Vn overlaps with that for PAI-1, and that the active conformation of PAI-1 blocks cell migration. Formation of a complex between PAI-1 and uPA causes loss of PAI-1 affinity for Vn and recovers cell migration (Stefansson & Lawrence, 1996). Although PAI-2 inhibits uPA, it does not acquire the same capability of PAI-1 to inhibit Vn-dependant cell migration as it does not bind Vn (Mikus *et al.*, 1993).

$\alpha2AP$ as well as other plasmin inhibitors such as bovine pancreas trypsin inhibitor (BPTI) and a urinary trypsin inhibitor (UTI) have been shown to inhibit tumor invasion (Mignatti *et al.*, 1986; Tsuboi & Rifkin, 1990; Meissauer *et al.*, 1991; Crowley *et al.*, 1993; Kobayashi *et al.*, 1994; Kobayashi *et al.*, 1994; Bianchi *et al.*, 1996). Although, inhibition of uPA and internalization of uPA-uPAR complex by physiological inhibitors should decrease invasion and metastasis, high tumor levels of PAI-1 in fact promote tumor progression. However, high levels of PAI-2 decrease tumor growth and metastasis (Croucher *et al.*, 2008). The internalization of the uPA/PAI-1 is mediated by the low density lipoprotein receptor-related protein (LRP) (Herz *et al.*, 1992). While the uPA/PAI-1 complex is degraded by lysosomes, uPAR and LRP are recycled back to the cell surface to concentrate ECM degradation at the leading edges, hence smooth the progress of endothelial and cancer cell motility (Nykjaer *et al.*, 1997; Prager *et al.*, 2004).

3   Extracellular matrix and membrane proteins associated with uPAR

As uPAR does not have a trans-membrane domain and is only fixed to membranes by GPI anchor, it uses the interaction with other proteins to trigger signal transductions. The crystal structure of uPAR in complex with both uPA and Vn revealed that uPA occupies the central cavity of the uPAR, whereas Vn binds at the outer side of the receptor (Huai *et al.*, 2008). Furthermore, it has been shown that the external receptor surface of uPAR is free to bind additional proteins (Llinas *et al.*, 2005). In addition, binding of uPA to its high-affinity receptor orchestrates uPAR interactions with other cellular components that play a critical role in varied patho-physiological and physiological processes (Mondino & Blasi, 2004; Romer *et al.*, 2004). The partner proteins of uPAR include several ECM and cellular proteins such as Vn, Kininogen, $\beta1$- $\beta2$- $\beta3$-integrins and epidermal growth factor receptor (EGFR). uPA system uses interaction with intracellular and extracellular proteins to modulate various functions (Mekkawy *et al.*, 2009;

Mekkawy *et al.*, 2010). These activities include proliferation, apoptosis, adhesion, migration and invasion at cellular level. In addition, uPA system contributes to degradation of BM and ECM, metastasis, angiogenesis as well as growth processes at tumor level (Mekkawy *et al.*, 2009).

3.1 Extracellular matrix proteins associated with uPAR

3.1.1 Vitronectin

Vitronectin is an important extracellular glycoprotein with a molecular weight of 65-75 kDa (Peterson, 1998). The N-terminal segment of Vn (43 amino acid residues) consists of a somatomedin-B (SMB) domain. Following SMB, there is a cell receptor binding site characterized by an Arg-Gly-Asp (RGD) sequence. Additionally, VN has four haemopexin-like domains (anti-cipated as putative haem-binding) and three heparin-binding domains (HBD) (Singh *et al.*, 2010). VN is synthesized in liver then circulated in blood plasma in a monomeric form (Preissner & Seiffert, 1998). The Vn is altered to a multimeric form in ECM (Barnes *et al.*, 1985; Hayashi *et al.*, 1985). Vn takes part in many biological functions including cell migration, adhesion and spreading, proliferation in addition to extracellular anchoring, fibrinolysis, hemostasis and immune defense (Schvartz *et al.*, 1999). The multimeric form binds to various members of uPA system including plasminogen (Gebb *et al.*, 1986), PAI-1 (Declerck *et al.*, 1988) and uPAR (Wei *et al.*, 1994). These interactions modulate the adhesion and motility of cancer cells. It has been found that domain I of uPAR is crucial in uPAR-mediated cellular binding to Vn (Sidenius & Blasi, 2000). However, all three domains of uPAR have been shown to take part in the interaction with Vn (Kanse *et al.*, 2004). Moreover, uPA has been found to increase the affinity of uPAR for Vn by regulating uPAR oligomerization (Wei *et al.*, 1994; Sidenius *et al.*, 2002). Vn can also form a ternary complex with suPAR/uPA. Such process accumulates proteolytic activity of uPA on cell surface and ECM; hence increases uPA activity by fivefold (Chavakis *et al.*, 1998). By using this mechanism, cancer cells can accelerate cell migration and tissue modification. This molecular structure of uPAR explains the observation of how uPAR can form a ternary complex with uPA and Vn. The uPAR epitope that is responsible for its interaction with Vn has been found to consist of two exposed loops. These loops connecting the central four stranded beta-sheet in uPAR domain I as well as a proximal region of the flexible linker peptide connecting uPAR domains I and II (Gardsvoll & Ploug, 2007).

Both uPAR and Vn levels have been found to be increased in serum of breast cancer patients (Cho *et al.*, 2010; Soydinc *et al.*, 2012). Vn has been also identified as a potential marker in breast cancer patients (Kim *et al.*, 2009; Kadowaki *et al.*, 2011). The components of ECM microenvironment play a fundamental role in cancer progression. Herein, members of uPA system interact with Vn to regulate cellular migration (Kanse *et al.*, 1996; Stahl & Mueller, 1997; Waltz *et al.*, 1997) as well as to initiate signaling pathways leading to cytoskeleton reorganization, improved cell adhesion and increased cell motility (Kjoller & Hall, 2001). PAI-1 has been found to compete directly with uPAR for binding to the somatomedin-B domain on the N-terminal of Vn (Deng *et al.*, 1996; Kanse *et al.*, 1996). In addition, PAI-1 was found to inhibit cell migration by competing with integrins for binding to Vn (Stefansson & Lawrence, 1996; Kjoller *et al.*, 1997). Moreover, PAI-1 has been found to promote adhesion to ECM and motility of breast cancer MDA-MB-435 cells in vitro. This promotion may clarify the linkage between PAI-1 and tumor metastasis (Waltz *et al.*, 1997; Palmieri *et al.*, 2002).

3.1.2   Kininogen

Human plasma kininogens is a key component of the plasma kallikrein-kinin system (Colman *et al.*, 1997). Human plasma kallikreins activate cleavage of high molecular weight kininogens (HK; 120 kDa) into a nicked kininogen consisting of two disulfide-linked 62 kDa and 56 kDa chains. This followed by another cleavage that yields a stable kinin-free protein (HKa) consisting of two disulfide-linked 62 kDa and 45 kDa chains with the loss of bradykinin (Mori & Nagasawa, 1981). Cell-associated kininogen can act as a receptor for plasma pre-kallikrein (Tait & Fujikawa, 1986; Tait & Fujikawa, 1987). Pre-kallikrein bound to kininogen is then converted to activated kallikrein on endothelial cell surface (Motta *et al.*, 1998). Kallikrein may also activate pro-urokinase bound to uPAR into active uPA (Lin *et al.*, 1997). It has been shown that human HK has a pro-angiogenic effect due to release of bradykinin (Colman *et al.*, 2003). In addition, bradykinin has also the capability to stimulate the release of the tissue PA (Smith *et al.*, 1985) and the vasodilator prostacyclin (Hong, 1980) as well as induction of endothelial cells hyperpolarization (Nakashima *et al.*, 1993).

A reduction of levels of HK has been observed in the serum (Kim *et al.*, 2009) and tissue samples (Gabrijelcic *et al.*, 1992) of breast cancer patients. HKa has been shown to bind at a site within DII and DIII of uPAR which is the same to or close to that which mediates the binding of Vn (Colman *et al.*, 1997). This observation may provide an explanation for the capability of HK to inhibit cell adhesion to Vn (Asakura *et al.*, 1992) and to increase uPAR activity (Motta *et al.*, 1998). The mechanism by which HKa inhibits uPAR-dependent cellular adhesion may mimic that of PAI-1 (Colman *et al.*, 1997) and may competes with uPAR for binding to the same region of the Vn somatomedin B domain (Deng *et al.*, 1996). Later, it has been shown that kininostatin, the functional domain of HKa, is linked to uPAR in the membrane rafts, by which it applies inhibitory influence on α5β3 integrin functions. This finding represents a new mechanism by which HKa exerts its anti-angiogenic activity (Wu *et al.*, 2007).

3.2   Membrane proteins associated with uPAR

3.2.1   Integrins

Integrins is a family of cellular receptors associated with the adhesion of the cell to the surrounding ECM. Integrins are heterodimers made of non-covalently associated 19 α-integrin and 8 β-integrin subunits (Caswell *et al.*, 2009). Each subunit of integrins consists of an extracellular N-terminal (700-1200 amino acid residues), a single trans-membrane domain, and a short cytoplasmic C-terminal domain (residues 5-65) called the tail (Hynes, 1992). The assembly of integrins and other focal adhesion related proteins was defined as the "integrin adhesome". Each integrin molecule in the adhesome has a capacity to interact with 8-10 partner proteins (Zaidel-Bar *et al.*, 2007).

A number of reports indicate that integrins interact with uPAR, and this interaction mediates several functions in development and disease. uPAR has been found to be associated with β2-integrin and Src-kinases in a multimeric receptor complex in human monocytes which suggests functional cooperation (Bohuslav *et al.*, 1995). In addition, interaction between β1-integrin and uPAR has been shown to affect intracellular pathways that regulate cell adhesion (Wei *et al.*, 1996; Wei *et al.*, 1999; Wei *et al.*, 2007). Moreover, uPA-dependent cell migration was found to be correlated with uPAR interaction with α5β1 and αvβ5 integrins. Such interaction could be involved in development, angiogenesis and tumor metastasis (Yebra *et al.*, 1996; Wang *et al.*, 2005). Interference with the uPAR/β1-integrins interaction has been found to impair integrins functions (Wang *et al.*, 2005). It has been confirmed that suPAR specifically binds to α4β1, α6β1, α9β1 and αvβ3 integrins on Chinese Hamster Ovary (CHO) cells in a cation-dependent manner (Tarui *et al.*, 2001). Additionally, anti-integrin and anti-uPAR antibodies have successfully inhibited the binding of suPAR to these integrins (Tarui *et al.*, 2001). These findings suggest that uPAR is an integrin ligand besides being an integrin-partner protein (Tarui *et al.*, 2001). Integrin α3 has been identified as a molecular marker of cells undergoing epithelial–mesenchymal transition (EMT) and of cancer cells with aggressive phenotypes (Shirakihara *et al.*, 2013). In addition, several clinical reports have linked higher expression of integrins, particularly ß1-integrin subfamily, to the development and metastasis of cancer cells as well as poor prognosis in patients with breast cancer (Friedrichs *et al.*, 1995; Zutter *et al.*, 1995; Perou *et al.*, 2000; Vogetseder *et al.*, 2013). In metastatic MDA-MB-231 breast cancer cells, the adhesive and proteolytic actions are firmly associated with β1 integrin/uPAR complexes, and that complexes are involved in tumor progression in vivo (van der Pluijm *et al.*, 2001). Further, a sequence in uPAR DIII of uPAR (residues 240–248) has been found to bind α5β1 integrin, to control tumor growth (Chaurasia *et al.*, 2006), and to manage cancer cell invasion in vitro and progression in vivo (Tang *et al.*, 2008).

3.2.2   EGFR

EGFR is one of four homologous trans-membrane receptors that intermediates the responses to a family of growth factors. EGFR is a 170 kDa glycoprotein having an extracellular N-terminal containing the ligand-binding domain and a single hydrophobic trans-membrane region. EGFR also has an intracellular C-terminal domain containing tyrosine residues that intermediate EGFR signal transduction (Jorissen *et al.*, 2003). EGFR stimulation can lead to cell proliferation (Zyzak *et al.*, 1994), survival (Moro *et al.*, 1998) and migration (Frey *et al.*, 2004). Despite the fact that the expression of EGFR has been observed in all types of breast cancer, it has been found to be higher in basal and triple-negative breast cancer (Nielsen *et al.*, 2004; Hoadley *et al.*, 2007; Rakha *et al.*, 2009; Duffy *et al.*, 2012). EGFR expression has been linked to early relapse and poor prognosis in breast cancer patients (Sainsbury *et al.*, 1987; Salomon *et al.*, 1995). Thus, targeting of EGFR signaling in breast cancer has been evaluated in several studies (Masuda *et al.*, 2012).

The main signaling pathways activated by EGFR are mediated through PI3K-AKT and ERK-MAPK pathways resulting in several biologic functions (Barton *et al.*, 2010). EGFR is crucial for uPAR-mediated functions. uPAR uses EGFR to transfer the signal via ERK/MAPK signal transduction (Liu *et al.*, 2002; Jo *et al.*, 2003), and EGFR inhibitors are able to block the signal transduction generated by uPA, implicating that EGFR connects uPAR to ERK/MAPK (Jo *et al.*, 2003). Moreover, both EGFR and uPAR are co-involved in modulating tumor invasion through a mechanism involving Src and MMPs in breast cancer MCF-7 cells (Guerrero *et al.*, 2004). Furthermore, EGF was found to stimulate uPAR expression and cell invasiveness in a range of carcinoma cells (Liu *et al.*, 2002; Shiratsuchi *et al.*, 2002; Unlu & Leake, 2003). Additionally, uPA secretion and p56lck-induced cell motility are mediated by activation of EGFR/ERK pathways in both highly invasive (MDA-MB-231) and less invasive (MCF-7) breast cancer cell lines (Mahabeleshwar *et al.*, 2004). Interestingly, a significant correlation has been observed between EGFR and uPAR expression in human breast cancer tissues (Magkou *et al.*, 2008; Berg *et al.*, 2012). Moreover, independent uPAR signaling to ERK pathway has been found responsive to the EGFR tyrosine kinase inhibitors, Erlotinib and Gefitinib in breast cancer MCF-7 cells (Eastman *et al.*, 2012).

Conversely, other reports showed that uPAR is also required for EGFR-mediated functions. In two uPA-stimulated breast cancer cell lines, proliferation was totally suppressed when EGFR expression is blocked (Jo *et al.*, 2005). In addition, EGF mitogenic activity was blocked by uPAR gene silencing that interrupts uPAR-dependent cell signaling in MDA-MB-231 breast cancer cells (Jo *et al.*, 2007). Furthermore, EGF-mediated migration in ovarian cancer cells is associated with decreased internalization and increased surface expression of uPAR (Henic *et al.*, 2006). Both anti-uPAR and anti-EGFR inhibitors have been shown to inhibit cell migration in response to uPA and to EGF (Henic *et al.*, 2006). The incorporated down-regulation of uPAR together with inhibition of EGFR has been shown to induce a synergistic anti-tumor effect in vitro (Abu-Ali *et al.*, 2008). Moreover, the uPAR-deficient mouse keratinocytes failed to produce EGFR-dependent laminin-5 with interruption of cell migration (D'Alessio *et al.*, 2008).

4   Clinical relevance of uPA system in breast cancer

Owing to the association of components of uPA system to the pathogenesis of breast cancer, many of these components have been identified as prognostic factors (Grondahl-Hansen *et al.*, 1993; Rosenquist *et al.*, 1993; Janicke *et al.*, 1994; Benraad *et al.*, 1996; Manders *et al.*, 2004; Manders *et al.*, 2004; Offersen *et al.*, 2008). Here, a number of positive clinical studies will be highlighted. Pedersen et al., were the first to show the relationship between the level of uPA/PAI-1 complex and survival in breast cancer patients (Pedersen *et al.*, 2000). Levels of uPA/PAI-1 complex in tissues from 576 patients with lymph node-negative (N0) invasive breast carcinoma using Enzyme-linked immunosorbent assay (ELISA) were found to be significantly associated with poor overall survival (OS) (Manders *et al.*, 2004). Foekens *et al.* (2000) have determined the value of uPA, uPAR, PAI-1 and PAI-2 by ELISA as potential prognostic markers of relapse-free survival (RFS) and poor OS in 2780 patients with primary invasive breast cancer. The first interim analysis of a 4.5 year randomized trial Chemo-N0 (1993-1998) confirmed the reported prognostic value of uPA and PAI-1 in 556 N0 breast cancer patients by ELISA. This method identified patients at high risk of disease recurrence who could benefit from adjuvant chemotherapy (Janicke *et al.*, 2001). Harbeck *et al.* (2002) have also used ELISA to determine the prognostic value of uPA and PAI-1 levels in primary cancer tissues from 3424 breast cancer patients. They have suggested that risk of relapse as well as response to adjuvant chemotherapy and endocrine therapy can be determined using these biomarkers. Additionally, the combination of PAI-1 and uPA gave the best risk discrimination assessment in N0 breast cancer patients (n = 125; 6-year median follow-up) (Harbeck *et al.*, 1999). Later, the clinical relevance of the uPA and PAI-1 levels was confirmed using ELISA. Their levels have been found to support risk-adapted individualized therapy choice in N0 breast cancer patients (n = 269) without adjuvant systemic therapy (Harbeck *et al.*, 2002). Another pooled analysis of tumors from 8377 N0 breast cancer patients have been conducted by the European Organization for Research and Treatment of Cancer–Receptor and Biomarker Group (EORTC-RBG) using different immunoassays including ELISA, Luminometric Immuno Assay (LIA), and protein assays. The data showed that higher uPA and PAI-1 values were independently associated with poor RFS and OS in both node-positive and node-negative patients. In addition, the study verified a strong connection between high levels of uPA and PAI-1 in tumor tissue extracts and poor prognosis of N0 breast cancer patients (Look *et al.*, 2002). Additionally, a long-term follow up of more than 10 years showed uPA/PAI-1 levels to have a strong prognostic significance in 118 N0 breast cancer patients independent of HER2 status using ELISA (Zemzoum *et al.*, 2003). Later, a 7.5-year follow-up study verified the linkage between higher levels of uPA and PAI-1 to aggressiveness of invasive breast cancer. The value of PAI-1 as an independent prognostic biomarker was confirmed for the overall group of breast cancer patients as well as in the subgroup of node-positive patients (Jelisavac-Cosic *et al.*, 2011). Recently, a ten-year analysis of the prospective multicenter Chemo-N0 (1993-1998) trial used ELISA tests in extracts of fresh/frozen primary tumor tissues to evaluate the clinical efficacy of a uPA and PAI-1 biomarkers. The trial validated the ASCO-recommended biomarkers uPA and PAI-1 for risk assessment and therapy decision making in NO breast cancer patients (Harbeck *et al.*, 2013).

In 2002, the German Working Group for Gynecological Oncology (AGO) recommended uPA and PAI-1 with the highest level of evidence as new risk-group assessment factors in NO breast cancer patients (Harris *et al.*, 2007). In 2007, the American Society of Clinical Oncology (ASCO) has recommended the tumor levels of uPA and PAI-1 as markers in patients with early stage NO breast cancer. Levels of uPA and PAI-1 measured by ELISA on a minimum of 300 mg of fresh or frozen breast cancer tissue were considered as the most highly validated breast cancer biomarkers that carried the highest level of evidence for risk assessment in NO breast cancer. Immunohistochemical analysis for uPA and PAI-1 has been found to be inaccurate. Low tumor levels of uPA and PAI-1 were linked to low risk of recurrence. Consequently, minimal extra benefit may be acquired from chemotherapy (Harris *et al.*, 2007). The prognostic significance of ELISA using smaller samples has not been authenticated either (Schmitt *et al.*, 2006).

5   Future directions

Since breast cancer over-express several components of the uPA system, more recently, numerous therapies that target the uPA system are under development. This is mainly because the uPA system provides attractive sites for quenching and hence, renders the cancer cells less capable of carrying out its tumor promotion role. Using computational three dimensional chemistry, numerous molecules have been identified to serve as potential drugs for therapeutic blocking of uPA system in breast cancer cells and hence interfere with invasion, migration and adhesion (Wang *et al.*, 2011). Other therapies involving the targeting of uPAR with antagonistic recombinant human antibodies are in development (LeBeau *et al.*, 2013), whilst RNAi mediated down-regulation of uPAR has also been investigated (Li *et al.*, 2010). Additionally, a number of recombinant toxins were capable of specifically targeting uPA-expressing tumor cells including non–small cell lung cancer, pancreatic cancer, acute myeloid leukemia, and basal-like breast cancer (Abi-Habib *et al.*, 2004; Abi-Habib *et al.*, 2006). The progress in the field of targeted therapy such as development of bi-specific targeted therapy for both EGFR and uPAR in head and neck cancers (Waldron *et al.*, 2012) will most probably pave towards the development of further therapies for breast cancer. There are also some need therapeutic agents that are currently in clinical development. For example, Upamostat (Mesupron®; the amidoxime-prodrug of the active metabolite WX-UK1) is currently in clinical trial as an anti-metastatic and non-cytotoxic agent for the treatment of pancreatic and breast cancer (Froriep *et al.*, 2013; Heinemann *et al.*, 2013).

Finally, the measurement of the biomarkers uPA and PAI-1 using ELISA on a of 300mg of fresh or frozen tumor tissue has been validated and recommended for therapy assessment in NO breast cancer patients. In addition, targeting the uPA system will eventually open up new roads for the successful treatment of breast cancer. This would enable patients to receive more effective therapies; and clinicians would also be able to treat patients more effectively, culminating in mutual benefit between the patient and the clinician. Like most targeted therapies, it is premature to arrive at any definitive conclusion on the success of such therapies as experience tells that targeted therapies for cancer, although hypothetically provide a successful path, in reality does not offer a complete cure since tumor cells often develop resistance to such therapies.

References

Abi-Habib, R. J., Liu, S., Bugge, T. H., Leppla, S. H. & Frankel, A. E. (2004). A urokinase-activated recombinant diphtheria toxin targeting the granulocyte-macrophage colony-stimulating factor receptor is selectively cytotoxic to human acute myeloid leukemia blasts. Blood 104(7): 2143-2148.

Abi-Habib, R. J., Singh, R., Liu, S., Bugge, T. H., Leppla, S. H. & Frankel, A. E. (2006). A urokinase-activated recombinant anthrax toxin is selectively cytotoxic to many human tumor cell types. Mol Cancer Ther 5(10): 2556-2562.

Abu-Ali, S., Fotovati, A. & Shirasuna, K. (2008). Tyrosine-kinase inhibition results in EGFR clustering at focal adhesions and consequent exocytosis in uPAR down-regulated cells of head and neck cancers. Mol Cancer 7: 47.

Anderson, B. O., Yip, C. H., Ramsey, S. D., Bengoa, R., Braun, S., Fitch, M., Groot, M., Sancho-Garnier, H., Tsu, V. D., Global Summit Health Care, S. & Public Policy, P. (2006). Breast cancer in limited-resource countries: health care systems and public policy. Breast J 12 Suppl 1: S54-69.

Andolfo, A., English, W. R., Resnati, M., Murphy, G., Blasi, F. & Sidenius, N. (2002). Metalloproteases cleave the urokinase-type plasminogen activator receptor in the D1-D2 linker region and expose epitopes not present in the intact soluble receptor. Thromb Haemost 88(2): 298-306.

Andreasen, P. A., Egelund, R. & Petersen, H. H. (2000). The plasminogen activation system in tumor growth, invasion, and metastasis. Cell Mol Life Sci 57(1): 25-40.

Asakura, S., Hurley, R. W., Skorstengaard, K., Ohkubo, I. & Mosher, D. F. (1992). Inhibition of cell adhesion by high molecular weight kininogen. J Cell Biol 116(2): 465-476.

Barnes, D. W., Reing, J. E. & Amos, B. (1985). Heparin-binding properties of human serum spreading factor. J Biol Chem 260(16): 9117-9122.

Barton, S., Starling, N. & Swanton, C. (2010). Predictive molecular markers of response to epidermal growth factor receptor(EGFR) family-targeted therapies. Curr Cancer Drug Targets 10(8): 799-812.

Beaufort, N., Leduc, D., Rousselle, J. C., Magdolen, V., Luther, T., Namane, A., Chignard, M. & Pidard, D. (2004). Proteolytic regulation of the urokinase receptor/CD87 on monocytic cells by neutrophil elastase and cathepsin G. J Immunol 172(1): 540-549.

Beaufort, N., Leduc, D., Rousselle, J. C., Namane, A., Chignard, M. & Pidard, D. (2004). Plasmin cleaves the juxtamembrane domain and releases truncated species of the urokinase receptor (CD87) from human bronchial epithelial cells. FEBS Lett 574(1-3): 89-94.

Behrendt, N., Ploug, M., Patthy, L., Houen, G., Blasi, F. & Dano, K. (1991). The ligand-binding domain of the cell surface receptor for urokinase-type plasminogen activator. J Biol Chem 266(12): 7842-7847.

Behrendt, N., Ronne, E. & Dano, K. (1996). Domain interplay in the urokinase receptor. Requirement for the third domain in high affinity ligand binding and demonstration of ligand contact sites in distinct receptor domains. J Biol Chem 271(37): 22885-22894.

Behzadian, M. A., Windsor, L. J., Ghaly, N., Liou, G., Tsai, N. T. & Caldwell, R. B. (2003). VEGF-induced paracellular permeability in cultured endothelial cells involves urokinase and its receptor. FASEB J 17(6): 752-754.

Benraad, T. J., Geurts-Moespot, J., Grondahl-Hansen, J., Schmitt, M., Heuvel, J. J., de Witte, J. H., Foekens, J. A., Leake, R. E., Brunner, N. & Sweep, C. G. (1996). Immunoassays (ELISA) of urokinase-type plasminogen activator (uPA): report of an EORTC/BIOMED-1 workshop. Eur J Cancer 32A(8): 1371-1381.

Berg, D., Wolff, C., Malinowsky, K., Tran, K., Walch, A., Bronger, H., Schuster, T., Hofler, H. & Becker, K. F. (2012). Profiling signalling pathways in formalin-fixed and paraffin-embedded breast cancer tissues reveals cross-talk between EGFR, HER2, HER3 and uPAR. J Cell Physiol 227(1): 204-212.

Bergmann, S., Rohde, M., Preissner, K. T. & Hammerschmidt, S. (2005). The nine residue plasminogen-binding motif of the pneumococcal enolase is the major cofactor of plasmin-mediated degradation of extracellular matrix, dissolution of fibrin and transmigration. Thromb Haemost 94(2): 304-311.

Bianchi, E., Ferrero, E., Fazioli, F., Mangili, F., Wang, J., Bender, J. R., Blasi, F. & Pardi, R. (1996). Integrin-dependent induction of functional urokinase receptors in primary T lymphocytes. J Clin Invest 98(5): 1133-1141.

Bohuslav, J., Horejsi, V., Hansmann, C., Stockl, J., Weidle, U. H., Majdic, O., Bartke, I., Knapp, W. & Stockinger, H. (1995). Urokinase plasminogen activator receptor, beta 2-integrins, and Src-kinases within a single receptor complex of human monocytes. J Exp Med 181(4): 1381-1390.

Carrell, R. W. & Boswell, D. R. (1986). Serpins: the superfamily of plasma serine proteinase inhibitors. Proteinase inhibitors. S. Barrett, Elsevier Science: 403-420.

Castellino, F. J. & Ploplis, V. A. (2005). Structure and function of the plasminogen/plasmin system. Thromb Haemost 93(4): 647-654.

Caswell, P. T., Vadrevu, S. & Norman, J. C. (2009). Integrins: masters and slaves of endocytic transport. Nat Rev Mol Cell Biol 10(12): 843-853.

Chaurasia, P., Aguirre-Ghiso, J. A., Liang, O. D., Gardsvoll, H., Ploug, M. & Ossowski, L. (2006). A region in urokinase plasminogen receptor domain III controlling a functional association with alpha5beta1 integrin and tumor growth. J Biol Chem 281(21): 14852-14863.

Chavakis, T., Kanse, S. M., Yutzy, B., Lijnen, H. R. & Preissner, K. T. (1998). Vitronectin concentrates proteolytic activity on the cell surface and extracellular matrix by trapping soluble urokinase receptor-urokinase complexes. Blood 91(7): 2305-2312.

Cho, W., Jung, K. & Regnier, F. E. (2010). Sialylated Lewis x antigen bearing glycoproteins in human plasma. J Proteome Res 9(11): 5960-5968.

Collen, D. (2001). Ham-Wasserman lecture: role of the plasminogen system in fibrin-homeostasis and tissue remodeling. Hematology Am Soc Hematol Educ Program: 1-9.

Collen, D. & Lijnen, H. R. (1991). Basic and clinical aspects of fibrinolysis and thrombolysis. Blood 78(12): 3114-3124.

Colman, R. W., Pixley, R. A., Najamunnisa, S., Yan, W., Wang, J., Mazar, A. & McCrae, K. R. (1997). Binding of high molecular weight kininogen to human endothelial cells is mediated via a site within domains 2 and 3 of the urokinase receptor. J Clin Invest 100(6): 1481-1487.

Colman, R. W., Pixley, R. A., Sainz, I. M., Song, J. S., Isordia-Salas, I., Muhamed, S. N., Powell, J. A., Jr. & Mousa, S. A. (2003). Inhibition of angiogenesis by antibody blocking the action of proangiogenic high-molecular-weight kininogen. J Thromb Haemost 1(1): 164-170.

Croucher, D. R., Saunders, D. N., Lobov, S. & Ranson, M. (2008). Revisiting the biological roles of PAI2 (SERPINB2) in cancer. Nat Rev Cancer 8(7): 535-545.

Crowley, C. W., Cohen, R. L., Lucas, B. K., Liu, G., Shuman, M. A. & Levinson, A. D. (1993). Prevention of metastasis by inhibition of the urokinase receptor. Proc Natl Acad Sci U S A 90(11): 5021-5025.

Cunningham, O., Andolfo, A., Santovito, M. L., Iuzzolino, L., Blasi, F. & Sidenius, N. (2003). Dimerization controls the lipid raft partitioning of uPAR/CD87 and regulates its biological functions. EMBO J 22(22): 5994-6003.

D'Alessio, S., Gerasi, L. & Blasi, F. (2008). uPAR-deficient mouse keratinocytes fail to produce EGFR-dependent laminin-5, affecting migration in vivo and in vitro. J Cell Sci 121(Pt 23): 3922-3932.

Declerck, P. J., Demol, M., Alessi, M. C., Baudner, S., Paques, E. P., Preissner, K. T., Mullerberghaus, G. & Collen, D. (1988). Purification and Characterization of a Plasminogen-Activator Inhibitor-1 Binding-Protein from Human-Plasma - Identification as a Multimeric Form of S-Protein (Vitronectin). J Biol Chem 263(30): 15454-15461.

del Zoppo, G. J. (2010). Plasminogen activators in ischemic stroke: introduction. Stroke 41(10 Suppl): S39-41.

Deng, G., Curriden, S. A., Wang, S., Rosenberg, S. & Loskutoff, D. J. (1996). Is plasminogen activator inhibitor-1 the molecular switch that governs urokinase receptor-mediated cell adhesion and release? J Cell Biol 134(6): 1563-1571.

Deng, G., Royle, G., Wang, S., Crain, K. & Loskutoff, D. J. (1996). Structural and functional analysis of the plasminogen activator inhibitor-1 binding motif in the somatomedin B domain of vitronectin. J Biol Chem 271(22): 12716-12723.

Duffy, M. J., McGowan, P. M. & Crown, J. (2012). Targeted therapy for triple-negative breast cancer: where are we? Int J Cancer 131(11): 2471-2477.

Durand, M. K., Bodker, J. S., Christensen, A., Dupont, D. M., Hansen, M., Jensen, J. K., Kjelgaard, S., Mathiasen, L., Pedersen, K. E., Skeldal, S., Wind, T. & Andreasen, P. A. (2004). Plasminogen activator inhibitor-I and tumour growth, invasion, and metastasis. Thromb Haemost 91(3): 438-449.

Eastman, B. M., Jo, M., Webb, D. L., Takimoto, S. & Gonias, S. L. (2012). A transformation in the mechanism by which the urokinase receptor signals provides a selection advantage for estrogen receptor-expressing breast cancer cells in the absence of estrogen. Cell Signal 24(9): 1847-1855.

Ehrlich, H. J., Gebbink, R. K., Keijer, J., Linders, M., Preissner, K. T. & Pannekoek, H. (1990). Alteration of serpin specificity by a protein cofactor. Vitronectin endows plasminogen activator inhibitor 1 with thrombin inhibitory properties. J Biol Chem 265(22): 13029-13035.

Foekens, J. A., Peters, H. A., Look, M. P., Portengen, H., Schmitt, M., Kramer, M. D., Brunner, N., Janicke, F., Meijer-van Gelder, M. E., Henzen-Logmans, S. C., van Putten, W. L. & Klijn, J. G. (2000). The urokinase system of plasminogen activation and prognosis in 2780 breast cancer patients. Cancer Res 60(3): 636-643.

Foekens, J. A., Schmitt, M., van Putten, W. L., Peters, H. A., Kramer, M. D., Janicke, F. & Klijn, J. G. (1994). Plasminogen activator inhibitor-1 and prognosis in primary breast cancer. J Clin Oncol 12(8): 1648-1658.

Frey, M. R., Golovin, A. & Polk, D. B. (2004). Epidermal growth factor-stimulated intestinal epithelial cell migration requires Src family kinase-dependent p38 MAPK signaling. J Biol Chem 279(43): 44513-44521.

Friedrichs, K., Ruiz, P., Franke, F., Gille, I., Terpe, H. J. & Imhof, B. A. (1995). High Expression Level of Alpha-6 Integrin in Human Breast-Carcinoma Is Correlated with Reduced Survival. Cancer Res 55(4): 901-906.

Froriep, D., Clement, B., Bittner, F., Mendel, R. R., Reichmann, D., Schmalix, W. & Havemeyer, A. (2013). Activation of the anti-cancer agent upamostat by the mARC enzyme system. Xenobiotica 43(9): 780-784.

Fukao, H., Ueshima, S., Okada, K. & Matsuo, O. (1997). The role of the pericellular fibrinolytic system in angiogenesis. Jpn J Physiol 47(2): 161-171.

Gabrijelcic, D., Svetic, B., Spaic, D., Skrk, J., Budihna, J. & Turk, V. (1992). Determination of cathepsins B, H, L and kininogen in breast cancer patients. Agents Actions Suppl 38 (Pt 2): 350-357.

Gardsvoll, H., Dano, K. & Ploug, M. (1999). Mapping part of the functional epitope for ligand binding on the receptor for urokinase-type plasminogen activator by site-directed mutagenesis. J Biol Chem 274(53): 37995-38003.

Gardsvoll, H. & Ploug, M. (2007). Mapping of the vitronectin-binding site on the urokinase receptor: involvement of a coherent receptor interface consisting of residues from both domain I and the flanking interdomain linker region. J Biol Chem 282(18): 13561-13572.

Gebb, C., Hayman, E. G., Engvall, E. & Ruoslahti, E. (1986). Interaction of vitronectin with collagen. J Biol Chem 261(35): 16698-16703.

Gondi, C. S., Kandhukuri, N., Dinh, D. H., Gujrati, M. & Rao, J. S. (2007). Down-regulation of uPAR and uPA activates caspase-mediated apoptosis and inhibits the PI3K/AKT pathway. Int J Oncol 31(1): 19-27.

Grondahl-Hansen, J., Christensen, I. J., Rosenquist, C., Brunner, N., Mouridsen, H. T., Dano, K. & Blichert-Toft, M. (1993). High levels of urokinase-type plasminogen activator and its inhibitor PAI-1 in cytosolic extracts of breast carcinomas are associated with poor prognosis. Cancer Res 53(11): 2513-2521.

Guerrero, J., Santibanez, J. F., Gonzalez, A. & Martinez, J. (2004). EGF receptor transactivation by urokinase receptor stimulus through a mechanism involving Src and matrix metalloproteinases. Exp Cell Res 292(1): 201-208.

Harbeck, N., Dettmar, P., Thomssen, C., Berger, U., Ulm, K., Kates, R., Hofler, H., Janicke, F., Graeff, H. & Schmitt, M. (1999). Risk-group discrimination in node-negative breast cancer using invasion and proliferation markers: 6-year median follow-up. Br J Cancer 80(3-4): 419-426.

Harbeck, N., Kates, R. E., Look, M. P., Meijer-Van Gelder, M. E., Klijn, J. G., Kruger, A., Kiechle, M., Janicke, F., Schmitt, M. & Foekens, J. A. (2002). Enhanced benefit from adjuvant chemotherapy in breast cancer patients classified high-risk according to urokinase-type plasminogen activator (uPA) and plasminogen activator inhibitor type 1 (n = 3424). Cancer Res 62(16): 4617-4622.

Harbeck, N., Kates, R. E. & Schmitt, M. (2002). Clinical relevance of invasion factors urokinase-type plasminogen activator and plasminogen activator inhibitor type 1 for individualized therapy decisions in primary breast cancer is greatest when used in combination. J Clin Oncol 20(4): 1000-1007.

Harbeck, N., Schmitt, M., Meisner, C., Friedel, C., Untch, M., Schmid, M., Sweep, C. G., Lisboa, B. W., Lux, M. P., Beck, T., Hasmuller, S., Kiechle, M., Janicke, F. & Thomssen, C. (2013). Ten-year analysis of the prospective multicentre Chemo-N0 trial validates American Society of Clinical Oncology (ASCO)-recommended biomarkers uPA and PAI-1 for therapy decision making in node-negative breast cancer patients. Eur J Cancer.

Harris, L., Fritsche, H., Mennel, R., Norton, L., Ravdin, P., Taube, S., Somerfield, M. R., Hayes, D. F. & Bast, R. C., Jr. (2007). American Society of Clinical Oncology 2007 update of recommendations for the use of tumor markers in breast cancer. J Clin Oncol 25(33): 5287-5312.

Hayashi, M., Akama, T., Kono, I. & Kashiwagi, H. (1985). Activation of vitronectin (serum spreading factor) binding of heparin by denaturing agents. J Biochem 98(4): 1135-1138.

Heinemann, V., Ebert, M. P., Laubender, R. P., Bevan, P., Mala, C. & Boeck, S. (2013). Phase II randomised proof-of-concept study of the urokinase inhibitor upamostat (WX-671) in combination with gemcitabine compared with gemcitabine alone in patients with non-resectable, locally advanced pancreatic cancer. Br J Cancer 108(4): 766-770.

Henic, E., Sixt, M., Hansson, S., Hoyer-Hansen, G. & Casslen, B. (2006). EGF-stimulated migration in ovarian cancer cells is associated with decreased internalization, increased surface expression, and increased shedding of the urokinase plasminogen activator receptor. Gynecol Oncol 101(1): 28-39.

Herz, J., Clouthier, D. E. & Hammer, R. E. (1992). Ldl Receptor-Related Protein Internalizes and Degrades Upa-Pai-1 Complexes and Is Essential for Embryo Implantation. Cell 71(3): 411-421.

Hoadley, K. A., Weigman, V. J., Fan, C., Sawyer, L. R., He, X., Troester, M. A., Sartor, C. I., Rieger-House, T., Bernard, P. S., Carey, L. A. & Perou, C. M. (2007). EGFR associated expression profiles vary with breast tumor subtype. BMC Genomics 8: 258.

Hong, S. L. (1980). Effect of bradykinin and thrombin on prostacyclin synthesis in endothelial cells from calf and pig aorta and human umbilical cord vein. Thromb Res 18(6): 787-795.

Horowitz, J. C., Rogers, D. S., Simon, R. H., Sisson, T. H. & Thannickal, V. J. (2008). Plasminogen activation induced pericellular fibronectin proteolysis promotes fibroblast apoptosis. Am J Respir Cell Mol Biol 38(1): 78-87.

Huai, Q., Zhou, A., Lin, L., Mazar, A. P., Parry, G. C., Callahan, J., Shaw, D. E., Furie, B., Furie, B. C. & Huang, M. (2008). Crystal structures of two human vitronectin, urokinase and urokinase receptor complexes. Nat Struct Mol Biol 15(4): 422-423.

Huber, R. & Carrell, R. W. (1989). Implications of the three-dimensional structure of alpha 1-antitrypsin for structure and function of serpins. Biochemistry 28(23): 8951-8966.

Hynes, R. O. (1992). Integrins: versatility, modulation, and signaling in cell adhesion. Cell 69(1): 11-25.

Janicke, F., Pache, L., Schmitt, M., Ulm, K., Thomssen, C., Prechtl, A. & Graeff, H. (1994). Both the cytosols and detergent extracts of breast cancer tissues are suited to evaluate the prognostic impact of the urokinase-type plasminogen activator and its inhibitor, plasminogen activator inhibitor type 1. Cancer Res 54(10): 2527-2530.

Janicke, F., Prechtl, A., Thomssen, C., Harbeck, N., Meisner, C., Untch, M., Sweep, C. G., Selbmann, H. K., Graeff, H., Schmitt, M. & German, N. S. G. (2001). Randomized adjuvant chemotherapy trial in high-risk, lymph node-negative breast cancer patients identified by urokinase-type plasminogen activator and plasminogen activator inhibitor type 1. J Natl Cancer Inst 93(12): 913-920.

Jelisavac-Cosic, S., Sirotkovic-Skerlev, M., Kulic, A., Jakic-Razumovic, J., Kovac, Z. & Vrbanec, D. (2011). Prognostic significance of urokinase-type plasminogen activator (uPA) and plasminogen activator inhibitor (PAI-1) in patients with primary invasive ductal breast carcinoma - a 7.5-year follow-up study. Tumori 97(4): 532-539.

Jemal, A., Bray, F., Center, M. M., Ferlay, J., Ward, E. & Forman, D. (2011). Global cancer statistics. CA Cancer J Clin 61(2): 69-90.

Jo, M., Thomas, K. S., Marozkina, N., Amin, T. J., Silva, C. M., Parsons, S. J. & Gonias, S. L. (2005). Dynamic assembly of the urokinase-type plasminogen activator signaling receptor complex determines the mitogenic activity of urokinase-type plasminogen activator. J Biol Chem 280(17): 17449-17457.

Jo, M., Thomas, K. S., O'Donnell, D. M. & Gonias, S. L. (2003). Epidermal growth factor receptor-dependent and -independent cell-signaling pathways originating from the urokinase receptor. J Biol Chem 278(3): 1642-1646.

Jo, M., Thomas, K. S., Takimoto, S., Gaultier, A., Hsieh, E. H., Lester, R. D. & Gonias, S. L. (2007). Urokinase receptor primes cells to proliferate in response to epidermal growth factor. Oncogene 26(18): 2585-2594.

Jorissen, R. N., Walker, F., Pouliot, N., Garrett, T. P. J., Ward, C. W. & Burgess, A. W. (2003). Epidermal growth factor receptor: mechanisms of activation and signalling. Exp Cell Res 284(1): 31-53.

Kadowaki, M., Sangai, T., Nagashima, T., Sakakibara, M., Yoshitomi, H., Takano, S., Sogawa, K., Umemura, H., Fushimi, K., Nakatani, Y., Nomura, F. & Miyazaki, M. (2011). Identification of vitronectin as a novel serum marker for early breast cancer detection using a new proteomic approach. J Cancer Res Clin Oncol 137(7): 1105-1115.

Kanse, S. M., Chavakis, T., Kuo, A., Bdeir, K., Cines, D. B. & Preissner, K. T. (2004). Variability in the expression of urokinase receptor (CD87) mutants on cells: relevance to cell adhesion. Cell Biochem Funct 22(4): 257-264.

Kanse, S. M., Kost, C., Wilhelm, O. G., Andreasen, P. A. & Preissner, K. T. (1996). The urokinase receptor is a major vitronectin-binding protein on endothelial cells. Exp Cell Res 224(2): 344-353.

Kim, B. K., Lee, J. W., Park, P. J., Shin, Y. S., Lee, W. Y., Lee, K. A., Ye, S., Hyun, H., Kang, K. N., Yeo, D., Kim, Y., Ohn, S. Y., Noh, D. Y. & Kim, C. W. (2009). The multiplex bead array approach to identifying serum biomarkers associated with breast cancer. Breast Cancer Res 11(2): R22.

Kjoller, L. & Hall, A. (2001). Rac mediates cytoskeletal rearrangements and increased cell motility induced by urokinase-type plasminogen activator receptor binding to vitronectin. J Cell Biol 152(6): 1145-1157.

Kjoller, L., Kanse, S. M., Kirkegaard, T., Rodenburg, K. W., Ronne, E., Goodman, S. L., Preissner, K. T., Ossowski, L. & Andreasen, P. A. (1997). Plasminogen activator inhibitor-1 represses integrin- and vitronectin-mediated cell migration independently of its function as an inhibitor of plasminogen activation. Exp Cell Res 232(2): 420-429.

Kobayashi, H., Fujie, M., Shinohara, H., Ohi, H., Sugimura, M. & Terao, T. (1994). Effects of urinary trypsin inhibitor on the invasion of reconstituted basement membranes by ovarian cancer cells. Int J Cancer 57(3): 378-384.

Kobayashi, H., Shinohara, H., Ohi, H., Sugimura, M., Terao, T. & Fujie, M. (1994). Urinary trypsin inhibitor (UTI) and fragments derived from UTI by limited proteolysis efficiently inhibit tumor cell invasion. Clin Exp Metastasis 12(2): 117-128.

Laskowski, M., Jr. & Kato, I. (1980). Protein inhibitors of proteinases. Annu Rev Biochem 49: 593-626.

Laug, W. E., Cao, X. R., Yu, Y. B., Shimada, H. & Kruithof, E. K. (1993). Inhibition of invasion of HT1080 sarcoma cells expressing recombinant plasminogen activator inhibitor 2. Cancer Res 53(24): 6051-6057.

LeBeau, A. M., Duriseti, S., Murphy, S. T., Pepin, F., Hann, B., Gray, J. W., VanBrocklin, H. F. & Craik, C. S. (2013). Targeting uPAR with antagonistic recombinant human antibodies in aggressive breast cancer. Cancer Res 73(7): 2070-2081.

Li, C., Cao, S., Liu, Z., Ye, X., Chen, L. & Meng, S. (2010). RNAi-mediated downregulation of uPAR synergizes with targeting of HER2 through the ERK pathway in breast cancer cells. Int J Cancer 127(7): 1507-1516.

Liang, O. D., Bdeir, K., Matz, R. L., Chavakis, T. & Preissner, K. T. (2003). Intermolecular contact regions in urokinase plasminogen activator receptor. J Biochem 134(5): 661-666.

Lijnen, H. R. (2001). Elements of the fibrinolytic system. Ann N Y Acad Sci 936: 226-236.

Lin, Y., Harris, R. B., Yan, W., McCrae, K. R., Zhang, H. & Colman, R. W. (1997). High molecular weight kininogen peptides inhibit the formation of kallikrein on endothelial cell surfaces and subsequent urokinase-dependent plasmin formation. Blood 90(2): 690-697.

Liu, D., Aguirre Ghiso, J., Estrada, Y. & Ossowski, L. (2002). EGFR is a transducer of the urokinase receptor initiated signal that is required for in vivo growth of a human carcinoma. Cancer Cell 1(5): 445-457.

Llinas, P., Le Du, M. H., Gardsvoll, H., Dano, K., Ploug, M., Gilquin, B., Stura, E. A. & Menez, A. (2005). Crystal structure of the human urokinase plasminogen activator receptor bound to an antagonist peptide. EMBO J 24(9): 1655-1663.

Lomholt, A. F., Hoyer-Hansen, G., Nielsen, H. J. & Christensen, I. J. (2009). Intact and cleaved forms of the urokinase receptor enhance discrimination of cancer from non-malignant conditions in patients presenting with symptoms related to colorectal cancer. Br J Cancer 101(6): 992-997.

Look, M. P., van Putten, W. L., Duffy, M. J., Harbeck, N., Christensen, I. J., Thomssen, C., Kates, R., Spyratos, F., Ferno, M., Eppenberger-Castori, S., Sweep, C. G., Ulm, K., Peyrat, J. P., Martin, P. M., Magdelenat, H., Brunner, N., Duggan, C., Lisboa, B. W., Bendahl, P. O., Quillien, V., Daver, A., Ricolleau, G., Meijer-van Gelder, M. E., Manders, P., Fiets, W. E., Blankenstein, M. A., Broet, P., Romain, S., Daxenbichler, G., Windbichler, G., Cufer, T., Borstnar, S., Kueng, W., Beex, L. V., Klijn, J. G., O'Higgins, N., Eppenberger, U., Janicke, F., Schmitt, M. & Foekens, J. A. (2002). Pooled analysis of prognostic impact of urokinase-type plasminogen activator and its inhibitor PAI-1 in 8377 breast cancer patients. J Natl Cancer Inst 94(2): 116-128.

Magkou, C., Nakopoulou, L., Zoubouli, C., Karali, K., Theohari, I., Bakarakos, P. & Giannopoulou, I. (2008). Expression of the epidermal growth factor receptor (EGFR) and the phosphorylated EGFR in invasive breast carcinomas. Breast Cancer Res 10(3): R49.

Mahabeleshwar, G. H., Das, R. & Kundu, G. C. (2004). Tyrosine kinase, p56lck-induced cell motility, and urokinase-type plasminogen activator secretion involve activation of epidermal growth factor receptor/extracellular signal regulated kinase pathways. J Biol Chem 279(11): 9733-9742.

Manders, P., Tjan-Heijnen, V. C., Span, P. N., Grebenchtchikov, N., Foekens, J. A., Beex, L. V. & Sweep, C. G. (2004). Predictive impact of urokinase-type plasminogen activator: plasminogen activator inhibitor type-1 complex on the efficacy of adjuvant systemic therapy in primary breast cancer. Cancer Res 64(2): 659-664.

Manders, P., Tjan-Heijnen, V. C., Span, P. N., Grebenchtchikov, N., Geurts-Moespot, A., van Tienoven, D. T., Beex, L. V. & Sweep, F. C. (2004). Complex of urokinase-type plasminogen activator with its type 1 inhibitor predicts poor outcome in 576 patients with lymph node-negative breast carcinoma. Cancer 101(3): 486-494.

Manders, P., Tjan-Heijnen, V. C., Span, P. N., Grebenchtchikov, N., Geurts-Moespot, A. J., van Tienoven, D. T., Beex, L. V. & Sweep, F. C. (2004). The complex between urokinase-type plasminogen activator (uPA) and its type-1 inhibitor (PAI-I) independently predicts response to first-line endocrine therapy in advanced breast cancer. Thromb Haemost 91(3): 514-521.

Masuda, H., Zhang, D., Bartholomeusz, C., Doihara, H., Hortobagyi, G. N. & Ueno, N. T. (2012). Role of epidermal growth factor receptor in breast cancer. Breast Cancer Res Treat 136(2): 331-345.

Meijer-van Gelder, M. E., Look, M. P., Peters, H. A., Schmitt, M., Brunner, N., Harbeck, N., Klijn, J. G. & Foekens, J. A. (2004). Urokinase-type plasminogen activator system in breast cancer: association with tamoxifen therapy in recurrent disease. Cancer Res 64(13): 4563-4568.

Meissauer, A., Kramer, M. D., Hofmann, M., Erkell, L. J., Jacob, E., Schirrmacher, V. & Brunner, G. (1991). Urokinase-type and tissue-type plasminogen activators are essential for in vitro invasion of human melanoma cells. Exp Cell Res 192(2): 453-459.

Mekkawy, A. H., De Bock, C. E., Lin, Z., Morris, D. L., Wang, Y. & Pourgholami, M. H. (2010). Novel protein interactors of urokinase-type plasminogen activator receptor. Biochem Biophys Res Commun 399(4): 738-743.

Mekkawy, A. H., Morris, D. L. & Pourgholami, M. H. (2009). Urokinase plasminogen activator system as a potential target for cancer therapy. Future Oncol 5(9): 1487-1499.

Mignatti, P., Robbins, E. & Rifkin, D. B. (1986). Tumor Invasion through the Human Amniotic Membrane - Requirement for a Proteinase Cascade. Cell 47(4): 487-498.

Mikus, P., Urano, T., Liljestrom, P. & Ny, T. (1993). Plasminogen-activator inhibitor type 2 (PAI-2) is a spontaneously polymerising SERPIN. Biochemical characterisation of the recombinant intracellular and extracellular forms. Eur J Biochem 218(3): 1071-1082.

Mondino, A. & Blasi, F. (2004). uPA and uPAR in fibrinolysis, immunity and pathology. Trends Immunol 25(8): 450-455.

Montuori, N., Rossi, G. & Ragno, P. (1999). Cleavage of urokinase receptor regulates its interaction with integrins in thyroid cells. FEBS Lett 460(1): 32-36.

Montuori, N., Visconte, V., Rossi, G. & Ragno, P. (2005). Soluble and cleaved forms of the urokinase-receptor: degradation products or active molecules? Thromb Haemost 93(2): 192-198.

Mori, K. & Nagasawa, S. (1981). Studies on human high molecular weight (HMW) kininogen. II. Structural change of HMW kininogen by the action of human plasma kallikrein. J Biochem 89(5): 1465-1473.

Moro, L., Venturino, M., Bozzo, C., Silengo, L., Altruda, F., Beguinot, L., Tarone, G. & Defilippi, P. (1998). Integrins induce activation of EGF receptor: role in MAP kinase induction and adhesion-dependent cell survival. EMBO J 17(22): 6622-6632.

Motta, G., Rojkjaer, R., Hasan, A. A., Cines, D. B. & Schmaier, A. H. (1998). High molecular weight kininogen regulates prekallikrein assembly and activation on endothelial cells: a novel mechanism for contact activation. Blood 91(2): 516-528.

Mueller, B. M., Yu, Y. B. & Laug, W. E. (1995). Overexpression of plasminogen activator inhibitor 2 in human melanoma cells inhibits spontaneous metastasis in scid/scid mice. Proc Natl Acad Sci U S A 92(1): 205-209.

Nakashima, M., Mombouli, J. V., Taylor, A. A. & Vanhoutte, P. M. (1993). Endothelium-dependent hyperpolarization caused by bradykinin in human coronary arteries. J Clin Invest 92(6): 2867-2871.

Nielsen, T. O., Hsu, F. D., Jensen, K., Cheang, M., Karaca, G., Hu, Z., Hernandez-Boussard, T., Livasy, C., Cowan, D., Dressler, L., Akslen, L. A., Ragaz, J., Gown, A. M., Gilks, C. B., van de Rijn, M. & Perou, C. M. (2004). Immunohistochemical and clinical characterization of the basal-like subtype of invasive breast carcinoma. Clin Cancer Res 10(16): 5367-5374.

Nykjaer, A., Conese, M., Christensen, E. I., Olson, D., Cremona, O., Gliemann, J. & Blasi, F. (1997). Recycling of the urokinase receptor upon internalization of the uPA:serpin complexes. EMBO J 16(10): 2610-2620.

Offersen, B. V., Alsner, J., Ege Olsen, K., Riisbro, R., Brunner, N., Sorensen, F. B., Sorensen, B. S., Schlemmer, B. O. & Overgaard, J. (2008). A comparison among HER2, TP53, PAI-1, angiogenesis, and proliferation activity as prognostic variables in tumours from 408 patients diagnosed with early breast cancer. Acta Oncol 47(4): 618-632.

Palmieri, D., Lee, J. W., Juliano, R. L. & Church, F. C. (2002). Plasminogen activator inhibitor-1 and -3 increase cell adhesion and motility of MDA-MB-435 breast cancer cells. J Biol Chem 277(43): 40950-40957.

Pedersen, A. N., Christensen, I. J., Stephens, R. W., Briand, P., Mouridsen, H. T., Dano, K. & Brunner, N. (2000). The complex between urokinase and its type-1 inhibitor in primary breast cancer: relation to survival. Cancer Res 60(24): 6927-6934.

Perou, C. M., Sorlie, T., Eisen, M. B., van de Rijn, M., Jeffrey, S. S., Rees, C. A., Pollack, J. R., Ross, D. T., Johnsen, H., Akslen, L. A., Fluge, O., Pergamenschikov, A., Williams, C., Zhu, S. X., Lonning, P. E., Borresen-Dale, A. L., Brown, P. O. & Botstein, D. (2000). Molecular portraits of human breast tumours. Nature 406(6797): 747-752.

Petersen, L. C., Lund, L. R., Nielsen, L. S., Dano, K. & Skriver, L. (1988). One-chain urokinase-type plasminogen activator from human sarcoma cells is a proenzyme with little or no intrinsic activity. J Biol Chem 263(23): 11189-11195.

Peterson, C. B. (1998). Binding sites on native and multimeric vitronectin exhibit similar affinity for heparin the influence of self-association and multivalence on ligand binding. Trends Cardiovasc Med 8(3): 124-131.

Ploug, M. (1998). Identification of specific sites involved in ligand binding by photoaffinity labeling of the receptor for the urokinase-type plasminogen activator. Residues located at equivalent positions in uPAR domains I and III participate in the assembly of a composite ligand-binding site. Biochemistry 37(47): 16494-16505.

Ploug, M. (2003). Structure-function relationships in the interaction between the urokinase-type plasminogen activator and its receptor. Curr Pharm Des 9(19): 1499-1528.

Poliakov, A., Tkachuk, V., Ovchinnikova, T., Potapenko, N., Bagryantsev, S. & Stepanova, V. (2001). Plasmin-dependent elimination of the growth-factor-like domain in urokinase causes its rapid cellular uptake and degradation. Biochem J 355(Pt 3): 639-645.

Potempa, J., Korzus, E. & Travis, J. (1994). The serpin superfamily of proteinase inhibitors: structure, function, and regulation. J Biol Chem 269(23): 15957-15960.

Prager, G. W., Breuss, J. M., Steurer, S., Olcaydu, D., Mihaly, J., Brunner, P. M., Stockinger, H. & Binder, B. R. (2004). Vascular endothelial growth factor receptor-2-induced initial endothelial cell migration depends on the presence of the urokinase receptor. Circ Res 94(12): 1562-1570.

Prager, G. W., Mihaly, J., Brunner, P. M., Koshelnick, Y., Hoyer-Hansen, G. & Binder, B. R. (2009). Urokinase mediates endothelial cell survival via induction of the X-linked inhibitor of apoptosis protein. Blood 113(6): 1383-1390.

Preissner, K. T. & Seiffert, D. (1998). Role of vitronectin and its receptors in haemostasis and vascular remodeling. Thromb Res 89(1): 1-21.

Rabbani, S. A., Gladu, J., Mazar, A. P., Henkin, J. & Goltzman, D. (1997). Induction in human osteoblastic cells (SaOS2) of the early response genes fos, jun, and myc by the amino terminal fragment (ATF) of urokinase. J Cell Physiol 172(2): 137-145.

Rakha, E. A., Elsheikh, S. E., Aleskandarany, M. A., Habashi, H. O., Green, A. R., Powe, D. G., El-Sayed, M. E., Benhasouna, A., Brunet, J. S., Akslen, L. A., Evans, A. J., Blamey, R., Reis-Filho, J. S., Foulkes, W. D. & Ellis, I. O. (2009). Triple-negative breast cancer: distinguishing between basal and nonbasal subtypes. Clin Cancer Res 15(7): 2302-2310.

Resnati, M., Guttinger, M., Valcamonica, S., Sidenius, N., Blasi, F. & Fazioli, F. (1996). Proteolytic cleavage of the urokinase receptor substitutes for the agonist-induced chemotactic effect. EMBO J 15(7): 1572-1582.

Riccio, A., Grimaldi, G., Verde, P., Sebastio, G., Boast, S. & Blasi, F. (1985). The human urokinase-plasminogen activator gene and its promoter. Nucleic Acids Res 13(8): 2759-2771.

Riisbro, R., Stephens, R. W., Brunner, N., Christensen, I. J., Nielsen, H. J., Heilmann, L. & von Tempelhoff, G. F. (2001). Soluble urokinase plasminogen activator receptor in preoperatively obtained plasma from patients with gynecological cancer or benign gynecological diseases. Gynecol Oncol 82(3): 523-531.

Roldan, A. L., Cubellis, M. V., Masucci, M. T., Behrendt, N., Lund, L. R., Dano, K., Appella, E. & Blasi, F. (1990). Cloning and expression of the receptor for human urokinase plasminogen activator, a central molecule in cell surface, plasmin dependent proteolysis. EMBO J 9(2): 467-474.

Romer, J., Nielsen, B. S. & Ploug, M. (2004). The urokinase receptor as a potential target in cancer therapy. Curr Pharm Des 10(19): 2359-2376.

Rosenquist, C., Thorpe, S. M., Dano, K. & Grondahl-Hansen, J. (1993). Enzyme-linked immunosorbent assay of urokinase-type plasminogen activator (uPA) in cytosolic extracts of human breast cancer tissue. Breast Cancer Res Treat 28(3): 223-229.

Sainsbury, J. R., Farndon, J. R., Needham, G. K., Malcolm, A. J. & Harris, A. L. (1987). Epidermal-growth-factor receptor status as predictor of early recurrence of and death from breast cancer. Lancet 1(8547): 1398-1402.

Salomon, D. S., Brandt, R., Ciardiello, F. & Normanno, N. (1995). Epidermal growth factor-related peptides and their receptors in human malignancies. Crit Rev Oncol Hematol 19(3): 183-232.

Schmitt, M., Sturmheit, A. S., Welk, A., Schnelldorfer, C. & Harbeck, N. (2006). *Procedures for the quantitative protein determination of urokinase and its inhibitor, PAI-1, in human breast cancer tissue extracts by ELISA. Methods Mol Med 120: 245-265.*

Schvartz, I., Seger, D. & Shaltiel, S. (1999). *Vitronectin. Int J Biochem Cell Biol 31(5): 539-544.*

Shevde, L. A. & Welch, D. R. (2003). *Metastasis suppressor pathways--an evolving paradigm. Cancer Lett 198(1): 1-20.*

Shirakihara, T., Kawasaki, T., Fukagawa, A., Semba, K., Sakai, R., Miyazono, K., Miyazawa, K. & Saitoh, M. (2013). *Identification of integrin alpha3 as a molecular marker of cells undergoing EMT and of cancer cells with aggressive phenotypes. Cancer Sci.*

Shiratsuchi, T., Ishibashi, H. & Shirasuna, K. (2002). *Inhibition of epidermal growth factor-induced invasion by dexamethasone and AP-1 decoy in human squamous cell carcinoma cell lines. J Cell Physiol 193(3): 340-348.*

Sidenius, N., Andolfo, A., Fesce, R. & Blasi, F. (2002). *Urokinase regulates vitronectin binding by controlling urokinase receptor oligomerization. J Biol Chem 277(31): 27982-27990.*

Sidenius, N. & Blasi, F. (2000). *Domain 1 of the urokinase receptor (uPAR) is required for uPAR-mediated cell binding to vitronectin. FEBS Lett 470(1): 40-46.*

Siegel, R., Naishadham, D. & Jemal, A. (2013). *Cancer statistics, 2013. CA Cancer J Clin 63(1): 11-30.*

Singh, B., Su, Y. C. & Riesbeck, K. (2010). *Vitronectin in bacterial pathogenesis: a host protein used in complement escape and cellular invasion. Mol Microbiol 78(3): 545-560.*

Smith, D., Gilbert, M. & Owen, W. G. (1985). *Tissue plasminogen activator release in vivo in response to vasoactive agents. Blood 66(4): 835-839.*

Soeda, S., Oda, M., Ochiai, T. & Shimeno, H. (2001). *Deficient release of plasminogen activator inhibitor-1 from astrocytes triggers apoptosis in neuronal cells. Brain Res Mol Brain Res 91(1-2): 96-103.*

Soydinc, H. O., Duranyildiz, D., Guney, N., Derin, D. & Yasasever, V. (2012). *Utility of serum and urine uPAR levels for diagnosis of breast cancer. Asian Pac J Cancer Prev 13(6): 2887-2889.*

Stahl, A. & Mueller, B. M. (1994). *Binding of urokinase to its receptor promotes migration and invasion of human melanoma cells in vitro. Cancer Res 54(11): 3066-3071.*

Stahl, A. & Mueller, B. M. (1997). *Melanoma cell migration on vitronectin: regulation by components of the plasminogen activation system. Int J Cancer 71(1): 116-122.*

Steeg, P. S. (2003). *Metastasis suppressors alter the signal transduction of cancer cells. Nat Rev Cancer 3(1): 55-63.*

Stefansson, S. & Lawrence, D. A. (1996). *The serpin PAI-1 inhibits cell migration by blocking integrin alpha V beta 3 binding to vitronectin. Nature 383(6599): 441-443.*

Stefansson, S., McMahon, G. A., Petitclerc, E. & Lawrence, D. A. (2003). *Plasminogen activator inhibitor-1 in tumor growth, angiogenesis and vascular remodeling. Curr Pharm Des 9(19): 1545-1564.*

Stein, P. E. & Carrell, R. W. (1995). *What do dysfunctional serpins tell us about molecular mobility and disease? Nat Struct Biol 2(2): 96-113.*

Stepanova, V. V. & Tkachuk, V. A. (2002). *Urokinase as a multidomain protein and polyfunctional cell regulator. Biochemistry (Mosc) 67(1): 109-118.*

Tait, J. F. & Fujikawa, K. (1986). *Identification of the binding site for plasma prekallikrein in human high molecular weight kininogen. A region from residues 185 to 224 of the kininogen light chain retains full binding activity. J Biol Chem 261(33): 15396-15401.*

Tait, J. F. & Fujikawa, K. (1987). *Primary structure requirements for the binding of human high molecular weight kininogen to plasma prekallikrein and factor XI. J Biol Chem 262(24): 11651-11656.*

Tang, C. H., Hill, M. L., Brumwell, A. N., Chapman, H. A. & Wei, Y. (2008). *Signaling through urokinase and urokinase receptor in lung cancer cells requires interactions with beta1 integrins. J Cell Sci 121(Pt 22): 3747-3756.*

Tarui, T., Mazar, A. P., Cines, D. B. & Takada, Y. (2001). Urokinase-type plasminogen activator receptor (CD87) is a ligand for integrins and mediates cell-cell interaction. J Biol Chem 276(6): 3983-3990.

Travis, J. & Salvesen, G. S. (1983). Human plasma proteinase inhibitors. Annu Rev Biochem 52: 655-709.

Tsuboi, R. & Rifkin, D. B. (1990). Bimodal Relationship between Invasion of the Amniotic Membrane and Plasminogen-Activator Activity. Int J Cancer 46(1): 56-60.

Unlu, A. & Leake, R. E. (2003). The effect of EGFR-related tyrosine kinase activity inhibition on the growth and invasion mechanisms of prostate carcinoma cell lines. Int J Biol Markers 18(2): 139-146.

van der Pluijm, G., Sijmons, B., Vloedgraven, H., van der Bent, C., Drijfhout, J. W., Verheijen, J., Quax, P., Karperien, M., Papapoulos, S. & Lowik, C. (2001). Urokinase-receptor/integrin complexes are functionally involved in adhesion and progression of human breast cancer in vivo. Am J Pathol 159(3): 971-982.

Vassalli, J. D., Baccino, D. & Belin, D. (1985). A cellular binding site for the Mr 55,000 form of the human plasminogen activator, urokinase. J Cell Biol 100(1): 86-92.

Verde, P., Stoppelli, M. P., Galeffi, P., Di Nocera, P. & Blasi, F. (1984). Identification and primary sequence of an unspliced human urokinase poly(A)+ RNA. Proc Natl Acad Sci U S A 81(15): 4727-4731.

Vogetseder, A., Thies, S., Ingold, B., Roth, P., Weller, M., Schraml, P., Goodman, S. L. & Moch, H. (2013). alphav-Integrin isoform expression in primary human tumors and brain metastases. Int J Cancer.

Waldron, N. N., Oh, S. & Vallera, D. A. (2012). Bispecific targeting of EGFR and uPAR in a mouse model of head and neck squamous cell carcinoma. Oral Oncol 48(12): 1202-1207.

Waltz, D. A., Natkin, L. R., Fujita, R. M., Wei, Y. & Chapman, H. A. (1997). Plasmin and plasminogen activator inhibitor type 1 promote cellular motility by regulating the interaction between the urokinase receptor and vitronectin. J Clin Invest 100(1): 58-67.

Wang, F., Li, J., Sinn, A. L., Knabe, W. E., Khanna, M., Jo, I., Silver, J. M., Oh, K., Li, L., Sandusky, G. E., Sledge, G. W., Nakshatri, H., Jones, D. R., Pollok, K. E. & Meroueh, S. O. (2011). Virtual screening targeting the urokinase receptor, biochemical and cell-based studies, synthesis, pharmacokinetic characterization, and effect on breast tumor metastasis. J Med Chem 54(20): 7193-7205.

Wang, X. Q., Sun, P. & Paller, A. S. (2005). Gangliosides inhibit urokinase-type plasminogen activator (uPA)-dependent squamous carcinoma cell migration by preventing uPA receptor/alphabeta integrin/epidermal growth factor receptor interactions. J Invest Dermatol 124(4): 839-848.

Wei, Y., Lukashev, M., Simon, D. I., Bodary, S. C., Rosenberg, S., Doyle, M. V. & Chapman, H. A. (1996). Regulation of integrin function by the urokinase receptor. Science 273(5281): 1551-1555.

Wei, Y., Tang, C. H., Kim, Y., Robillard, L., Zhang, F., Kugler, M. C. & Chapman, H. A. (2007). Urokinase receptors are required for alpha 5 beta 1 integrin-mediated signaling in tumor cells. J Biol Chem 282(6): 3929-3939.

Wei, Y., Waltz, D. A., Rao, N., Drummond, R. J., Rosenberg, S. & Chapman, H. A. (1994). Identification of the urokinase receptor as an adhesion receptor for vitronectin. J Biol Chem 269(51): 32380-32388.

Wei, Y., Yang, X., Liu, Q., Wilkins, J. A. & Chapman, H. A. (1999). A role for caveolin and the urokinase receptor in integrin-mediated adhesion and signaling. J Cell Biol 144(6): 1285-1294.

Wu, Y., Rizzo, V., Liu, Y., Sainz, I. M., Schmuckler, N. G. & Colman, R. W. (2007). Kininostatin associates with membrane rafts and inhibits alpha(v)beta3 integrin activation in human umbilical vein endothelial cells. Arterioscler Thromb Vasc Biol 27(9): 1968-1975.

Yebra, M., Parry, G. C., Stromblad, S., Mackman, N., Rosenberg, S., Mueller, B. M. & Cheresh, D. A. (1996). Requirement of receptor-bound urokinase-type plasminogen activator for integrin alphavbeta5-directed cell migration. J Biol Chem 271(46): 29393-29399.

Zaidel-Bar, R., Milo, R., Kam, Z. & Geiger, B. (2007). A paxillin tyrosine phosphorylation switch regulates the assembly and form of cell-matrix adhesions. J Cell Sci 120(Pt 1): 137-148.

Zemzoum, I., Kates, R. E., Ross, J. S., Dettmar, P., Dutta, M., Henrichs, C., Yurdseven, S., Hofler, H., Kiechle, M., Schmitt, M. & Harbeck, N. (2003). *Invasion factors uPA/PAI-1 and HER2 status provide independent and complementary information on patient outcome in node-negative breast cancer. J Clin Oncol 21(6): 1022-1028.*

Zutter, M. M., Santoro, S. A., Staatz, W. D. & Tsung, Y. L. (1995). *Re-expression of the alpha 2 beta 1 integrin abrogates the malignant phenotype of breast carcinoma cells. Proc Natl Acad Sci U S A 92(16): 7411-7415.*

Zyzak, L. L., MacDonald, L. M., Batova, A., Forand, R., Creek, K. E. & Pirisi, L. (1994). *Increased levels and constitutive tyrosine phosphorylation of the epidermal growth factor receptor contribute to autonomous growth of human papillomavirus type 16 immortalized human keratinocytes. Cell Growth Differ 5(5): 537-547.*

Current Involvement and Clinical Relevance of Non-coding RNA Dysregulated Expression in Neuroblastoma

Duncan Ayers
Department of Pathology
Faculty of Medicine & Surgery
University of Malta, Malta
Faculty of Medical and Human Sciences
The University of Manchester, United Kingdom

John Carabott
Faculty of Health Sciences
University of Malta, Malta

1   Neuroblastoma

1.1   Introduction

Neuroblastoma is the most frequent extra-cranial solid tumour occurring in infancy with an estimated incidence of 1 in 7000 live birth cases (Malis 2013). It is considered as the most common cancer diagnosed during the first years of life with a mean age of diagnosis at 17 months (London *et al.* 2005). In paediatric oncology, neuroblastoma accounts for 12% of cancer deaths and about 4% of malignancies in patients (Smith *et al.* 2010). Evidence corroborates that the tumour arises from neural-crest tissue through incomplete commitment of developing precursor cells, primordial cells of the sympathetic nervous system (Hoehner *et al.* 1996). Being an extracranial tumour of the sympathetic nervous system, the adrenal medulla and paraspinal ganglia are mostly affected and therefore neuroblastoma commonly manifests as mass lesions in the neck, chest, abdomen or pelvis (Maris 2010).

Clinically, neuroblastoma is highly variable, ranging from patients presenting with an asymptomatic mass, primary tumours that cause morbidity as a consequence of local invasion, or widely metastasised tumours leading to disseminated disease (Maris 2010).

Consequently, treatment varies greatly depending on risk stratification, varying from a wait-and-see approach to aggressive multimodal therapy. Moreover, prediction of patient outcome in terms of prognosis differs from a 40% survival rate - despite a combination of surgery, chemotherapy and radiotherapy - to spontaneous regression with minimal or no treatment (Maris *et al.* 2007). Vis-a-vis all human cancers, neuroblastoma exhibits the highest propensity to spontaneously and completely regress (Yamamoto *et al.* 1998). The disproportionate difference in severe morbidity and mortality compared to spontaneous regression makes it appreciable why neuroblastoma is considered a 'phenomenon' by clinicians and scientists alike.

1.2   Clinical Presentation

The majority of neuroblastoma cases, 65% of primary tumours, arise in the abdomen with half of these originating in the adrenal medulla (Maris *et al.* 2007). Following the abdomen, the most common sites are the neck, chest and pelvis (London *et al.* 2005). As can be expected from a diverse tumour, presenting signs and symptoms vary in different cases and are dependent on site of primary tumour, absence or presence of metastasis, or presence of paraneoplastic syndromes. Clinically, three categories are normally distinguished albeit all share considerable overlap, namely localized, metastatic and 4S NB (Maris *et al.* 2007). These clinical categories are designated by utilization of the Shimada Classification system (Shimada *et al.* 1984).

1.3   Genetics & Biological Variability

Occurrence of neuroblastoma is predominantly a sporadic process but in 1-2% of cases a family history has been associated with the tumour (Kushner *et al.* 1986). Due to the presence of hereditary cases, researchers presumed to discover a unifying tumour suppressor gene responsible for neuroblastoma tumourigenesis. Only in 2008, did the anaplastic lymphoma kinase (ALK) oncogene link most familial neuroblastomas (Mossé *et al.* 2008). Germline single nucleotide polymorphisms (SNPs) resulted in gain-of-function mutations in the tyrosine kinase moiety of ALK (Mossé *et al.* 2008). As a consequence, constitutive activation of the tyrosine kinase led to a premalignant state. Nonetheless, ALK mutations are somatically acquired in up to 15% of sporadic neuroblastoma (Mossé *et al.* 2008).

Sporadic neuroblastoma is thought to arise from multiple mutations, which in themselves may be common, but their association increases the susceptibility of the primordial cell to undergo tumourigenesis (Maris 2010). Genome wide association studies (GWAs) have identified a few genes and chromosomal regions that are elevated in neuroblastoma patients as opposed to controls (Capasso et al. 2009; Maris et al. 2008). Nonetheless, these abnormalities are considered relatively common DNA variations (Maris 2010), further corroborating the absence of a singular identified event in neuroblastoma tumourigenesis as yet. Most interestingly is the recent concept that paediatric malignancies exhibit less somatic mutations with respect to adult cancers (Parsons et al. 2011).

The singular, most predictive finding in neuroblastoma biology is the amplification of the MYCN oncogene which is greatly linked to a poor outcome (Brodeur et al. 1987). Gene amplification is one of the most profound pathways for tumourigenesis by activation of proto-oncogenes into oncogenes (Schwab et al. 2003). MYCN amplification is observed in 20% of primary tumours and strongly raises the risk group of otherwise favourable localised tumours or 4S disease (Brodeur et al. 1984).

Correlating with MYCN amplification, deletion of the short arm of chromosome 1 (1p) is highly associated with advanced disease stage (White et al. 1995). 1p deletions coexist with MYCN amplification and are identified in 25-35% of neuroblastoma (Maris et al. 2007). Till the present day, the genes responsible for the pathogenesis of neuroblastoma have not been identified in the 1p region, albeit some speculate that this could be due to loss of heterozygosity (Maris et al. 2007). Another high risk feature, but whose presence is not exhibited in tumours with MYCN amplification, is the allelelic loss of 11q-presenting in up to 45% of primary tumours (Plantaz et al. 2001).

The DNA content is also a relevant prognostic indicator and can be of either two forms in neuroblastoma. A hyperdiploid, almost triploid, karyotype is associated with a better prognosis since this has been found in less aggressive tumours which exhibit gross mitotic defects (Maris et al. 2007). More aggressive tumours, on the contrary, have genomic, not mitotic, stability defects thus exhibiting near-diploid DNA content (Brodeur 2003).

Despite all these aberrations, including rearrangements and large chromosomal amplifications and losses, it is now being thought that the most profound effects of neuroblastoma tumourigenesis are based on epigenetics, with defects being likely in DNA methylation and acetylation which regulate the transcriptome (Cole & Maris 2012).

1.4   Treatment

Neuroblastoma tumours are heterogenous, with some tumours being highly aggressive whereas others show spontaneous regression without treatment. Tumours with favourable prognostic markers as determined by the current risk stratification have been given progressively less therapeutic intensity over the years (Maris 2010). Below, brief treatment protocols are described based on risk group stratification of neuroblastoma cases.

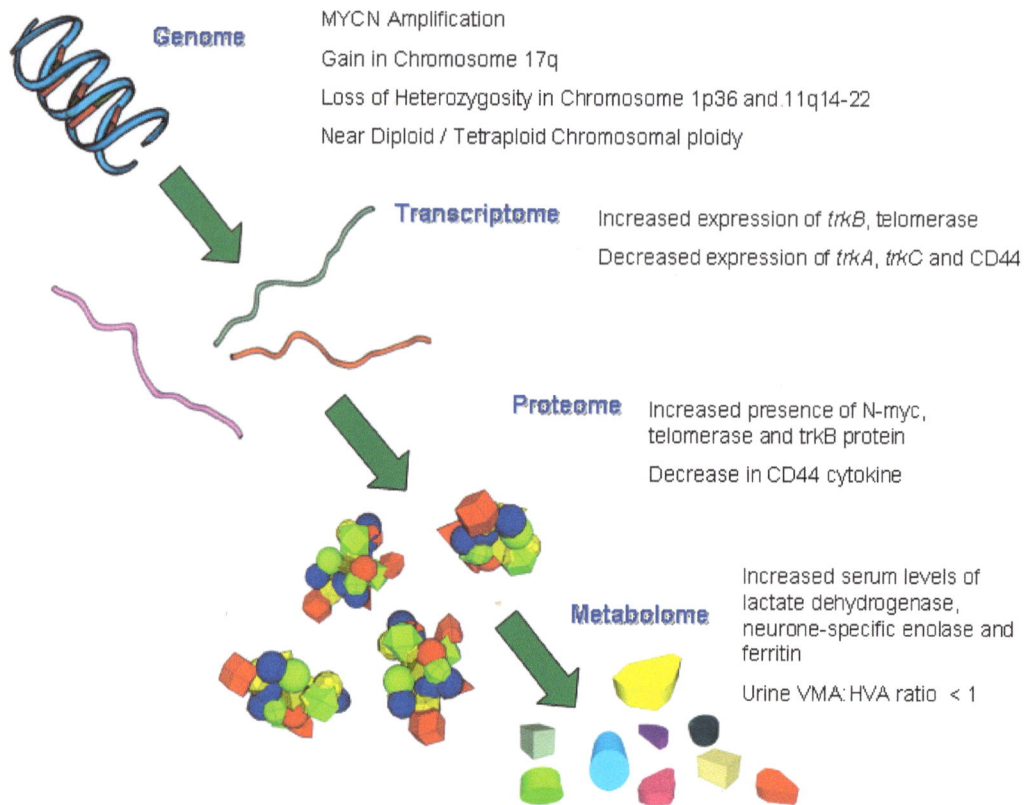

Genome
MYCN Amplification
Gain in Chromosome 17q
Loss of Heterozygosity in Chromosome 1p36 and 11q14-22
Near Diploid / Tetraploid Chromosomal ploidy

Transcriptome
Increased expression of *trkB*, telomerase
Decreased expression of *trkA*, *trkC* and CD44

Proteome
Increased presence of N-myc, telomerase and trkB protein
Decrease in CD44 cytokine

Metabolome
Increased serum levels of lactate dehydrogenase, neurone-specific enolase and ferritin
Urine VMA:HVA ratio < 1

Figure 1: Outline of the multiple factors affecting NB progression. Such factors are identified at various stages of protein synthesis and processing. Additionally, many of such factors, such as MYCN amplification and chromosome 17q gains, are currently utilized in the oncology clinic as markers for NB tumour aggressiveness (Logan *et al.* 2010).

Low-Risk Disease

Research has shown that Stage 1 disease can be almost entirely, more than 95% survival rate, cured with surgery alone (Perez *et al.* 2000). Nevertheless, Stage 1 or 2 disease with MYCN amplification may pose a dilemma as to whether surgery alone is sufficient (Cohn *et al.* 1995). Newborns with localised small masses are safely observed to allow for spontaneous remission and prevent unnecessary surgery, since these rarely progress to advanced disease (Weinstein *et al.* 2003). As a rule of thumb, the first approach to low-risk neuroblastoma is removal of the primary tumour and keep chemotherapy as a last resort to prevent acute and long-term morbidity related to the treatment (Weinstein *et al.* 2003).

Intermediate-Risk Disease

This risk group is the most difficult to classify with the current risk stratification as it exhibits the most heterogeneity when limited prognostic markers are used for the stratification. Approach to moderate risk disease is a combination of low-dose chemotherapy and surgery whenever possible to de-bulk as much tumour mass (Maris 2010). Chemotherapy given to intermediate-risk patients are a combination of cyclo-phosphamide and doxorubicin in four cycles (Weinstein *et al.* 2003). Patients with INSS stage 3 disease demonstrating biologically favourable features, an intermediate risk group, are spared radical surgery and radiotherapy even when there is presence of gross residual tumour (Kushner *et al.* 1996).

4S Disease

4S disease is typically a low or intermediate risk group. Low risk group show non-aggressive markers such as MYCN single copies, hyper-diploid karyotype and favourable histology (Maris *et al.* 2007). These infants have a survival probability of 85% to 92% (Nickerson *et al.* 2000). Infants younger than two months with swift hepatomegaly progression, however, may show symptoms of respiratory compromise that requires dealing with (Nickerson *et al.* 2000). Another facet of stage 4S is similar to that of classic stage 4 with rapid tumour progression and relapse and is therefore treated as a high-risk group (Nickerson *et al.* 2000).

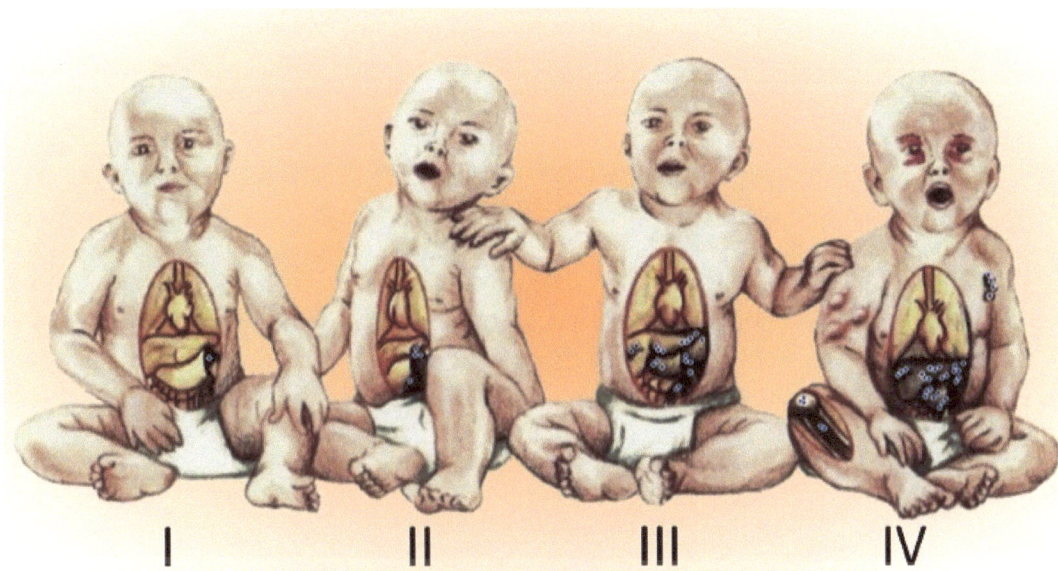

Figure 2: Overview of neuroblastoma tumour progression stages, according to the International Neuroblastoma Staging System. In Stage I the tumour is highly localized and can be removed surgically.Stage II neuroblastoma describes a localized tumour with incomplete or no gross excision and spread to neighbouring lymph nodes. In Stage III the tumour spreads beyond the midline (vertebral column) with possible distal lymph node affliction. Stage IV represents extensive tumour metastases into varying regions such as the liver, bone, bone marrow and skin.

High-Risk Disease

Survival for children presenting with high-risk neuroblastoma has not improved much over the past couple of decades, with cure rates remaining considerably low (Weinstein *et al.* 2003). Intensification of therapy at the induction phase (Cheung & Heller 1991), myeloablative therapy followed by stem cell transplant and improved supportive care are thought to be the reason behind an observable improvement in treatment of high-risk neuroblastoma (Weinstein *et al.* 2003). The treatment follows three phases: induction and consolidation phases of remission, followed by maintenance to eradicate minimal residual disease (Maris 2010). Multiple drug agents are used for induction therapy and at high doses since this has been shown to increase the response rate and overall survival (Cheung & Heller 1991). The multi-drug regimen typically used entails of cycles of cisplatin and etoposide alternating with vincristine, doxorubicin and cyclophosphamide (Kushner *et al.* 1994).

2   miRNAs

The advent of RNA interference (RNAi) technology in the late 1990s has brought with it a major change in perspective regarding the factors affecting gene regulatory processes in most living organisms. In particular, the fact that the non-coding regions of the transcriptome actually do play very active roles in multiple cellular functions such as gene regulation, has re-written known dogma on this field.

Essential components of the RNAi pathway are micro RNAs (miRNAs), consisting of endogenously produced 70 base-long, stem-loop structures (pre-miRNAs) that are cleared by the Dicer enzyme to form the active miRNAs (Graves & Zeng 2012). Such individual miRNAs are consequently taken up by the RNA interference silencing complex (RISC) and the resultant complex (in mammals) normally binds to the 3' untranslated region (UTR) of the target transcript, with resultant post-transcriptional gene silencing through inhibition of ribosomal translation (Graves & Zeng 2012)(See Figure 3). A more detailed account of miRNA processing is described in Figure 3, however the readers are advised to consult other literature sources regarding highly detailed research on miRNA processing as this book chapter focuses on the clinical relevance of miRNAs.

Since their discovery twenty years ago, a plethora of studies have linked dys-regulated expression of individual / networks of miRNAs with a wide spectrum of human disease conditions, including cancer (Caroli *et al.* 2013; P.-S. Chen *et al.* 2012; Farazi *et al.* 2013; Iorio & Croce 2012; Matejuk *et al.* 2013; Pan *et al.* 2013; Papaconstantinou *et al.* 2013; Pogribny & Beland 2013; Shen *et al.* 2012; Thounaojam *et al.* 2013).

The direct influences of miRNA up-regulation induces down-regulation of target genes that are vital to specific cellular pathways which, in turn, become aberrant and therefore lead to and/or exacerbate the disease condition (Iorio & Croce 2012). In addition, the down-regulation of miRNAs that are known to prevent or regulate the onset/progression of particular disease conditions is another method by which miRNAs influence pathogenesis and progression (Iorio & Croce 2012). In the context of cancer, miRNAs directly exacerbating tumour progression and aggressiveness are termed as oncomirs (Iorio & Croce 2012). Currently, the most notable oncomir, being implicated in a spectrum of human cancer conditions, is oncomiR-21 (Chusorn *et al.* 2013; Hua *et al.* 2012; Huang *et al.* 2013; Reis *et al.* 2012). Conversely, miRNAs associated with a good prognosis in cancer are termed as tumour suppressor miRNAs, and, once dysregulated, can also exacerbate tumour progression (Iorio & Croce 2012). Examples of tumour suppressor miRNAs include miR-206, miR-375 and miR-874 (Jung *et al.* 2013; Kesanakurti *et al.* 2013; Zhou *et al.* 2013).

Initial reports concerning the clinical influence of miRNAs in NB date back to 2008, whereby functional screening studies have identified miR-34a as a tumour suppressor miRNA (Cole *et al.* 2008). In addition, miR-34a was found to be down-regulated in NB tumours having loss of 1p36 heterozygosity (Welch *et al.* 2007) and that this specific miRNA has the capacity to directly down-regulate MYCN expression (Wei *et al.* 2008). Other screening studies in the same year reported, through miRNA microarray screening of an inducible SH-EP MYCN cell line model, that MYCN possesses regulatory properties on a spectrum of miRNAs, including the polycistron miR-17-92 and miR-221 (Schulte *et al.* 2008).

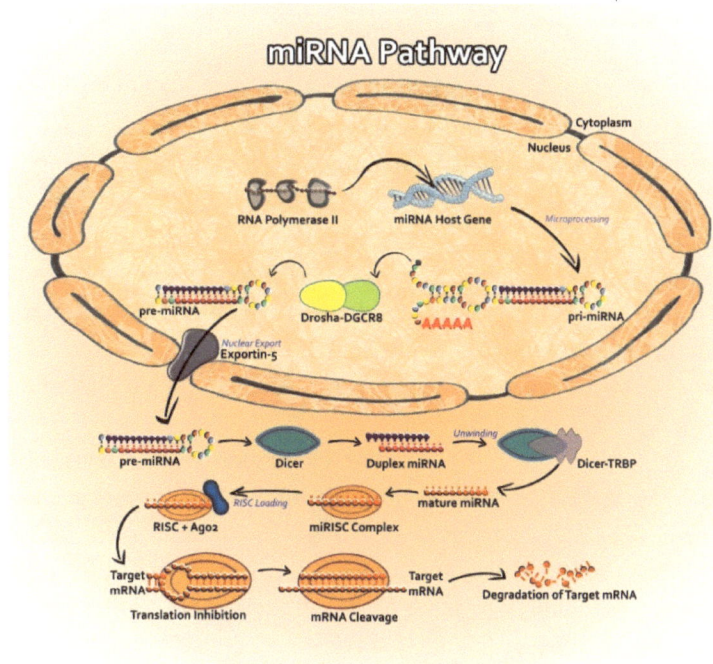

Figure 3: Summary of the miRNA biogenesis pathway (Wilson *et al.* 2009). The pre-miRNA generated form the endogenous, miRNA host gene within the nucleus is actively transported into the cytoplasm and cleaved by the Dicer enzyme. This leaves a miRNA duplex molecule that binds to the RNA interference silencing complex (RISC). Ultimately, attachment of the complex through the miRNA guide strand sequence, mainly on the 3' un-translated region of the target, leads to inhibition of translation processes by ribosomes in humans. In other cases, if the miRNA guide strand binds to target coding regions, this results in mRNA cleavage and resultant degradation of the target transcript.

Further studies elucidated that MYCN – induced miRNA expression allowed for global down-regulation of key genes involved in pathways that are commonly linked to NB tumour aggression (P Mestdagh, Fredlund, Pattyn, Schulte, *et al.* 2010; Bray *et al.* 2009). In 2009, another tumour suppressor miRNA, miR-125b, was also found to play an important part in the regulation of NB progression by directing the level of neuroblast differentiation within such tumours through the down-regulatory effect on a subset of 164 recognised target genes (Le *et al.* 2009). Similarly, miR-128 was highlighted as a tumour suppressor miRNA, since when over-expressed it induced a reduction in NB invasive properties and motility due to the consequent down-regulation of the neuroblast motility proteins Reelin and DCX (Evangelisti *et al.* 2009).

Furthermore, the rapid development of miRNA-specific microarray technologies allowed for the identification of cancer-specific and NB-specific miRNA dys-regulation profiles that could serve as useful diagnostic biomarker signatures within the clinical setting (Wei *et al.* 2009).

Evidence for the key oncogenic roles of the miR-17-92 polycistron in NB tumour progression was brought to light in 2010, whereby it was elucidated that such a miRNA polycistron was linked to multiple cancer-related phenotypes such as cellular adhesion properties, cell proliferation and RAS-signalling (Pieter Mestdagh *et al.* 2010). This study ultimately indicated over-expression of the component miRNAs of the miR-17-92 miRNA polycistron as an overall marker for poor prognosis in NB cases, especially due to the additional down-regulatory effects on target genes in the TGF-ß signaling pathway (Pieter Mestdagh *et al.* 2010).

Additional oncogenic miRNAs identified in the same year included miR-9 (Khew-Goodall & Goodall 2010; Ma *et al.* 2010). This miRNA was found to be induced by MYCN and/or MYC over-expression and is a major metastasis promotor, primarily due to its down-regulatory effects on the metastasis-regulating E-cadherin protein (Ma *et al.* 2010). The miR-9 oncomir was also linked to breast cancer metastasis (Almeida *et al.* 2010).

In the 2010-2011 period, other tumour suppressor miRNAs were identified, such as miR-10a, miR-10b and miR-184 (Meseguer *et al.* 2011; Foley *et al.* 2010). Other tumour suppressor miRNAs such as let-7 and miR-101 were identified to directly target MYCN expression (Buechner *et al.* 2011). Functional evidence was also gathered for the validation of miR-542-5p as a reliable tumour suppressor miRNA in NB (Bray *et al.* 2011).

Additional screening studies for global miRNA expression profile analyses were performed and resulted in the identification of 46 confirmed dys-regulated miRNAs and that such signature miRNA expression profiles can be utilized as a novel prediction method for prognosis in clinical NB cases (Schulte, Schowe, *et al.* 2010). Other similar studies involved the novel next generation sequencing technologies and have also demonstrated to highlight signature miRNA expression profiles that can be utilized in the clinic for patient stratification purposes (Schulte, Marschall, *et al.* 2010).

Recent evidence has brought to light the epigenetic (DNA methylation) regulatory mechanisms that are responsible for the induction of down-regulated expression of 67 miRNAs in NB which in turn affect the expression of known NB oncogenes (Das *et al.* 2013).

Chemoresistance properties of NB tumours are also influenced by means of miRNA dys-regulatory effects, although present evidence to prove this is still in its infancy. Recent research has highlighted the impact of miR-204 in enhancing the chemosensitivity properties of NB cell lines to cisplatin, through over-expression of the miRNA by means of mimic molecules (Ryan *et al.* 2012). Another study has demonstrated that the oncomir miR-21 contributes to cisplatin resistance in NB cell lines following tumour exposure to the conventional chemotherapeutic agent (Y. Chen *et al.* 2012).

An interesting premise for miRNA roles in NB would be that of miRNA signature expression profiles leading to the onset of spontaneous regression of the tumour, resulting in a marked increase in patient survival probabilities. However, at present, there is no scientific literature which has yet been published that depicts such occurrences.

3   Long non-coding RNAs (lncRNAs)

The lncRNA segment of the genome constitutes the largest family of non-protein-coding RNAs with an estimated list of approximately 10,000 lncRNAs already identified (Derrien *et al.* 2012). The hallmark characteristics of lncRNAs consist of RNA Polymerase II transcripts having a length of over 200 nucleotides and such transcripts do not contain any open reading frame (Kornienko *et al.* 2013). The functional activities of lncRNAs are widespread (see Figure 4), though these can be summarized as being positive / negative regulations of gene expression at either the transcriptional or post-transcriptional level (Kornienko *et al.* 2013).

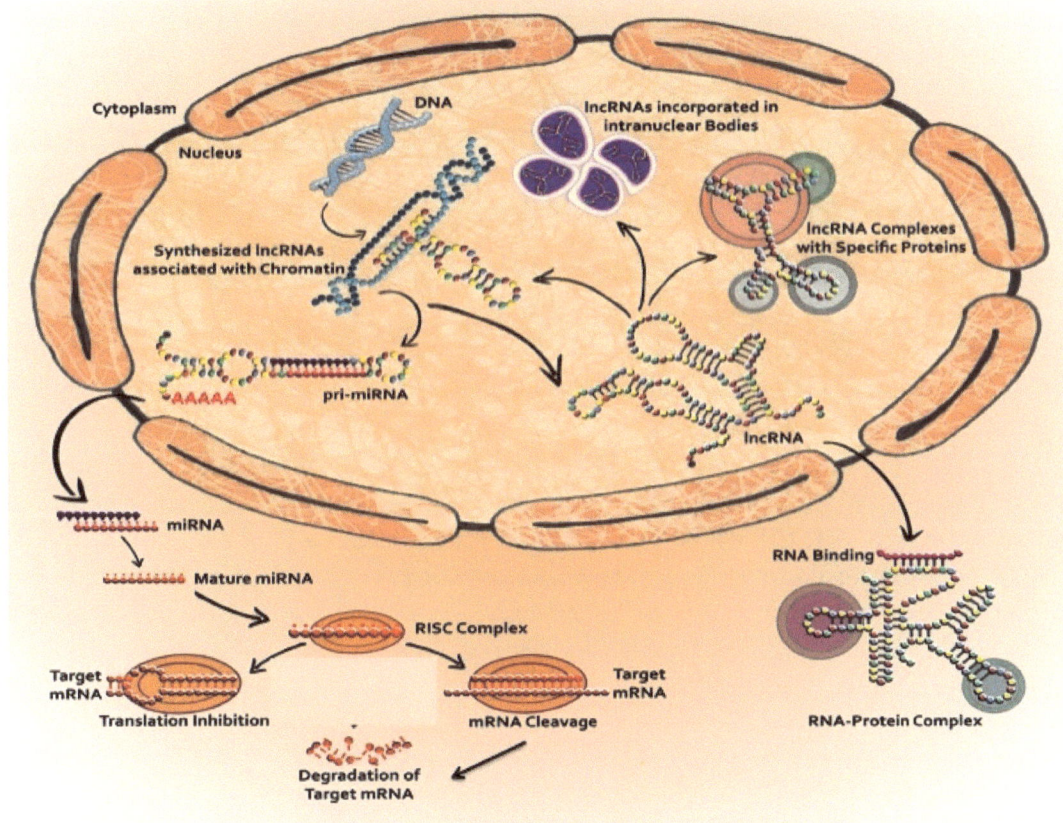

Figure 4: Overview of known lncRNA functional roles (Hirano 2013). LncRNA activities can be described as cis- or trans-acting, depending on the lncRNA target site being located on the individual lncRNA host chromosome (cis-acting) or other chromosome (trans-acting).

Evidence for the influences of lncRNAs in human disease condition pathogenesis and disease progression are being constantly uncovered (Hirano 2013; Guil & Esteller 2012; Taft *et al.* 2010). Presently, there are at least 19 lncRNAs that have been highlighted to possess oncogenic or tumour suppressive properties (H. Zhang *et al.* 2013). From this list, five lncRNAs have been validated to act as prognostic biomarkers (H. Zhang *et al.* 2013).

The lncRNA H19 has been demonstrated to act as a tumour suppressor biomarker as it can control the metastatic properties of hepatocellular carcinoma (HCC), unless its expression is down-regulated (L. Zhang *et al.* 2013). The expression ratio of H19 in intra- and peri-tumoural samples in HCC can be therefore utilized as a prognostic test for HCC metastasis progression (L. Zhang *et al.* 2013).

Another representative lncRNA oncogenic biomarker is MALAT-1, which has been identified to be implicated in lung adenocarcinoma metastasis (Gutschner *et al.* 2013). In addition, recent studies have also identified and validated the use of MALAT-1 as a novel diagnostic biomarker and drug target in castration-resistant prostate carcinoma (Ren, Wang, *et al.* 2013; Ren, Liu, *et al.* 2013). Furthermore, MALAT-1 was found to be up-regulated in laryngeal squamous cell carcinoma and metastatic bladder cancer (Feng *et al.* 2012; Ying *et al.* 2012).

The homeobox antisense intergenic RNA (HOTAIR) lncRNA has also been extensively studied and identified to be associated with tumour progression. HOTAIR was recently found to be up-regulated in gastric adenocarcinoma tissues and also as free circulating lncRNA in plasma samples from gastric cancer patients (Hajjari *et al.* 2013; Arita *et al.* 2013). Knockdown of HOTAIR was also confirmed to decrease the level or tumour invasion and additionally revert epithelial-to-mesenchymal transition properties in gastric cancer and therefore places HOTAIR as a novel prognostic biomarker for such a tumour model (Xu *et al.* 2013). In addition to gastric adenocarcinoma, HOTAIR has been highlighted to have up-regulated expression and associated with metastasis in several other tumour models including melanoma, non-small cell lung cancer, oesophageal squamous cell, ovarian and hepatocellular carcinomas (Tang *et al.* 2013; Nakagawa *et al.* 2013; Lv *et al.* 2013; Cui *et al.* 2013; Ishibashi *et al.* 2013). The above scientific evidence all suggests HOTAIR to be a useful prognostic biomarker for poor survival within such tumour model cases presented in the oncology clinic.

Presently, the level of scientific publications focusing on the influences of lncRNAs in NB is still limited. However, there are indications that the MYCN oncogene in NB has the capacity to affect the expression of multiple lncRNAs such as transcribed ultra-conserved regions (T-UCRs) and non coding RNA expressed in aggressive NB (ncRANs) (Buechner & Einvik 2012).

A 28 T-UCR expression profile signature has already been correlated with good prognosis in non-infantile metastatic NB (Buechner & Einvik 2012). In addition, another 7 T-UCR expression profile signature was identified to be up-regulated in MYCN-amplified NB tumour samples (P Mestdagh, Fredlund, Pattyn, Rihani, *et al.* 2010; Buechner & Einvik 2012).

4   Conclusions

Following the scientific evidence illustrated above, it is certainly not a matter of dispute that non-coding RNA classes are emerging as novel key players in the intertwined network of gene regulatory pathways, this being particular with respect to tumourigenesis and progression within multiple human cancer conditions – including neuroblastoma. An undoubtedly interesting concept would be the possibility that individual miRNAs and/or lncRNAs can act as both oncogenic and tumour suppressor molecular key players, depending on separate upstream regulator activations according to the environmental and/or disease status of the individual tumour cell. Sadly, there is no evidence present in the literature at the time of writing of this chapter to confirm such a hypothesis.

Consequently, current perspectives for neuroblastoma and other tumour model research is that unique miRNA and lncRNA expression signatures will be identified and validated for multiple tumour phenotypic characteristics such as metastatic potential, differentiation properties and chemoresistance to name but a few. Ultimately, such validated signatures can be utilized as a fast and effective diagnostic tool in the oncology clinic, uncovering crucial information on the status and nature of the tumour within any individual patient, therefore empowering the clinician to decide the ideal therapeutic course of action to take by bearing in mind the exact nature of the tumour due to such translational research approaches. Presently, there already exist several free, online analytical database web tools for the investigation of miRNA expression profiling data (miRNA Bodymap, Ghent University, Belgium) and as a detailed repository for all validated lncRNAs (lncipedia, Ghent University, Belgium) to aid in identifying non-coding RNAs of clinical importance – both as a diagnostic measure and as potentially novel drug targets (Mestdagh *et al.* 2011; Volders *et al.* 2013).

In addition, non-coding RNAs that have been confirmed as oncogenic can be considered as drug targets for novel translational therapies. The recent advances in nanoparticle technology can be utilized for the deployment of antagonist molecules for oncogenic non-coding RNAs within target tumour tissues.

The long-term future for the exploitation of miRNAs and lncRNAs for translational cancer medicine certainly looks bright and the day will soon come where non-coding RNA diagnostics will form part of the routine diagnostic tools performed daily within the oncology clinic, which will unlock the potentially life-saving information required for treating the cancer afflicted patients effectively with minimal adverse effects.

Acknowledgements

The authors would like to thank Mr. Anton Abela (Faculty of Medicine & Surgery, University of Malta, Malta) for preparing figures 2-4 illustrated in this chapter.

References

Almeida, M.I., Reis, R.M. & Calin, G.A., 2010. MYC-microRNA-9-metastasis connection in breast cancer. Cell research, 20(6), pp.603–604.

Arita, T. et al., 2013. Circulating Long Non-coding RNAs in Plasma of Patients with Gastric Cancer. Anticancer research, 33(8), pp.3185–3193.

Bray, I. et al., 2011. MicroRNA-542-5p as a novel tumor suppressor in neuroblastoma. Cancer letters, 303(1), pp.56–64.

Bray, I. et al., 2009. Widespread dysregulation of MiRNAs by MYCN amplification and chromosomal imbalances in neuroblastoma: association of miRNA expression with survival. PloS one, 4(11), p.e7850.

Brodeur, G.M. et al., 1984. Amplification of N-myc in untreated human neuroblastomas correlates with advanced disease stage. Science (New York, N.Y.), 224(4653), pp.1121–1124.

Brodeur, G.M. et al., 1987. Consistent N-myc copy number in simultaneous or consecutive neuroblastoma samples from sixty individual patients. Cancer research, 47(16), pp.4248–4253.

Brodeur, G.M., 2003. Neuroblastoma: biological insights into a clinical enigma. Nature reviews. Cancer, 3(3), pp.203–216.

Buechner, J. et al., 2011. Tumour-suppressor microRNAs let-7 and mir-101 target the proto-oncogene MYCN and inhibit cell proliferation in MYCN-amplified neuroblastoma. British journal of cancer, 105(2), pp.296–303.

Buechner, J. & Einvik, C., 2012. N-myc and noncoding RNAs in neuroblastoma. Molecular cancer research: MCR, 10(10), pp.1243–1253.

Capasso, M. et al., 2009. Common variations in BARD1 influence susceptibility to high-risk neuroblastoma. Nature genetics, 41(6), pp.718–723.

Caroli, A. et al., 2013. Potential therapeutic role of microRNAs in ischemic heart disease. Journal of cardiology, 61(5), pp.315–320.

Chen, P.-S., Su, J.-L. & Hung, M.-C., 2012. Dysregulation of microRNAs in cancer. Journal of biomedical science, 19, p.90.

Chen, Y. et al., 2012. Micro-RNA-21 regulates the sensitivity to cisplatin in human neuroblastoma cells. Journal of pediatric surgery, 47(10), pp.1797–1805.

Cheung, N.V. & Heller, G., 1991. Chemotherapy dose intensity correlates strongly with response, median survival, and median progression-free survival in metastatic neuroblastoma. Journal of clinical oncology: official journal of the American Society of Clinical Oncology, 9(6), pp.1050–1058.

Chusorn, P. et al., 2013. Overexpression of microRNA-21 regulating PDCD4 during tumorigenesis of liver fluke-associated cholangiocarcinoma contributes to tumor growth and metastasis. Tumour biology: the journal of the International Society for Oncodevelopmental Biology and Medicine, 34(3), pp.1579–1588.

Cohn, S.L. et al., 1995. Lack of correlation of N-myc gene amplification with prognosis in localized neuroblastoma: a Pediatric Oncology Group study. Cancer research, 55(4), pp.721–726.

Cole, K.A. et al., 2008. A functional screen identifies miR-34a as a candidate neuroblastoma tumor suppressor gene. Molecular cancer research: MCR, 6(5), pp.735–742.

Cole, K.A. & Maris, J.M., 2012. New strategies in refractory and recurrent neuroblastoma: translational opportunities to impact patient outcome. Clinical cancer research: an official journal of the American Association for Cancer Research, 18(9), pp.2423–2428.

Cui, L. et al., 2013. [Expression of long non-coding RNA HOTAIR mRNA in ovarian cancer]. Sichuan da xue xue bao. Yi xue ban = Journal of Sichuan University. Medical science edition, 44(1), pp.57–59.

Das, S. et al., 2013. Modulation of neuroblastoma disease pathogenesis by an extensive network of epigenetically regulated microRNAs. Oncogene, 32(24), pp.2927–2936.

Derrien, T. et al., 2012. The GENCODE v7 catalog of human long noncoding RNAs: analysis of their gene structure, evolution, and expression. Genome research, 22(9), pp.1775–1789.

Evangelisti, C. et al., 2009. MiR-128 up-regulation inhibits Reelin and DCX expression and reduces neuroblastoma cell motility and invasiveness. FASEB journal: official publication of the Federation of American Societies for Experimental Biology, 23(12), pp.4276–4287.

Farazi, T.A. et al., 2013. MicroRNAs in human cancer. Advances in experimental medicine and biology, 774, pp.1–20.

Feng, J. et al., 2012. Expression of long non-coding ribonucleic acid metastasis-associated lung adenocarcinoma transcript-1 is correlated with progress and apoptosis of laryngeal squamous cell carcinoma. Head & neck oncology, 4(2), p.46.

Foley, N.H. et al., 2010. MicroRNA-184 inhibits neuroblastoma cell survival through targeting the serine/threonine kinase AKT2. Molecular cancer, 9, p.83.

Graves, P. & Zeng, Y., 2012. Biogenesis of mammalian microRNAs: a global view. Genomics, proteomics & bioinformatics, 10(5), pp.239–245.

Guil, S. & Esteller, M., 2012. Cis-acting noncoding RNAs: friends and foes. Nature structural & molecular biology, 19(11), pp.1068–1075.

Gutschner, T. et al., 2013. The noncoding RNA MALAT1 is a critical regulator of the metastasis phenotype of lung cancer cells. Cancer research, 73(3), pp.1180–1189.

Hajjari, M. et al., 2013. Up-regulation of HOTAIR long non-coding RNA in human gastric adenocarcinoma tissues. Medical oncology (Northwood, London, England), 30(3), p.670.

Hirano, T., 2013. Is CCDC26 a Novel Cancer-Associated Long-Chain Non-Coding RNA? In Y. Siregar, ed. Oncogene and Cancer - From Bench to Clinic. InTech. Available at: http://www.intechopen.com/books/oncogene-and-cancer-from-bench-to-clinic/is-ccdc26-a-novel-cancer-associated-long-chain-non-coding-rna- [Accessed July 30, 2013].

Hoehner, J.C. et al., 1996. A developmental model of neuroblastoma: differentiating stroma-poor tumors' progress along an extra-adrenal chromaffin lineage. Laboratory investigation; a journal of technical methods and pathology, 75(5), pp.659–675.

Hua, D. et al., 2012. A catalogue of glioblastoma and brain MicroRNAs identified by deep sequencing. Omics: a journal of integrative biology, 16(12), pp.690–699.

Huang, Y.-H. et al., 2013. Thyroid hormone regulation of miR-21 enhances migration and invasion of hepatoma. Cancer research, 73(8), pp.2505–2517.

Iorio, M.V. & Croce, C.M., 2012. Causes and consequences of microRNA dysregulation. Cancer journal (Sudbury, Mass.), 18(3), pp.215–222.

Ishibashi, M. et al., 2013. Clinical significance of the expression of long non-coding RNA HOTAIR in primary hepatocellular carcinoma. Oncology reports, 29(3), pp.946–950.

Jung, H.M. et al., 2013. Tumor suppressor miR-375 regulates MYC expression via repression of CIP2A coding sequence through multiple miRNA-mRNA interactions. Molecular biology of the cell, 24(11), pp.1638–1648.

Kesanakurti, D. et al., 2013. Suppression of tumor cell invasiveness and in vivo tumor growth by microRNA-874 in non-small cell lung cancer. Biochemical and biophysical research communications, 434(3), pp.627–633.

Khew-Goodall, Y. & Goodall, G.J., 2010. Myc-modulated miR-9 makes more metastases. Nature cell biology, 12(3), pp.209–211.

Kornienko, A.E. et al., 2013. Gene regulation by the act of long non-coding RNA transcription. BMC biology, 11, p.59.

Kushner, B.H. et al., 1994. Highly effective induction therapy for stage 4 neuroblastoma in children over 1 year of age. Journal of clinical oncology: official journal of the American Society of Clinical Oncology, 12(12), pp.2607–2613.

Kushner, B.H. et al., 1996. Survival from locally invasive or widespread neuroblastoma without cytotoxic therapy. Journal of clinical oncology: official journal of the American Society of Clinical Oncology, 14(2), pp.373–381.

Kushner, B.H., Gilbert, F. & Helson, L., 1986. Familial neuroblastoma. Case reports, literature review, and etiologic considerations. Cancer, 57(9), pp.1887–1893.

Le, M.T.N. et al., 2009. MicroRNA-125b promotes neuronal differentiation in human cells by repressing multiple targets. Molecular and cellular biology, 29(19), pp.5290–5305.

Logan, J.A. et al., 2010. Systems biology and modeling in neuroblastoma: practicalities and perspectives. Expert review of molecular diagnostics, 10(2), pp.131–145.

London, W.B. et al., 2005. Evidence for an age cutoff greater than 365 days for neuroblastoma risk group stratification in the Children's Oncology Group. Journal of clinical oncology: official journal of the American Society of Clinical Oncology, 23(27), pp.6459–6465.

Lv, X.-B. et al., 2013. Long noncoding RNA HOTAIR is a prognostic marker for esophageal squamous cell carcinoma progression and survival. PloS one, 8(5), p.e63516.

Ma, L. et al., 2010. miR-9, a MYC/MYCN-activated microRNA, regulates E-cadherin and cancer metastasis. Nature cell biology, 12(3), pp.247–256.

Malis, J., 2013. Clinical Presentation of Neuroblastoma. In H. Shimada, ed. Neuroblastoma. InTech. Available at: http://www.intechopen.com/books/neuroblastoma/clinical-presentation-of-neuroblastoma [Accessed June 20, 2013].

Maris, J.M. et al., 2008. Chromosome 6p22 locus associated with clinically aggressive neuroblastoma. The New England journal of medicine, 358(24), pp.2585–2593.

Maris, J.M. et al., 2007. Neuroblastoma. Lancet, 369(9579), pp.2106–2120.

Maris, J.M., 2010. Recent advances in neuroblastoma. The New England journal of medicine, 362(23), pp.2202–2211.

Matejuk, A. et al., 2013. MicroRNAs and Tumor Vasculature Normalization: Impact on Anti-Tumor Immune Response. Archivum immunologiae et therapiae experimentalis.

Meseguer, S. et al., 2011. MicroRNAs-10a and -10b contribute to retinoic acid-induced differentiation of neuroblastoma cells and target the alternative splicing regulatory factor SFRS1 (SF2/ASF). The Journal of biological chemistry, 286(6), pp.4150–4164.

Mestdagh, P, Fredlund, E., Pattyn, F., Rihani, A., et al., 2010. An integrative genomics screen uncovers ncRNA T-UCR functions in neuroblastoma tumours. Oncogene, 29(24), pp.3583–3592.

Mestdagh, P, Fredlund, E., Pattyn, F., Schulte, J.H., et al., 2010. MYCN/c-MYC-induced microRNAs repress coding gene networks associated with poor outcome in MYCN/c-MYC-activated tumors. Oncogene, 29(9), pp.1394–1404.

Mestdagh, P. et al., 2011. The microRNA body map: dissecting microRNA function through integrative genomics. Nucleic acids research, 39(20), p.e136.

Mestdagh, Pieter et al., 2010. The miR-17-92 microRNA cluster regulates multiple components of the TGF-β pathway in neuroblastoma. Molecular cell, 40(5), pp.762–773.

Mossé, Y.P. et al., 2008. Identification of ALK as a major familial neuroblastoma predisposition gene. Nature, 455(7215), pp.930–935.

Nakagawa, T. et al., 2013. Large noncoding RNA HOTAIR enhances aggressive biological behavior and is associated with short disease-free survival in human non-small cell lung cancer. Biochemical and biophysical research communications, 436(2), pp.319–324.

Nickerson, H.J. et al., 2000. Favorable biology and outcome of stage IV-S neuroblastoma with supportive care or minimal therapy: a Children's Cancer Group study. Journal of clinical oncology: official journal of the American Society of Clinical Oncology, 18(3), pp.477–486.

Pan, H.-W., Li, S.-C. & Tsai, K.-W., 2013. MicroRNA dysregulation in gastric cancer. Current pharmaceutical design, 19(7), pp.1273–1284.

Papaconstantinou, I. et al., 2013. The role of variations within microRNA in inflammatory bowel disease. European journal of gastroenterology & hepatology, 25(4), pp.399–403.

Parsons, D.W. et al., 2011. The genetic landscape of the childhood cancer medulloblastoma. Science (New York, N.Y.), 331(6016), pp.435–439.

Perez, C.A. et al., 2000. Biologic variables in the outcome of stages I and II neuroblastoma treated with surgery as primary therapy: a children's cancer group study. Journal of clinical oncology: official journal of the American Society of Clinical Oncology, 18(1), pp.18–26.

Plantaz, D. et al., 2001. Comparative genomic hybridization (CGH) analysis of stage 4 neuroblastoma reveals high frequency of 11q deletion in tumors lacking MYCN amplification. International journal of cancer. Journal international du cancer, 91(5), pp.680–686.

Pogribny, I.P. & Beland, F.A., 2013. Role of microRNAs in the regulation of drug metabolism and disposition genes in diabetes and liver disease. Expert opinion on drug metabolism & toxicology, 9(6), pp.713–724.

Reis, S.T. et al., 2012. miR-21 may acts as an oncomir by targeting RECK, a matrix metalloproteinase regulator, in prostate cancer. BMC urology, 12, p.14.

Ren, S., Wang, F., et al., 2013. Long non-coding RNA metastasis associated in lung adenocarcinoma transcript 1 derived miniRNA as a novel plasma-based biomarker for diagnosing prostate cancer. European journal of cancer (Oxford, England: 1990).

Ren, S., Liu, Y., et al., 2013. Long Noncoding RNA MALAT-1 is a New Potential Therapeutic Target for Castration-Resistant Prostate Cancer. The Journal of urology.

Ryan, J. et al., 2012. MicroRNA-204 increases sensitivity of neuroblastoma cells to cisplatin and is associated with a favourable clinical outcome. British journal of cancer, 107(6), pp.967–976.

Schulte, J.H., Schowe, B., et al., 2010. Accurate prediction of neuroblastoma outcome based on miRNA expression profiles. International journal of cancer. Journal international du cancer, 127(10), pp.2374–2385.

Schulte, J.H., Marschall, T., et al., 2010. Deep sequencing reveals differential expression of microRNAs in favorable versus unfavorable neuroblastoma. Nucleic acids research, 38(17), pp.5919–5928.

Schulte, J.H. et al., 2008. MYCN regulates oncogenic MicroRNAs in neuroblastoma. International journal of cancer. Journal international du cancer, 122(3), pp.699–704.

Schwab, M. et al., 2003. Neuroblastoma: biology and molecular and chromosomal pathology. The lancet oncology, 4(8), pp.472–480.

Shen, N. et al., 2012. MicroRNAs--novel regulators of systemic lupus erythematosus pathogenesis. Nature reviews. Rheumatology, 8(12), pp.701–709.

Shimada, H. et al., 1984. Histopathologic prognostic factors in neuroblastic tumors: definition of subtypes of ganglioneuroblastoma and an age-linked classification of neuroblastomas. Journal of the National Cancer Institute, 73(2), pp.405–416.

Smith, M.A. et al., 2010. Outcomes for children and adolescents with cancer: challenges for the twenty-first century. Journal of clinical oncology: official journal of the American Society of Clinical Oncology, 28(15), pp.2625–2634.

Taft, R.J. et al., 2010. Non-coding RNAs: regulators of disease. The Journal of pathology, 220(2), pp.126–139.

Tang, L. et al., 2013. Long Noncoding RNA HOTAIR Is Associated with Motility, Invasion, and Metastatic Potential of Metastatic Melanoma. BioMed research international, 2013, p.251098.

Thounaojam, M.C., Kaushik, D.K. & Basu, A., 2013. MicroRNAs in the brain: it's regulatory role in neuroinflammation. Molecular neurobiology, 47(3), pp.1034–1044.

Volders, P.-J. et al., 2013. LNCipedia: a database for annotated human lncRNA transcript sequences and structures. Nucleic acids research, 41(Database issue), pp.D246–251.

Wei, J.S. et al., 2009. microRNA profiling identifies cancer-specific and prognostic signatures in pediatric malignancies. Clinical cancer research: an official journal of the American Association for Cancer Research, 15(17), pp.5560–5568.

Wei, J.S. et al., 2008. The MYCN oncogene is a direct target of miR-34a. Oncogene, 27(39), pp.5204–5213.

Weinstein, J.L., Katzenstein, H.M. & Cohn, S.L., 2003. Advances in the diagnosis and treatment of neuroblastoma. The oncologist, 8(3), pp.278–292.

Welch, C., Chen, Y. & Stallings, R.L., 2007. MicroRNA-34a functions as a potential tumor suppressor by inducing apoptosis in neuroblastoma cells. Oncogene, 26(34), pp.5017–5022.

White, P.S. et al., 1995. A region of consistent deletion in neuroblastoma maps within human chromosome 1p36.2-36.3. Proceedings of the National Academy of Sciences of the United States of America, 92(12), pp.5520–5524.

Wilson, R. et al., 2009. Does RNA interference provide new hope for control of chronic hepatitis B infection? Antiviral therapy, 14(7), pp.879–889.

Xu, Z.-Y. et al., 2013. Knockdown of Long Non-coding RNA HOTAIR Suppresses Tumor Invasion and Reverses Epithelial-mesenchymal Transition in Gastric Cancer. International journal of biological sciences, 9(6), pp.587–597.

Yamamoto, K. et al., 1998. Spontaneous regression of localized neuroblastoma detected by mass screening. Journal of clinical oncology: official journal of the American Society of Clinical Oncology, 16(4), pp.1265–1269.

Ying, L. et al., 2012. Upregulated MALAT-1 contributes to bladder cancer cell migration by inducing epithelial-to-mesenchymal transition. Molecular bioSystems, 8(9), pp.2289–2294.

Zhang, H. et al., 2013. Long non-coding RNA: a new player in cancer. Journal of hematology & oncology, 6(1), p.37.

Zhang, L. et al., 2013. Epigenetic activation of the MiR-200 family contributes to H19-mediated metastasis suppression in hepatocellular carcinoma. Carcinogenesis, 34(3), pp.577–586.

Zhou, J. et al., 2013. miR-206 is down-regulated in breast cancer and inhibits cell proliferation through the up-regulation of cyclinD2. Biochemical and biophysical research communications, 433(2), pp.207–212.

The Clinical Significance and Biology of Thymidine Kinase 1

Melissa M. Alegre
Microbiology and Molecular Biology
Brigham Young University, USA

Richard A. Robison
Microbiology and Molecular Biology
Brigham Young University, USA

Kim L. O'Neill
Microbiology and Molecular Biology
Brigham Young University, USA

1   Introduction

Cancer is a complex disease and remains the second leading cause of death overall (Siegel *et al.*, 2013). Our knowledge of the biochemical pathways that contribute to malignancy is ever increasing. As we understand more cancer biology, we also identify relevant clinical indicators of malignancy called biomarkers. One class of biomarkers of particular note have been proliferation markers including thymidine kinase 1 (TK1), Ki-67, and proliferating cell nuclear antigen (PCNA). Ki-67 is the most prominent and widely used proliferation marker, although its relevance is limited to immunohistochemical assessment (Dowsett *et al.*, 2011). However, several studies indicate that TK1 may be a more accurate proliferation marker than either Ki-67 or PCNA in non-small cell, breast, and colorectal carcinomas (He *et al.*, 2004; Mao *et al.*, 2005; Mao *et al.*, 2002; Wu *et al.*, 2000). In addition to TK1's potential as a histological biomarker, TK1 is useful as a diagnostic and prognostic serological biomarker. In recent years, TK1 has also been used as an imaging tool in positron emission tomography (PET). The diversity of TK1's clinical applications and its apparent advantage over other proliferation markers warrants a closer look into its biology and clinical relevance. In fact, experts have estimated that "in the next 5-10 years [2013-2018] it may be presumed that thymidine kinase will become a part of the recommended procedures for follow-up in most haematological malignancies and in solid tumors" (Topolcan & Holubec, 2008). As a result, this review seeks to highlight these recent advances which have propelled TK1 forward into clinical view.

2   Biology of TK1

2.1   TK1 and TK2 Isoforms

There are two isoenzymes of thymidine kinase: TK1 and TK2. Initially TK1 was identified as TK-fetal while TK2 was identified as TK-adult due to their prevalence in fetal or adult tissue, respectively (Madec *et al.*, 1988; Munch-Petersen, 1990). TK1 (TK-fetal) was overexpressed in fetal tissue as well as several types of tumors, including breast, colon, lung, and a variety of haematological malignancies (Catalano *et al.*, 1989; De Blasio *et al.*, 1990; Madec *et al.*, 1988; Munch-Petersen, 1990; Musto *et al.*, 1989; Weber *et al.*, 1990). TK2 (TK-adult) was found at stable levels in adult tissues and did not fluctuate with the cell cycle (He *et al.*, 1991). This is primarily because TK2 is directed to the mitochondria by a 40 amino acid leader sequence, and is responsible for maintaining dTTP pools in the mitochondria, independent of the cell cycle (Saada *et al.*, 2001; Wang & Eriksson, 2000). Apart from their basic function of maintaining dTTP pools, TK1 and TK2 vary considerably in their basic biology and their relationship to disease. Since TK2 does not play a prominent role in malignancy and is thoroughly reviewed elsewhere, the remainder of this review will focus on TK1 (Munch-Petersen, 2010; Priego *et al.*, 2012).

2.2   TK1 Function

During DNA synthesis, nucleotides are either synthesized de novo or through the salvage pathway where they are recycled from intracellular and extracellular sources. TK1 is one of two major salvage pathway kinases responsible for maintaining the cellular nucleotide pool (Reichard, 1988). TK1 is primarily responsible for the phosphorylation of deoxythymidine (dT). Its product, dTMP, is then subsequently phosphorylated and incorporated into the DNA as deoxythymidine triphosphate (dTTP) (Reichard, 1988). Expectedly, dTTP helps to regulate this process as it inhibits TK1, the rate-limiting step of this process (He,

Q. *et al.*, 2002; Munch-Petersen, 2009). Deoxycytidine kinase (dCK) is another salvage pathway kinase which primarily phosphorylates deoxycytidine in addition to deoxyadenosine and deoxyguanosine (Bohman & Eriksson, 1988; Reichard, 1988; Sarup & Fridland, 1987). In 2012, Austin *et al.* demonstrated that TK1 can help counteract dCK inactivation and restore deoxycytidine triphosphate (dCTP) levels, illustrating the complex and possibly redundant role of TK1 in maintaining the nucleotide pool balance (Austin *et al.*, 2012). Although adenosine triphosphate (ATP) and dT are the primary substrates of TK1, several thymidine analogs such as 3'-azido-2',3'dideoxythymidine (AZT), 3'-fluoro-2',3'dideoxythymidine (FLT) have also been utilized as TK1 substrates in clinical applications. One major advantage of AZT and FLT is the lack of confounding phosphorylation by TK2. Munch-Petersen et al. demonstrated that TK2 does not phosphorylate FLT and has a very poor capacity to phosphorylate AZT compared to its typical dT substrate (Eriksson *et al.*, 1991; Munch-Petersen *et al.*, 1991). The clinical applications of these substrates will be discussed in more depth in 3.1 TK1 Methods of Detection and 3.7 TK1 Imaging-Positron Emission Tomography (PET).

Under normal proliferating conditions, TK1 is regulated by the cell cycle (Kauffman & Kelly, 1991). TK1 levels are very low or barely detectable during G_1 phase and begin to increase during late G_1 phase (Wang *et al.*, 2001). TK1 levels peak during S phase at concentrations near 200 nM, at least 10-fold higher than levels during G_1 phase (Kauffman & Kelly, 1991; Munch-Petersen *et al.*, 1993; Mutahir *et al.*, 2013; Sherley & Kelly, 1988). Interestingly, Sherley *et al.* reported that under normal conditions, TK1 mRNA only increased 3-fold or less, compared to the 15-fold increase in protein levels, during the cell cycle (Sherley & Kelly, 1988). They also determined that the rate of [^{35}S] incorporation during S phase was 12-fold more efficient than during the G_1 phase (Sherley & Kelly, 1988). Indicating that the rapid increase in TK1 levels during S phase was a result of an increase in the efficiency of TK1 translation, rather than an increase in transcription. This finding is particularly interesting in light of a study by Chou et al. in which a 5'-untranslated region (5'UTR) allowed translation of TK1 mRNA to be cap-independent (Chou & Chang, 2001). Munch-Peterson et al. has since demonstrated that this rapid increase in TK1 is also a result of conversion from an inactive dimeric to the active tetrameric TK1 form (Munch-Petersen, 2010). On the other hand, Kauffman et al. reported that the rapid decrease in TK1 levels during the G_2 phase is primarily a result c-terminal dependent degradation (Kauffman & Kelly, 1991).

Closely associated with TK1's role in maintaining nucleotide pool balance throughout the cell cycle, is its role in DNA repair. Several studies confirm that TK1 levels increase as a result of DNA damage, especially following irradiation or chemotherapy (Chen, Eriksson, *et al.*, 2010; Haveman *et al.*, 2006; Kreder *et al.*, 2002). In 2010, Chen *et al.* further characterized the connection between TK1 and DNA damage by showing p53$^{-/-}$ tumor cells increased TK1 levels in response to DNA damage while p53 wildtype tumor cells did not (Chen, Eriksson, *et al.*, 2010). This connection between TK1 and p53 has been corroborated in other studies which report normal p53 function is required to maintain cell cycle dependent regulation of TK1, and upon p53 loss, there is a compensatory increase in TK1 (Radivoyevitch *et al.*, 2012; Schwartz *et al.*, 2004). Closer analysis of this connection revealed that the increase in TK1 levels following DNA damage is dependent on p21 (Chen, Eriksson, *et al.*, 2010). In fact, Huang *et al.* showed that the c-terminal domain of p21 interacts with TK1 and overexpression of TK1 prevents p21-dependent growth suppression (Huang & Chang, 2001). These results challenged the traditional role of TK1 in tumor cells. For example, Chen et al. determined that TK1 knockdown did not affect the growth of tumor cells, even though the levels of dTTP significantly decreased (p<0.01) (Chen, Eriksson, *et al.*, 2010). Their results support the conclusion that the primary role of TK1 in tumor cells is DNA repair rather than to provide sufficient dTTP levels for replication and growth. This conclusion is supported by several other studies which have shown that functional TK1, resulting in increased dTTP levels, is essential for DNA repair in tumor cells following treatment with an alkylating agent or radiation (al-Nabulsi *et al.*, 1994; Jeong *et al.*, 2004; McKenna *et al.*, 1985; Wakazono *et al.*, 1996). In this way, TK1 operates as a mechanism of resistance which promotes tumor cell survival.

Another surprising and obscure function of TK1 is its possible connection to the immune system. In an effort to understand the biological significance of TK1, Dobrovolsky *et al.* created TK1 knockout (TK $^{-/-}$) mice (Dobrovolsky *et al.*, 2003). These mice exhibited kidney abnormalities including sclerosis of kidney glomeruli, serous secretion by the salivary gland instead of mucous secretion, a significant decrease in splenic lymphocytes, abnormal lymphoid structure of the spleen, and occasional inflammation of the arteries (Dobrovolsky *et al.*, 2003). Given TK1's connection to proliferation, the cells most likely to be affected in TK1 knockout mice would be rapidly dividing cells or fetal cells. Interestingly, this was not the case, as the most pronounced changes were found in the kidney and salivary glands (Dobrovolsky *et al.*, 2003). The kidney abnormalities coincide with a report by Zaharevitz et al. indicating that mouse kidney cells preferentially rely on the nucleotide salvage pathway over de novo synthesis (Zaharevitz *et al.*, 1992). Similarly, Luo *et al.* reported that TK1 activity was 3-fold higher in normal human kidney cells compared to renal cell carcinoma (Luo *et al.*, 2009; Luo *et al.*, 2010). To date, this is the only human tissue in which TK1 is overexpressed in normal tissue compared to malignant tissue. Unfortunately, the mechanisms behind the TK1 knockout mice's kidney and salivary gland abnormalities are not understood, nor are the kidney's preferential use of the salvage pathway. On the other hand, the remaining phenotypic changes of the TK1 knockout mice indicate an attenuated or dysfunctional immune system (Dobrovolsky *et al.*, 2003). In particular, the cause of the significant decrease in splenic lymphocytes is not known but could be a result of either failure to activate or improper maturation (Dobrovolsky *et al.*, 2003). There is recent evidence that TK1 is overexpressed during hematopoiesis in normal human bone marrow indicating a potential role of TK1 in the maturation of lymphocytes (Alegre *et al.*, 2013). TK1 may also play a role in autoimmunological diseases, especially of the thyroid (Karbownik *et al.*, 2003; Schwartz *et al.*, 2004). In 2003, Karbownik *et al.* reported TK1 expression was 2-fold higher in leukocytes from patients with Hashimoto's and Graves' disease compared to healthy controls (Karbownik *et al.*, 2003). Although the connection between TK1 and the immune system is largely unexplored, it seems clear that it plays a significant role in maintaining normal immune function.

Overall, the biochemical role of TK1 is clear. In normal cells, TK1 is responsible for maintaining the dTTP nucleotide pool in a cell cycle-dependent manner. Additionally, TK1 plays an invaluable role in DNA repair and survival of tumor cells following DNA damage. The biological significance of TK1 is less understood and somewhat puzzling. Normal TK1 function is essential for proper development and function of the kidney and salivary gland although these mechanisms are not understood (Dobrovolsky *et al.*, 2003). TK1 also appears to be necessary for the normal function of the immune system and may play a role in its deregulation. Another unexplored and puzzling function of TK1 is its role in the circulatory system of cancer patients. TK1 is well-known for its elevation in the serum of cancer patients, which will be discussed in detail later. However, the mechanism by which TK1 enters the serum and its function in the serum has been largely unexplored. Perhaps, its function in the serum is connected to regulating the immune system. Further analyses are needed to understand this connection and its significance.

2.3   TK1 Structure

Human TK1 (hTK1) as a monomer, in its most basic structure, is 234 amino acids in length with a molecular weight of 25.5 kDa (Bradshaw & Deininger, 1984). TK1 adopts a variety of oligomeric forms although it is most commonly found as a dimer or tetramer, approximately 53 kDa and 100 kDa respectively (Munch-Petersen, 2009). In 1993, Munch-Petersen reported that the TK1 dimer was the low-efficiency form of the enzyme with a high Km (15 µM). On the other hand, the TK1 tetramer was a high-efficiency form with a low Km (0.7 µM) and was reported to have 30-fold increased efficiency compared to the dimer in catalyzing its phosphoryl transfer reaction (Munch-Petersen, 2009).

The crystallization of TK1 indicates that the tetrameric form is composed of a dimer of dimers (Segura-Pena, Lutz, *et al.*, 2007). As such, there are two distinct monomer-monomer interfaces labeled strong and weak. The weak interface is primarily stabilized indirectly by ATP, the donor molecule, while the strong interface is stabilized directly through many polar interactions (Segura-Pena, Lutz, *et al.*, 2007). Each monomeric subunit consists of an α/β-domain which is most similar to DNA binding proteins including RecA (Welin *et al.*, 2004). As TK1 catalyzes the conversion of dT to dTMP, the overall structure remains unaltered although Welin *et al.* reported two regions which do change conformation, the P loop and Lasso loop (Segura-Pena, Lichter, *et al.*, 2007; Welin *et al.*, 2004). These conformational changes occur independently and are only dependent on their respective substrates (Segura-Pena, Lichter, *et al.*, 2007). The P loop or flexible loop consists of residues Gly26-Ser33 in hTK1 and is where the phosphate donor, typically ATP, is held (Figure 1) (Birringer *et al.*, 2005; Welin *et al.*, 2004). When ATP binds, this P loop becomes rigid and forms an ordered β-hairpin structure (Segura-Pena, Lichter, *et al.*, 2007). An essential element of the P loop and ATP binding is stabilization by a magnesium ion (Segura-Pena, Lutz, *et al.*, 2007). This magnesium ion is surrounded by two phosphate groups of ATP, three water molecules, and a threonine residue (Segura-Pena, Lutz, *et al.*, 2007; Welin *et al.*, 2004).

```
              *   *      #                                    #
  1 mscinlptvl pgspsktrgq iqvilgpmfs gkstelmrrv rrfqiaqykc lvikyakdtr
                                             #     *
 61 ysssfcthdr ntmealpacl lrdvaqealg vavigidegq ffpdivefce amanagktvi
                                               #
121 vaaldgtfqr kpfgailnlv plaesvvklt avcmecfrea aytkrlgtek eveviggadk
181 yhsvcrlcyf kkasgqpagp dnkencpvpg kpgeavaark lfapqqilqc span
```

Figure 1: Human TK1 Structural Regions. The P loop (green) of human TK1, where ATP typically binds, consists of residues Gly26-Ser33. The lasso loop (red), where dT typically binds, consists of residues Leu166-Lys180. The Zinc binding motif (yellow) is located between Thr150-Lys191 and is stabilized by cysteines 153, 156, 185, and 188. During the phosphorylation reaction, the lasso loop stabilizes dT in a hydrophobic pocket (*) which consists of Leu24, Met28, and Phe101. The C5 of dT is bound by Thr163 (#), Glu98 (#) accepts a proton from 5'OH of dT while Lys32 (#) transfers a phosphate group to dT. The transitional state between dT and dTMP is stabilized by Arg60 (#).

On the other hand, the lasso loop consists of residues Leu166-Lys180 and is where the phosphate acceptor molecule, typically dT, is found (Welin *et al.*, 2004). Similar to the P loop, the binding of dT to the lasso loop is closely associated with a metal ion, zinc (Birringer *et al.*, 2005). This zinc-binding motif is located between residues Thr150-Lys191, and is held in place by four cysteines at residues 153, 156, 185, and 188 (Figure 1) (Birringer *et al.*, 2005). This situates zinc within 20 Å of the active site, highlighting its crucial role in TK1's phosphoryl transfer reaction (Welin *et al.*, 2004). The pivotal role of zinc is confirmed by Ishikawa et al. who reported that TK1 expression in rats fed a low-zinc diet was reduced by 50% and the percentage of cells in S phase was significantly reduced compared to controls (Ishikawa *et al.*, 2008). The actual phosphorylation reaction of TK1 requires coordination from several different residues (Figure 1). The lasso loop stabilizes dT in a hydrophobic pocket by Met28, Phe101, and Leu24, while the C5 of dT makes contact with Thr163 (Birringer *et al.*, 2005). Glu98 acts as a base which accepts a proton from the 5'OH of dT while Lys32 of the P loop transfers a phosphate group to this 5'OH of dT (Birringer *et al.*, 2005; Segura-Pena, Lutz, *et al.*, 2007). The transitional state during the conversion of dT to dTMP is stabilized by Arg60 (Welin *et al.*, 2004). The remarkable and unique component of TK1's reaction is that the backbone of the protein is involved in this reaction, rather than the side chains (Birringer *et al.*, 2005). This enables hTK1 to limit its substrates to ensure greater specificity unlike the herpes simplex virus TK which has a broad range of substrates and primarily uses side chains to catalyze its reaction (Birringer *et al.*, 2005).

In addition to inducing a conformational change at the monomeric level, ATP binding induces reversible TK1 tetramerization (Munch-Petersen *et al.*, 1993). In the presence of ATP, TK1 switches from a dimer to a tetramer (Kuroiwa *et al.*, 2000; Munch-Petersen *et al.*, 1993). In 2009, Munch-Petersen determined that this TK1 regulatory switch between the dimer and tetramer could occur with ATP, UTP, GTP or CTP indicating that the sugar and base were not involved in tetramerization, rather only the phosphate group was essential (Munch-Petersen, 2009). Although any of these nucleotides were sufficient to induce tetramerization, only ATP could act as a phosphate donor, indicating that ATP-dependent tetramerization and phosphorylation of dT are independent events (Munch-Petersen, 2009). In 2006, Zhu *et al.* reported that deletion of the c-terminal of TK1 did not effect this ATP-dependent tetramerization (Zhu *et al.*, 2006). On the other hand, Li *et al.* determined that serine-13 phosphorylation of TK1 disrupted ATP-induced tetramerization, (Li *et al.*, 2004). Additionally, Mutahir *et al.* demonstrated how the weak dimer interface is involved in this ATP-dependent regulatory switch. For example, they reported that this interface was composed of two antiparallel α1 helices in which there was only 7.5 Å separating the two dimers at the residues Phe29 and Ile45 (Mutahir *et al.*, 2013). A study by Segura-Pena *et al.* supported this conclusion in that two additional cysteine residues within the α1 helix, at the weak dimer interface, locked TK1 in the tetramer form (Segura-Pena, Lichter, *et al.*, 2007). In addition to causing tertiary structural changes, the binding of ATP can also induce the transformation of a closed, inactive tetramer to an open, catalytically active tetramer (Segura-Pena, Lichter, *et al.*, 2007). Sengura-Pena *et al.* reported that during this transformation, the weak dimer interface expands by almost 10% and rotates by 11 degrees (Segura-Pena, Lichter, *et al.*, 2007).

Interestingly, ATP is not the only mechanism by which this regulatory switch can be activated. In 2009, Munch-Petersen reported that the concentration of TK1 can also induce a dimer to tetramer switch, at concentrations higher than 0.2 mg/ml, regardless of ATP (Munch-Petersen, 2009). This confirms results by Birringer *et al.* who demonstrated that recombinant TK1 was exclusively found in the tetramer at concentrations ranging from 0.4-20 mg/ml (Birringer *et al.*, 2006). Munch-Petersen surprisingly showed TK1 remains as a tetramer at low concentrations (6μg/ml) when analyzed immediately but when the same sample was stored diluted for more than 2 weeks before analysis, TK1 existed as a dimer (Munch-Petersen, 2009). This illustrated that the dimer to tetramer switch is a very slow process which can help explain some discrepancies among other studies.

The dimer to tetramer switch of TK1 does not exist in all organisms and its study among various organisms hints at the structural evolution of TK1 (Mutahir *et al.*, 2013). In a study of the oligomeric structure of TK1 among ten organisms, Mutahir et al. determined that TK1 was only found as a dimer in bacteria, plant, and *Dictyostelium* while all vertebrates and *C. elegans* had tetrameric TK1. Therefore, they deduced that the origin of the TK1 tetramer occurred after the split between the animal and *Dictyostelium* lineages (Mutahir *et al.*, 2013). Furthermore, the regulatory switch from the TK1 dimer to tetramer did not exist in *C. elegans* and *Danio rerio* (zebrafish) and was only fully functional in birds and mammals (Mutahir *et al.*, 2013). This indicated that although the TK1 tetramer was present in all vertebrates, the TK1 regulatory switch from the dimer to tetramer originated with the warm-blooded vertebrate lineage (Mutahir *et al.*, 2013). Further work, including the testing of TK1 from more organisms, is still needed to understand the intricate mechanisms associated with the evolution of TK1's activities.

One intriguing and challenging hurdle in TK1's journey from bench-to-bedside has been its unique structure in malignancy. Initially, Karlstrom et al. reported that the majority of serum TK1 from leukemia patients had a molecular weight of approximately 730 kDa with only a small percentage at 58 kDa (Karlstrom, 1990). On the other hand, only the 58 kDa form could be found in proliferating HeLa cells (Karlstrom, 1990). Since then, Sharif *et al.* reported this high molecular weight form could be found in CEM cells, although the majority of TK1 was found in the 40-100 kDa fraction (Sharif, Kiran Kumar, *et al.*, 2012). They also confirmed earlier reports as they found that 90% of the TK1 in human leukemia serum was in this same high molecular weight form, 300-720 kDa (Sharif, Kiran Kumar, *et al.*, 2012). This high molecular weight form has made the detection of TK1 protein levels problematic for two major reasons. First, TK1 activity and protein levels do not correlate unless reducing agents are used, which also partially reduce immunoglobulins (He *et al.*, 2005; Sharif, Kiran Kumar, *et al.*, 2012). Additionally, recombinant TK1 does not reflect the same quaternary structure as serum TK1, making it difficult to use an appropriate TK1 positive control for immunoassays. Sharif et al. suggested that methionine and tyrosine residues of TK1, in addition to 7 of TK1's 11 cysteine residues, may contribute to the high molecular weight form of serum TK1. This conclusion was supported as they demonstrated that human serum TK1was found in oligomeric structures irrespective of reducing agents (Sharif, Kiran Kumar, *et al.*, 2012). It is also unclear as to whether this TK1 high molecular weight aggregate is a homo- or hetero-oligomer, indicating the possible existence of a protein binding partner.

Overall it can be seen that the structure of TK1 influences not only its function, but also its regulation and detection. A thorough understanding of the secondary structures and residues involved in TK1's phosphoryl transfer reaction enable us to design clinically relevant substrates such as AZT and FLT. TK1's structure can also help us design TK1 inhibitors which may re-sensitize otherwise resistant tumors. Additionally, a sound understanding of the structure of TK1 in malignancy will ultimately lead us to develop better methods of detection which could be used in the clinic. Finally, the structure of TK1 is particularly informative and essential in understanding the regulation of TK1 since post-translational modifications play a major role in its mechanism of control.

2.4   TK1 Mechanisms of control

TK1 is tightly regulated by the cell cycle. TK1 is found at very low levels in G_1 phase, peaks during S phase, and is degraded during late G_2/M phase (Kauffman & Kelly, 1991; Sherley & Kelly, 1988; Wang *et al.*, 2001). Phosphorylation is one common cell cycle mechanism which targets proteins for Skp, Cullin, F-box containing complex (SCF)-mediated degradation (Harper, 2002). Initially, Chang *et al.* reported that TK1 was heavily phosphorylated in rapidly dividing cells and partially hypo-phosphorylated in M phase-arrested cells, which suggested phosphorylation may play a role in TK1 regulation (Chang *et al.*, 1994; He *et al.*, 1996; Lin *et al.*, 2003). Additionally, Ke *et al.* demonstrated that phosphorylation of serine-13 targets TK1 for SCF-mediated degradation in yeast (Ke *et al.*, 2003). However, Ke *et al.* later determined that the APC/C-Cdh1 pathway is responsible for TK1 degradation in mammalian cells, not the SCF complex (Ke & Chang, 2004). This indicates that the cell cycle-dependent phosphorylation does not play a role in TK1 degradation (Ke & Chang, 2004). This APC/C-mediated degradation of TK1 explains the very low levels of TK1 at the beginning of the cell cycle, but it does not explain the rapid increase proceeding S phase. Munch-Petersen et al. has demonstrated that this rapid increase is mediated in part by the TK1 regulatory switch from an inactive dimer to an active tetramer (Munch-Petersen, 2009; Munch-Petersen *et al.*, 1995; Munch-Petersen *et al.*, 1993). During G_0 and G_1 phases, TK1 exists as a dimer with estimated concentrations at 0.03-0.09 µg/ml, much lower than the concentration which induces a dimer to tetramer switch (Munch-Petersen *et al.*, 1995; Munch-Petersen *et al.*, 1993). On the other hand, TK1 exists as a tetramer during S phase with estimated concentrations at 4-6 µg/ml (160-240 nM) (Munch-Petersen *et al.*, 1995; Munch-Petersen *et al.*, 1993). This transition is likely regulated by TK1 concentration during G_1 phase (since the concentration is so low), and ATP-dependent tetramerization is responsible for the increased TK1 activity during S phase (Munch-Petersen *et al.*, 1995). Interestingly, phosphorylation in rapidly dividing cells appears to play a role in this dimer to tetramer transition as well, rather than as a target for degradation (Li *et al.*, 2004). Li et al. demonstrated that serine-13 phosphorylation disrupts ATP-dependent tetramerization, and as a result, TK1 is preferentially found as an inactive dimer (Li *et al.*, 2004). Since cdc2 kinase phosphorylates serine-13 of TK1 during G_2/M phase, phosphorylation helps to regulate the tetramer to dimer switch and thus decrease TK1 activity following S phase (Chang *et al.*, 1998; Chang *et al.*, 1994).

Protein degradation plays an important role in maintaining appropriate levels of TK1 throughout the cell cycle, as briefly discussed previously. Closely associated with protein degradation is the half-life of TK1. Zhu et al. reported that a 44 amino acid deletion of TK1's c-terminus increased its half-life to 500 minutes, compared to 83 minutes for wild-type TK1 (Zhu *et al.*, 2006). This increased stability illustrated the crucial role of the c-terminus in TK1degradation. Similarly, Demeter et al. reported the half-life of TK1 from normal ovarian epithelial cells was 82 minutes compared to 36 minutes for that of malignant ovarian cells (Demeter *et al.*, 2001). Posch et al. showed that the unstable, decreased half-life (<60 minutes) of TK1 can also be a result of mutation of the binding sites for ATP or dT (Posch *et al.*, 2000). Although this may explain the decreased half-life in malignancy, these mutant TK1s did not increase with proliferation (Posch *et al.*, 2000). Further work is needed to understand the mechanism by which TK1 activity is increased in malignancy since it appears to be unstable in cancer cells compared to that in wildtype cells.

Under normal conditions, TK1 is polyubiquitinylated during the G_2/M phase which targets it for degradation by the APC/C pathway (Ke & Chang, 2004). Additionally, Ke et al. demonstrated that Cdh1 mutant inhibited TK1 degradation whereas a Cdc20 mutant had no significant effect on TK1 degradation, indicating that TK1 is degraded by the APC/C-Cdh1 complex (Ke & Chang, 2004). Cdh1 is the rate-limiting step for this degradation, as it binds to the KEN box (residues 203-205 of the c-terminal end of TK1) (Ke & Chang, 2004). This degradation process does not occur when dT is bound to TK1 (Ke *et al.*, 2007). In addition to acting as a control mechanism for degradation, dT-bound TK1 also reverses Cdh1-mediated expression of TK1(Ke *et al.*, 2007).

In addition to post-translational modifications such as ubiquitination or phosphorylation, TK1 is also subject to transcriptional regulation. The promoter region of TK1is suppressed by a G-quadruplex motif located between -13 and +8 relative to the transcription start site (Basundra *et al.*, 2010). Although this region controls TK1 expression generally, TK1's promoter also has regions responsible for cell cycle-dependent TK1 expression. For instance, initially the promoter region of TK1 (-441 to -63 relative to the transcriptional start site) was identified as the region responsible for cell cycle regulation (Kim, Y. K. et al., 1988). Subsequent analysis by Kim et al. determined that the minimum fragment which conferred cell cycle regulation was a 70 bp region between -133 and -64 which was named the cell cycle regulatory unit (CCRU) (Kim & Lee, 1991). Within this region, an inverted CCAAT sequence and one G-C rich motif were found between -84 and -64 (Kim & Lee, 1992). Kim et al. determined that without this 20 bp region, -84 to -64, the level of transcription dropped to barely detectable levels, indicating that this region acts as an enhancer element (Kim & Lee, 1992). Therefore, even though the actual cell cycle control element is found between -133 and -84, the enhancer element from -84 to -64 is also required for proper expression (Kim & Lee, 1992). Yi binding factor is known to regulate cell cycle-dependent TK1 expression in mice by binding to the Yi consensus sequence during late G_1/S phase (Dou et al., 1991). Similarly, a Yi-related sequence was identified in the human TK1 promoter between -109 and -84, which is important for cell cycle-dependent TK1 expression (Kim & Lee, 1992). Li et al. also determined that cyclin A and p33[cdk2] complexes were constitutively associated with this site, -109 to -84 (Kim et al., 1996; Li et al., 1993). Additionally the binding activity of the cyclin A/p107 complex was increased throughout the S phase and correlated to an increase in TK1 mRNA levels (Li et al., 1993). Another protein which is associated with cell cycle-dependent TK1 expression is CCAAT binding protein for TK gene (CBP/tk) (Pang & Chen, 1993). This protein binds to the CCAAT sequence located from -91 to -64 of the TK1 promoter, which is known to contribute to promoter strength (Good et al., 1995; Lipson et al., 1995; Mao, X. et al., 1995; Pang & Chen, 1993). NF-Y binding to the TK1 promoter is responsible for recruiting CBP/tk to the CCAAT sequence and Sp1 to the region -118 to -113 (Chang et al., 1999; Chang & Liu, 1994). The transcription and post-translational control of TK1 play an important role in maintaining normal TK1 function in a cell. It is through the deregulation of this process, that we begin to see its unregulated elevation in malignancy.

3   TK1 in Malignancy

TK1 has diagnostic, prognostic and therapeutic potential in malignancy. This is true for both TK1 found in the serum (sTK1) as well as TK1 expressed in tumor tissue. An understanding of TK1's various methods of detection is critical to understanding sTK1 diagnostic and prognostic potential.

3.1   TK1 Methods of Detection

The unique structure of sTK1, found in its high molecular weight form (300-720 kDa), has been a major challenge in developing a clinically relevant methods of detection. Furthermore, He et al. reported a puzzling observation in which malignant serum, high in TK1, diluted with normal serum reduced both TK1 concentration and activity more than expected (He et al., 2005). They also reported this same finding when malignant serum was diluted with BSA, indicating there is a factor in normal human and calf serum that destabilizes TK1 (He et al., 2005). Another puzzling and unique aspect of sTK1 is its long half-life. The half-life of TK1 is one hour in mouse EAT cells, four hours in HeLa cells, and a surprising 30 days in serum (He et al., 1991; He et al., 2000; Hengstschlager et al., 1994). The 30 day half-life of sTK1 has been confirmed for both breast cancer and gastric cancer (He et al., 2000; Zou et al., 2002). Clearly, the environment of sTK1 contributes to its unique structure and properties in ways that can't always be predicted by studying TK1 in cancer cells alone.

Consequently, the traditional method of quantifying TK1 is by measuring its activity using a radio-assay. For this assay, [^{3}H]-dT is phosphorylated using either ATP or CTP (O'Neill, K. L. *et al.*, 1986). [^{3}H]-dTMP then absorbs to ion exchange DE81 filter paper, is washed and radioactivity is measured. TK1 only utilizes ATP while TK2 utilizes both ATP and CTP, so the relative contribution of TK1 can be determined by using both ATP and CTP separately (Bristow *et al.*, 1988). In addition to these substrates, the reaction mixture varies slightly in its additives such as $MgCl_2$ and/or KCl, but a reducing agent, to break disulfide bonds, is crucial for the assay to ensure reliable, consistent results (O'Neill, K. L. *et al.*, 1986; Sharif, von Euler, *et al.*, 2012). In 2012, Sharif *et al.* optimized this traditional radioassay specifically for human sTK1 (Sharif, von Euler, *et al.*, 2012). They reported the area under the curve (AUC) was 0.94 with a sensitivity and specificity of 0.89 and 0.74 respectively (Sharif, von Euler, *et al.*, 2012). The traditional TK radioassay was commercialized and sold as a kit. Instead of [^{3}H]-dT, the kit utilizes [^{125}I]-deoxyuridine (Euler *et al.*, 2009). This same technology, slightly modified, is sold as either the radio-receptor analysis (RRA) kit (Immunotech, Czech Republic) or more commonly as the TK Prolifen assay or TK-REA (DiaSorin AB, Sweden) (Euler *et al.*, 2009; Span *et al.*, 2000; Votava *et al.*, 2007). Unfortunately, Svobodova *et al.* reported that sTK1 activity levels, using the RRA test, were significantly elevated in relatively few cases of 1087 cancer patients compared to healthy controls (Svobodova *et al.*, 2007). Despite the low cost of this test ($4/sample), these results should be interpreted with caution since they do not always reflect typical trends of TK1 in malignancy (Votava *et al.*, 2007). Today, the TK-REA kit is commonly used as a method of comparison for new ways to quantify TK1. For example, the TK-REA has been used in side-by-side comparisons with new assays especially the Liason, described later (Ohrvik *et al.*, 2004). On the other hand, the traditional, non-commercialized radioassay has been the standard method to determine TK1 activity since the late 1980's, and has also been used in several side-by-side comparisons (Luo *et al.*, 2009; McKenna *et al.*, 1988; O'Neill *et al.*, 1987; O'Neill *et al.*, 2001; O'Neill, K. L., Hoper, *et al.*, 1992; O'Neill, K. L., McKelvey, *et al.*, 1992; Robertson *et al.*, 1990; Thomas *et al.*, 1995). Unfortunately, there are several disadvantages of the traditional radioassay and TK-REA. For example, these tests are radioisotope-based, relatively expensive, time consuming, require specialized training and facilities, are relatively inconsistent, and have relatively low sensitivity (Zhang *et al.*, 2001).

Fortunately, in the late 1990's and early 2000's, anti-TK1 antibodies prompted the development of immunoassays which could be clinically applicable. TK1-specific antibodies proved problematic since TK1 is highly conserved among mammals (89-97% among humans, mice, and rabbits). Therefore, currently the only clinically robust antibodies are ones which bind the c-terminal fragment or the 24-amino acid active site called the lasso loop of TK1 (Euler & Eriksson, 2011). In 2001, Zhang *et al.* reported a TK1-specific monoclonal antibody which blocks the active site of TK1. This was later used to develop an enzyme-linked immunosorbent assay (ELISA) (Zhang *et al.*, 2001). This ELISA showed a strong correlation with the traditional radioassay and gave similar results without many of the disadvantages associated with the radioassay. The majority of clinical biomarkers today utilize a similar technique called a Sandwich ELISA. The Sandwich ELISA is highly specific and sensitive since it relies on two TK1-specific antibodies. In 2009, Carlsson *et al.* developed a Sandwich ELISA with AUC values of 0.56, 0.73, and 0.64 for postoperative, disease recurrence, and chemotherapy treated patients respectively (Carlsson *et al.*, 2009). AUC values for useful biomarkers are typically closer to 0.86 as is the case with CA 72-4, a biomarker for gastric cancer (Fernandez-Fernandez *et al.*, 1996). Unfortunately, this TK1 Sandwich ELISA has AUC values near 0.5, the value indicating the assay has no predictive power. Furthermore, the sensitivity and specificity of this assay were surprisingly low, indicating that it is not a clinically useful TK1 immunoassay (Carlsson *et al.*, 2009). As a result, no further studies have been conducted with this assay. There is still a need for a robust Sandwich ELISA which can be quickly integrated into the clinic to aid in diagnosis and prognosis of malignancy.

In order to circumvent the highly conserved nature of TK1 and make robust, high-affinity TK1 antibodies, Wu et al. developed a chicken polyclonal IgY antibody specific to the c-terminus of hTK1 (Wu *et al.*, 2003). This IgY TK1 antibody was used to develop a dot blot to quantify TK1 protein levels (TK1p) instead of TK1 activity (TK1a) (Wu *et al.*, 2003). This dot blot is highly sensitivity with the lowest detectable concentration of TK1p at 33.3 pg/ml (Wu *et al.*, 2003). In the past 10 years, this dot blot has been used in 14 studies including over 3,500 cancer patients and almost 70,000 healthy individuals (Chen *et al.*, 2011; Chen, Ying, *et al.*, 2010; Chen *et al.*, 2008; He *et al.*, 2010; He *et al.*, 2005; Kameyama *et al.*, 2011; Li *et al.*, 2005; Li *et al.*, 2010; Liu *et al.*, 2011; Pan *et al.*, 2010; Wu *et al.*, 2003; Xu *et al.*, 2008; Zhang *et al.*, 2006). In 2011, Chen *et al* reported the AUC of the dot blot for a healthy screen of 35,365 individuals was 0.96 (Chen *et al.*, 2011). They also reported that the specificity and sensitivity were 0.99 and 0.78 respectively, while only 0.8% of healthy city-dwellers had elevated sTK1 levels, which typically corresponded to pre-malignant conditions (Chen *et al.*, 2011). As of 2010, this dot blot has been commercialized, and the kit was approved by the Supervision Authority for Food and Medicine in China (Pan *et al.*, 2010). This commercialized, approved kit has been one of the biggest factors in propelling TK1 into clinical view during the past few years.

There have been several reports, including use of this commercial dot blot, which have demonstrated that TK1a and TK1p do not correlate (Kristensen *et al.*, 1994; Luo *et al.*, 2009; Sharif, Kiran Kumar, *et al.*, 2012). This has provided the rationale for some to focus on TK1a rather than TK1p. A focus on TK1a also circumvents the challenges associated with developing TK1 antibodies for immunoassays. As a result, Von Euler *et al.* developed a commercialized competitive ELISA to quantify TK1a using AZTMP antibodies (Euler *et al.*, 2009). This novel assay, currently referred to as the Liaison TK assay, simultaneously exploits the advantages of sensitivity and accuracy associated with an ELISA and negates the controversy regarding protein levels and activity. Although this assay is advantageous in that TK2 does not phosphorylate AZT, yielding no confounding TK2 activity, the Liaison TK assay has some disadvantages (Munch-Petersen *et al.*, 1991). For example, hTK1 is known to phosphorylate dT three times more efficiently than AZT (Eriksson *et al.*, 2002). Similarly, Sharif *et al.* reported that canine TK1 phosphorylated AZT three times more efficiently than hTK1 (Sharif, Kiran Kumar, *et al.*, 2012). This indicates that the Liason TK assay may be better suited for screening canine malignancies than human malignancies. In fact, many of the studies involving the Liaison TK assay have investigated canine malignancies (Euler *et al.*, 2009; Sharif, von Euler, *et al.*, 2012; Thamm *et al.*, 2012). Additionally, Ohrvik *et al.* demonstrated that the AZTMP antibodies can cross-react with endogenous antibodies in human serum (Ohrvik *et al.*, 2004). In comparison with other TK assays, the Liaison TK assay showed significant linear correlation with the TK REA (p<0.0001) (Euler *et al.*, 2009; Sharif, von Euler, *et al.*, 2012; von Euler *et al.*, 2006).

The Liaison TK assay, traditional TK assay, TK REA, and TK1 dot blot are among the most popular and well-established methods of detection for TK1. There have been a few other assays which have been developed either for commercial use or research purposes. The DiviTum kit (Biovica/Ronnerbol, Sweden) is another ELISA which measures TK activity, except it uses bromo-deoxyuridine as a substrate (Nisman *et al.*, 2013). DiviTum and Liaison TK assays are very similar although the DiviTum is a manual assay and the Liaison is automated. Nisman *et al.* demonstrated that both assays were correlated and had efficacy in predicting recurrence preoperatively in breast cancer patients (Nisman *et al.*, 2013). Similarly, the DiviTum assay is efficacious in renal cell carcinoma and non-small cell lung cancer in addition to breast cancer (Korkmaz *et al.*, 2013; Nisman, Yutkin, *et al.*, 2010). Faria *et al.* measured TK activity in hepatocellular carcinoma patients using liquid chromatography-MS/MS through the phosphorylation of FLT (Faria *et al.*, 2012). Alternatively, Tzeng *et al.* utilized capillary electrophoresis to separate and quantify dTMP following the traditional TK assay, negating the need for radioisotopes (Tzeng & Hung, 2005). On the other hand, some have developed methods to estimate protein concentrations while still circumventing the challenge of TK1 antibodies. Stalhandske et al. reported a PCR-based real-time assay in which they simultaneously measured both TK1 and dCK levels (Stalhandske *et al.*, 2013). These methods, although practical and valid, have not yet gained widespread popularity. Nevertheless, a thorough understanding of the various methods of TK1 detection, including their limits and strengths, will help shed light on potential discrepancies found as we explore the trends of TK1 in malignancy.

3.2   Serum-TK1 Diagnostic potential

Elevated sTK1in malignancy is a very early event. In 2008, Xu *et al.* reported 70% of pre-malignant cervical cancer cases were accompanied by elevated sTK1 protein levels (Xu *et al.*, 2008). Additionally, the mean age of pre-malignant cervical cancer patients was 10 years earlier, compared to cervical cancer patients (Xu *et al.*, 2008). There have been 3 large Chinese health screens which sought to determine sTK1p levels in healthy adults. In 2008, Chen *et al.* reported that in a health screen of 11,880 individuals, 0.5% had elevated sTK1p levels, using a previously determined cut off value of 2 pM (Chen *et al.*, 2008). Of the 0.5% with elevated sTK1, 83% reported malignancy-related diseases including benign or hyperplasia tissues (Chen *et al.*, 2008). Other malignancy-related diseases found to be associated with elevated sTK1p included proliferative tissue, fatty liver, inflammatory reactions and virus infections including hepatitis B. Similarly, a health screen involving 35,365 individuals revealed that 0.8% of urban-dwelling and 5.8% of oil-field workers had elevated sTK1p levels (Chen *et al.*, 2011). Of the individuals with elevated sTK1p, 8.8% developed new pre-malignancies or showed progression in existing pre-malignancies (Chen et al., 2011). Additionally, elevated sTK1p levels were associated with a 3-5 fold increased risk of developing malignancy within 5-72 months (Chen *et al.*, 2011). This was confirmed in another health screen of 8,135 individuals in which 1.1% had elevated sTK1p levels (Huang *et al.*, 2011). Huang *et al.* reported that of those with elevated sTK1p, one individual developed liver carcinoma within 13 months and five individuals showed malignancy-related disease progression within 19 months (Huang *et al.*, 2011). Overall, incidence of elevated sTK1p levels (>2pM) in healthy adults is low and is typically indicative of pre-malignant or malignancy-related diseases. sTK1 levels appear to play a valuable role in early detection of malignancy which may ultimately improve cancer mortality rates.

In addition to early detection, sTK1a and sTK1p levels are significantly elevated in a variety of haematological and solid tumors. Initially, sTK1a was studied primarily in haematological malignancies. Sharif *et al.* determined that sTK1 activity levels were significantly elevated in both chronic lymphocytic leukemia (CLL) and myelodysplastic syndrome (MDS), a type of preleukemia (Sharif, von Euler, *et al.*, 2012; Xu, W. *et al.*, 2009). In this study MDS sTK1 levels were the highest among the heamatological malignancy group (Sharif, von Euler, *et al.*, 2012). This coincides with an earlier study which reported that elevated sTK1a levels were indicative of progression of MDS into acute myeloid leukemia (AML) (Musto *et al.*, 1995). Significantly elevated sTK1a levels compared to healthy controls were also found in pre-treated acute lymphoblastic leukemia (ALL), non-Hodgkin lymphoma, and follicular lymphoma (O'Neill *et al.*, 2007; Pan *et al.*, 2010; Prochazka *et al.*, 2012). Although sTK1a levels were not initially thought to be a good indicator for solid tumors, we now know elevated sTK1 levels are significantly elevated compared to controls in virtually all solid tumors. This is true for malignant melanoma, systemic breast, preoperable primary breast, gastric, kidney, bladder, non-small cell lung (NSCLC), esophageal, cardiac, cervical, ovarian, colon, rectum, liver, head and neck, thyroid, and brain cancers, among others (Chen, Ying, et al., 2010; Elfagieh et al., 2012; Fujiwaki et al., 2001; He et al., 2005; He et al., 2000; Li et al., 2010; Liu et al., 2011; Nisman, Allweis, et al., 2010; Nisman, Yutkin, et al., 2010; Robertson et al., 1990; Thomas et al., 1995; Wu et al., 2013; Wu et al., 2003; Xu, W. et al., 2009; Zhang et al., 2006; Zou et al., 2002). Additionally, several studies have investigated whether there is a significant difference between benign and malignant tissue. He et al. reported in a study of 9 types of carcinoma tissue that sTK1 levels of pre-treated malignancy were significantly higher than either benign or noncancerous individuals (He et al., 2005). These findings, which indicate there is a significant difference in sTK1 levels in benign and malignant tissue, have been confirmed in several studies, although there is no significant difference in sTK1 levels between benign kidney and renal cell carcinoma (He et al., 2000; Nisman, Yutkin, et al., 2010; Xu et al., 2008). High sTK1 levels typically indicate a more advanced grade, stage, increased T-values, and increased tumor size (Chen, Eriksson, et al., 2010; Li et al., 2005; Li et al., 2010; Nisman, Allweis, et al., 2010). Although some studies have reported that sTK1 is associated with stage but not grade in tumors such as renal cell carcinoma, esophageal, cardiac, and bladder carcinoma (Li et al., 2010; Nisman, Yutkin, et al., 2010; Zhang et al., 2006). It is difficult to determine whether or not sTK1 levels in general correlate with grade in each of these carcinoma types, since this information was not always studied. A more thorough analysis of each cancer type is needed to determine if these results are specific to the cancer type or a result of the study's sample population. The overall trends of sTK1 levels and their early elevation among a wide variety of malignancies are clear. Over the years, many cancer biomarkers have been validated and show clinical promise. However, the unique ability of sTK1 to predict risk for malignancy months or even a year before the clinical manifestation of malignancy is an indispensable clinical tool.

3.3   Serum-TK1 Prognostic potential

In many haematological and solid tumors especially those for which sTK1 levels are significantly elevated, sTK1a and sTK1p is a prognostic factor. Responses to chemotherapy and/or surgery are often associated with sTK1 levels. For example, Zhang et al. compared preoperative sTK1p in bladder carcinoma patients with postoperative sTK1 levels at 1 week, 1, 3, and 6 months (Zhang et al., 2006). They reported sTK1p levels were 66% lower at 1 week postoperatively, reached normal levels (<2 pM) at 1month, and remained in the normal range until the study ended at 6 months (Zhang et al., 2006). Similarly, Li et al. reported in non-metastatic NSCLC patients, 1 month postoperative sTK1p levels decreased significantly by 45%, compared to preoperative sTK1 (Li et al., 2005). Conversely, they reported that sTK1p levels in metastatic NSCLC patients did not significantly change 1 month postoperative. This same trend was seen with metastatic and non-metastatic breast cancer surgery patients (He et al., 2000). Zou et al. saw the same significant decrease in postoperative sTK1 levels for gastric cancer although only sTK1p, not sTK1a, decreased (Liu et al., 2011; Zou et al., 2002).

Pre-treatment sTK1 levels have been shown to predict which patients are most likely to respond to treatment. Di Raimondo et al. demonstrated that 83% of CLL patients with complete response (CR) or partial response (PR) to fludarabine initially had sTK1a levels < 10 U/L. On the other hand, only 45% of the CLL patients with sTK1a levels ≤ 10 U/L had CR or PR, a significant difference compared to patients above this threshold (Di Raimondo et al., 2001). Alternatively, during chemotherapeutic treatment, sTK1 levels fluctuate depending on a patient's response. Robertson et al. tracked the sTK1a levels of 10 advanced breast cancer patients bimonthly during the first 6 months of their hormone therapy (Robertson et *al.*, 1990). Five patients responded positively to treatment with a resulting decline in their sTK1a levels while five patients progressed while on their treatment and showed increased sTK1a levels. Interestingly, Liu *et al.* reported no overall significant decrease in sTK1p of gastric patients after 1, 2, or 4 cycles of chemotherapy unless patients were sorted according to their response. Only those patients with either CR, PR or no recurrence had significantly decreased sTK1p levels after cycle 2 of chemotherapy, although the levels began to decline after cycle 1. The patients with either disease progression or recurrence during chemotherapy had increased sTK1p levels (Liu *et al.*, 2011). To determine what happens immediately after treatment, Pan *et al.* compared pre-treatment sTK1p levels to levels at day 1 and 28 of chemotherapy. They reported a significant increase in sTK1p levels at day 1 followed by a significant decrease correlated with response at day 28, at which time it reached normal sTK1p levels (Pan *et al.*, 2010). This peak in sTK1p during the first day after chemotherapy may be explained by TK1 being released from cancer cells as a result of cell death, which is an indication of effective treatment (Pan *et al.*, 2010). Di Raimondo *et al.* supported this conclusion as they showed sTK1a levels were correlated with those of beta2-microglobulin and lactate dehydrogenase, indicators of tumor cell turnover (Di Raimondo *et al.*, 2001). Xu *et al.* similarly reported that sTK1p levels in a variety of malignancies increased by 40-50% during the first month of treatment and subsequently decreased to normal levels (Xu *et al.*, 2008). The same trends in which sTK1a and sTK1p levels reflect response to treatment have been confirmed in many cancers including lung, esophageal, head and neck, thyroid, leukemia, and colon cancer (Chen, Ying, *et al.*, 2010; Topolcan *et al.*, 2005; Votava *et al.*, 2007).

In addition to cancer monitoring, sTK1 levels are indicative of survival. In CLL patients, high sTK1 levels were associated with a 22% survival rate compared with a 65% survival rate in patients with low sTK1 (Di Raimondo *et al.*, 2001; Fujiwaki *et al.*, 2001; Konoplev *et al.*, 2010). Similarly, in operable breast cancer patients high sTK1 is associated with shorter disease specific survival (DSS), local recurrence free survival (RFS) and distant relapse free interval (Broet *et al.*, 2001; Elfagieh *et al.*, 2012). In renal cell carcinoma and non-Hodgkin lymphoma high sTK1 indicated a lower 5-year RFS (Nisman, Yutkin, *et al.*, 2010; Pan *et al.*, 2010). Similarly, Liu *et al.* determined that monitoring sTK1 levels during the first 2 months of palliative treatment for advanced gastric cancer was more indicative of progression free survival (PFS) and RFS compared to initial baseline sTK1 (Liu *et al.*, 2011). In advanced breast cancer patients, the 5-year disease free survival (DFS) with high sTK1 was 21%, with a median of 23 months; while patients with low sTK1 had 56% DFS, with a median >30 months (Huang *et al.*, 2012). sTK1 was also able to subcategorize nonsmoldering CLL patients at risk for rapid disease progression. Hallek *et al.* reported nonsmoldering patients with high sTK1a had PFS as expected, 8 months. On the other hand, nonsmoldering patients with low sTK1a had a PFS of 49 months, more typical of smoldering CLL, which indicated that sTK1 was able to identify which nonsmoldering CLL patients were at risk for rapid progression (Hallek *et al.*, 1999).

Early detection of recurrence and elevated risk for recurrence are also associated with increased sTK1 levels. Generally, sTK1 levels are significantly higher, 50-60%, in patients with recurrent tumors compared with primary tumors (Li *et al.*, 2010; O'Neill *et al.*, 2007; Xu *et al.*, 2008). Huang *et al.* estimated that patients were 6-7 times more likely to get recurrence if sTK1p levels were high after neoadjuvant therapy (Huang *et al.*, 2012). He *et al.* also reported that 63% of breast cancer patients who recurred up to 18 months after surgery, had higher sTK1p but not elevated sTK1a (He *et al.*, 2006). In addition to indicating a risk for recurrence, sTK1 levels begin to rise months before the clinical manifestation of recurrent tumors. For example, Votava *et al.* reported that sTK1a began to elevate 1 month before a diagnosis of recurrence in childhood leukemia patients (Votava *et al.*, 2007). Svobodova *et al.* estimated that sTK1a levels increased at least 3 months before recurrence as detected by imaging methods, although the increase could be seen sometimes as early as 6 or 9 months before the clinical manifestation of recurrence (Svobodova *et al.*, 2007). Since recurrent tumors play a major role in cancer mortality, detecting recurrence through sTK1 levels several months earlier could help give clinicians an upper hand towards effective treatment.

Currently, there are nine FDA-approved cancer biomarkers including carcinoembryonic antigen (CEA), cancer antigen 15-3 (CA15-3), and cancer antigen 19-9 (CA19-9) (Rhea & Molinaro, 2011). CA15-3 is a breast cancer biomarker which is known for its poor sensitivity and specificity, but is approved for monitoring breast cancer treatment and recurrence (Rhea & Molinaro, 2011). CA15-3 and sTK1p levels were compared in breast cancer patients preoperatively and 3 months postoperatively (He *et al.*, 2006). sTK1p, but not CA15-3, was significantly increased with recurrence which indicated that sTK1 may be a better marker for breast cancer recurrence than CA15-3 (He *et al.*, 2006). Although CEA is primarily approved for colon cancer monitoring, it is also elevated in breast cancer patients (Chevinsky, 1991). Elfagieh *et al.* compared CEA, CA15-3, and sTK1 levels for breast cancer prognosis (Elfagieh *et al.*, 2012). They determined that increased levels of CEA, CA15-3, and sTK1 were found in 62%, 70%, and 78% of breast cancer patients respectively. They also reported a combined evaluation of all 3 biomarkers increased the sensitivity to 90%, which indicated that the most accurate diagnosis of breast cancer can be determined using all 3 biomarkers (Elfagieh *et al.*, 2012). In a comparison study of colon cancer, only sTK1a levels, not CEA or CA19-9 levels, changed during chemotherapy treatment (Topolcan *et al.*, 2005). Clearly, sTK1 levels provide more clinically relevant prognosis for monitoring cancer patients than several of the FDA-approved biomarkers currently in clinical use. Although sTK1 is also a worthy screening tool, its efficacy in cancer monitoring and prognosis fills a clinical need which may provide the driving force to propel TK1 into clinical use.

3.4   Tumor-TK1 Diagnostic potential

In addition to efficacy as a serum biomarker, TK1 has valuable potential as a means of diagnosis and prognosis in tumor tissue. TK1 expression in tumor tissue (tTK1) has repeatedly been shown to be a more relevant proliferation marker than PCNA. Although both TK1 and PCNA were overexpressed in malignant tissue compared with normal tissue, only TK1 was significantly increased with both grade and stage (Mao *et al.*, 2002; Wu *et al.*, 2000; Wu *et al.*, 2003). This was true for advanced breast, liver, thyroid, and colon cancer, although PCNA was associated with stage in colon cancer (Mao *et al.*, 2002; Wu *et al.*, 2000; Wu *et al.*, 2003). Ki67 and BrdU labeling are two other proliferation markers which have been compared with TK1. In 2009, Gasparri reported that TK1 expression during the cell cycle occurs earlier than either Ki67 or BrdU labeling, referred to as an activated G_1 state, which is high in TK1 and low in Ki67 (Gasparri *et al.*, 2009). Virtually all comparison studies reported a strong positive correlation between Ki67 and tTK1 expression in both malignant and pre-malignant conditions such as breast atypical ductal hyperplasia tissue (ADH), NSCLC, and infiltrating ductal breast carcinoma (Brockenbrough *et al.*, 2009; Guan *et al.*, 2009; He *et al.*, 2004). There are slight differences between Ki67 and tTK1 expression. Mao *et al.* reported a significant difference between tTK1 and Ki67 expression in lung adenocarcinoma tissue but not squamous cell carcinoma. In adenocarcinoma tissue, the significant increase of tTK1 expression resulted mostly from staining of stage 2 and grade 2 tumors (Mao *et al.*, 2005). Since there were also tumors which expressed Ki67 only, a combination of tTK1 and Ki67 was recommended for routine testing (Mao *et al.*, 2005). This recommendation was confirmed by He *et al.* who reported that the combination of tTK1 and Ki67 expression in breast carcinoma tissue detected the most tumors (He *et al.*,

2004). Zacchetti *et al.* ranked the proliferation markers according to their performance in breast tumors in this order PCNA<Ki67<BrdU labeling (Zacchetti *et al.*, 2003). Although this study did not include tTK1, tTK1 is elevated earlier in the cell cycle than Ki67 or BrdU, and can identify tumors which Ki67 misses, indicating that tTK1 may be a more accurate proliferation marker (Guan *et al.*, 2009).

Similar to sTK1 levels, tTK1 overexpression is an early event and can help identify pre-malignancies. Guan et al. demonstrated that tTK1 was positive in 80-90% of ADH, ductal carcinoma in situ (DCIS) and invasive ductal carcinoma (IDC) but only positive in less than 5% of usual ductal hyperplasia (UDH) (Guan *et al.*, 2009). This indicated that ADH, a pre-malignancy, was at increased risk for progression and was significantly higher in tTK1 expression compared to UDH (Guan *et al.*, 2009). The increase of TK1 early in the cell cycle, referred to as an activated G_1 state, is also indicative of the early increase of tTK1 (Gasparri *et al.*, 2009). Although the overexpression of tTK1 in pre-cancerous tissue has been confirmed, Alegre *et al.* demonstrated that tTK1 was not elevated in prostate hyperplasia tissue (Alegre *et al.*, 2012, 2013). However, since sTK1 is elevated in some cases of prostate hyperplasia, further work is needed to understand the clinical significance of elevated TK1 in prostate hyperplasia (Chen *et al.*, 2011; Huang *et al.*, 2011).

It is well established that tTK1 expression is significantly higher, compared to corresponding normal tissue, in breast, liver, thyroid, lung, colon, kidney, esophageal, uterine, prostate, and stomach cancer (Alegre *et al.*, 2013; Mao *et al.*, 2005; Mao *et al.*, 2002; Wu *et al.*, 2000; Wu *et al.*, 2003). Occasionally, the TK1 antibody used can affect the results of the study. Mao *et al.* found differences when NSCLC tissue was stained with a c-terminal mouse monoclonal (mAb) and c-terminal chicken anti-TK1 antibody (Mao *et al.*, 2005). Although there was not a significant difference in percentage of tTK1 positive tumors, the distribution of staining varied. The mAb primarily stained stage 2 and grade 2 tumors, with a decrease in tTK1 positive staining in more advanced tumors, while the chicken antibody showed the opposite result with the highest degree of staining in the more advanced tumors (Mao *et al.*, 2005). Although some reports using serum and tumor tissue have indicated that TK1 in kidney cancer is significantly elevated compared to normal tissue, Mizutani *et al.* reported tTK1 activity was 4 fold higher in normal kidney tissue compared to renal cell carcinoma (Mizutani *et al.*, 2003). In a subsequent study, they confirmed these findings and to date, this remains the only tissue reportedly higher in normal tissue than corresponding malignant tissue (Luo *et al.*, 2010). These discrepancies remain unclear although a thorough analysis of the differences among the antibodies used could shed light on this controversy. Nevertheless, standardization of scoring and a full characterization of the TK1 antibodies would enable clinicians to make needed comparisons as TK1 transitions from the bench to the bedside.

Recently a derivative of TK1 was also used to stain tumor tissue. XPA-210 is a c-terminal TK1 peptide fragment which includes amino acid 210 (Aufderklamm *et al.*, 2012). Typically tTK1 is a cytoplasmic marker, but XPA-210 expression as detected by a mAb, is located primarily in the nucleus which is more comparable to Ki67 (Gakis *et al.*, 2011). Although there have only been 3 studies involving XPA-210, the trends for prostate and renal cell carcinoma appear to confirm corresponding studies with tTK1 (Aufderklamm *et al.*, 2012; Gakis *et al.*, 2011; Kruck *et al.*, 2012). Regardless of which antibody or peptide fragment of TK1 is used, it remains clear that tTK1 is significantly overexpressed in a variety of tumor tissue, including some cases of pre-malignancy.

3.5 Tumor-TK1 Prognostic potential

tTK1 corresponds with sTK1 in that both have diagnostic and prognostic potential. Just as sTK1 correlated to survival, recurrence, and treatment, similar trends are seen with tTK1. Xu *et al.* reported that high tTK1 expression was associated with significantly worse 5 year survival in pT1 lung adenocarcinoma patients (Xu *et al.*, 2012). Additionally, Romain *et al.* reported tTK1 expression in node-negative breast cancer tumors was an independent factor for metastatic free survival and DFS (Romain *et al.*, 2000). Their subsequent study similarly reported high tTK1 increased the risk of developing distant recurrence and therefore, tTK1 was able to identify which node-negative patients were at a high risk for metastasis (Romain *et al.*, 2001). Aufderklamm *et al.* similarly reported that higher XPA-210, a fragment of TK1, was associated with shorter time to recurrence and metastasis (Aufderklamm *et al.*, 2012).

In addition to tTK1 expression, the TK1 activity of tumor tissue (tTK1a) is also associated with patient prognosis. Demeter *et al.* reported the activity of tTK1a was 12-fold higher in ovarian carcinoma, but Mizutani *et al.* reported only a 2-fold increase for bladder carcinoma relative to normal controls (Demeter *et al.*, 2001; Mizutani *et al.*, 2002). Mizutani *et al.* also showed that those with low tTK1a had longer RFS (Mizutani *et al.*, 2002). Similarly, O'Neill *et al.* reported that tTK1a levels in the initial primary breast tumor were associated with recurrence, in that those with recurrence also initially had significantly higher sTK1a levels (O'Neill, K. L., McKelvey, *et al.*, 1992). In a study by Foekens *et al.* the initial sTK1 activity level also affected the duration of response in advanced breast cancer (Foekens *et al.*, 2001). For tumors with low, intermediate or high tTK1a, the duration of response was 23, 15, and 13 months respectively (Foekens *et al.*, 2001). In renal cell carcinoma, the tTK1a levels are inversely associated with sensitivity to 5-fluorouracil (5FU), which is likely associated with TK1's role in DNA repair, as previously discussed (Mizutani *et al.*, 2003).

Unfortunately there is a need to correlate a patient's tTK1 and sTK1 levels to determine if they are redundant. Both sTK1 and tTK1 generally share the same trends in diagnosis and prognosis. TK1 levels are elevated very early including in pre-malignancy in both serum and tumor tissue. Additionally, increased TK1 in serum and tumor is associated with worse prognosis and disease progression including recurrence. Finally, serum and tumor TK1 appear more accurate and indicative of patient prognosis when compared with other biomarkers including proliferation markers. The efficacy and utility of monitoring TK1 levels both in malignant and healthy individuals remains clear.

3.6 TK1 Therapeutic potential

Although the primary clinical value of TK1 is in its diagnostic and prognostic potential, TK1 also has therapeutic potential. TK1 plays an intricate role in DNA repair and maintaining dTTP levels, as discussed previously. Franciullino *et al.* demonstrated that overexpression of TK1 leads to desensitization of tumor cells to 5FU (Fanciullino *et al.*, 2006). Somewhat surprisingly, they also showed that TK1 does not limit the production of 5FU-monophosphate, indicating as previously discussed, that TK1 is involved in DNA repair. Due to the redundant nature of TK1, Di Cresce *et al.* targeted both TK1 and thymidylate synthase (TS), the salvage and de novo pathways respectively, with siRNA which successfully re-sensitized tumors to 5FU treatment (Di Cresce *et al.*, 2011). A study by Wakazono *et al.* demonstrated that a decrease in dTTP levels made tumor cells hypersensitive to treatment with alkylating agents (Wakazono *et al.*, 1996). Since TK1 and TS both contribute to dTTP levels, this appears to explain the importance simultaneous knockdown of TK1 and TS to re-sensitize tumors.

TK1 is also used in gene therapy although instead of hTK1, herpes simplex virus TK (HSV-TK) is utilized. A virus-based vector delivers the HSV-TK to gliomas or other tumors in connection with ganciclovir treatment, a harmless prodrug (Zhang *et al.*, 2010). HSV-TK acts as a suicide gene by cleaving ganciclovir into a toxic compound (Zhang *et al.*, 2010). This system works for a variety of tumors and has been reviewed thoroughly elsewhere (Oh *et al.*, 2010). Since HSV-TK varies considerably from human TK1 in structure, function and characteristics in malignancy, we will not discuss it further in this review.

3.7   TK1 Imaging: Positron Emission Tomography (PET)

PET imaging is a clinical tool used to help determine tumor metabolism. Flurodeoxyglucose (FDG) is the approved substrate for PET imaging. Unfortunately, FDG-PET is limited in that metabolism is complex and FDG only assesses one aspect of cellular metabolism (Shields, 2012). In an effort to understand more about tumor proliferation to enable more accurate prognosis, 3'-deoxy-3'-fluorothymidine (FLT) and other substrates were created (Agarwal *et al.*, 2013; Bading & Shields, 2008; Struthers *et al.*, 2010). Katz *et al.* reported that FLT, but not FDG, predicted response to TRAIL and sorafenib treatment in tumors with functional p53 (Katz *et al.*, 2011).

FLT is phosphorylated by TK1, producing FLT-MP which is then trapped in cells. Unfortunately, FLT-PET is not currently in clinical use. This is most likely because there is tremendous controversy regarding whether FLT uptake into cells correlates with proliferation, measured by TK1 and/or Ki67 levels. Shinomiya *et al.* recommended that FLT should not be used as a measure of proliferation since FLT phosphorylation did not reflect either tTK1 expression or tTK1 mRNA levels (Shinomiya *et al.*, 2013). Zhang *et al.* agreed as they reported low FLT uptake with corresponding high TK1 and Ki67 expression in tumor tissue (Zhang, C. C. *et al.*, 2012). Several others have agreed that either TK1 or Ki67 expression is not associated with FLT uptake (Benz *et al.*, 2012; Lee *et al.*, 2011; McKinley *et al.*, 2013). Conversely, Brockenbrough *et al.* reported that FLT uptake was correlated with tTK1 and Ki67 expression but not tTK1a (Brockenbrough *et al.*, 2011). Still others have reported FLT uptake strongly correlated with tTK1a and/or tTK1 expression (Barthel *et al.*, 2005; Kameyama *et al.*, 2011; Rasey *et al.*, 2002). McKinley *et al.* has tried to reconcile this controversy. They reported that FLT uptake corresponds with tumor proliferation, as a function of thymidine salvage pathway utilization, but not general proliferation as measured by Ki67 expression (McKinley *et al.*, 2013). Furthermore, FLT uptake did not distinguish between tumors which primarily utilized the thymidine salvage pathway (TK1) and those which utilized the de novo thymidine pathway (McKinley *et al.*, 2013).

Despite the numerous studies which have shown FLT-PET's prognostic potential and possible advantages over FDG-PET, we still do not adequately understand the connection between proliferation and FLT-PET. Unless resolved with a clear consensus, this controversy will continue to bar FLT-PET from being utilized clinically.

4   Conclusion

Overall, TK1 is a clinically relevant cancer biomarker which is significantly elevated in serum and tissue of cancer patients. Structurally, TK1 is primarily found as an active tetramer or dimer of dimers. As an active tetramer, TK1 is responsible for converting dT to dTMP in a cell-cycle dependent manner. By extension, TK1 is also responsible for maintaining adequate dTTP levels for DNA synthesis. In tumor cells TK1 plays a pivotal role in DNA repair and affects a tumor's sensitivity to chemotherapy treatment. During the cell cycle, TK1 rapidly increases in late G_1 and peaks in S phase. This rapid increase is primarily due to ATP availability and a concentration-dependent dimer to tetramer switch. Following the S phase peak, TK1 is rapidly degraded by the APC/C-Cdh1 complex which recognizes a KEN box on the c-terminus of TK1.

In malignancy, TK1 exits the cell as a very stable, high molecular weight form which appears to be a TK1 aggregate, 3-7 times larger than active TK1. TK1 is significantly elevated early in the progression of normal cells to malignancy. In fact, in serum and tumors, TK1 is found elevated in some cases of pre-cancer. Furthermore, TK1 is elevated in serum and tumor tissue of virtually all types of cancer. In addition to the diagnostic potential of TK1, TK1 also has beneficial prognostic potential. In particular, high sTK1 or tTK1 levels are associated with worse prognosis, including shorter survival and an increased risk for recurrence. In fact, sTK1 elevates 1-9 months prior to the clinical manifestation of recurrence. As a tool for monitoring a patient's response to treatment, sTK1 decreases significantly in patients with complete response or partial response. On the other hand, sTK1 continues to increase in patients who continue to see disease progression or recurrence. In addition to diagnostic and prognostic potential, TK1 also has therapeutic potential. Although most of its current therapeutic application lies with HSV-TK as a suicide gene, TK1 can also be used as a means of re-sensitizing tumors to chemotherapeutic agents. Finally, TK1 is also used as a potential imaging tool through FLT-PET, as a means of determining the extent of a tumor's proliferation. Clearly, TK1 has vast clinical potential, especially as a screening and monitoring tool for cancer patients. As more accurate and robust methods of detection for TK1 arise, TK1 will no doubt be a powerful clinical tool in the coming years.

References

Agarwal, H. K., McElroy, C. A., Sjuvarsson, E., Eriksson, S., Darby, M. V., & Tjarks, W. (2013). Synthesis of N3-substituted carboranyl thymidine bioconjugates and their evaluation as substrates of recombinant human thymidine kinase 1. European Journal of Medicinal Chemistry, 60, 456-468.

al-Nabulsi, I., Takamiya, Y., Voloshin, Y., Dritschilo, A., Martuza, R. L., & Jorgensen, T. J. (1994). Expression of thymidine kinase is essential to low dose radiation resistance of rat glioma cells. Cancer Res, 54(21), 5614-5617.

Alegre, M. M., Robison, R. A., & O'Neill, K. L. (2012). Thymidine Kinase 1 Upregulation Is an Early Event in Breast Tumor Formation. J Oncol, 2012, 575647.

Alegre, M. M., Robison, R. A., & O'Neill, K. L. (2013). Thymidine Kinase 1: A Universal Marker for Cancer. Cancer and Clinical Oncology, 2(1), 159-167.

Aufderklamm, S., Hennenlotter, J., Todenhoefer, T., Gakis, G., Schilling, D., Vogel, U., . . . Schwentner, C. (2012). XPA-210: a new proliferation marker determines locally advanced prostate cancer and is a predictor of biochemical recurrence. World J Urol, 30(4), 547-552.

Austin, W. R., Armijo, A. L., Campbell, D. O., Singh, A. S., Hsieh, T., Nathanson, D., . . . Radu, C. G. (2012). Nucleoside salvage pathway kinases regulate hematopoiesis by linking nucleotide metabolism with replication stress. J Exp Med, 209(12), 2215-2228.

Bading, J. R., & Shields, A. F. (2008). Imaging of cell proliferation: status and prospects. J Nucl Med, 49 Suppl 2, 64S-80S.

Barthel, H., Perumal, M., Latigo, J., He, Q., Brady, F., Luthra, S. K., . . . Aboagye, E. O. (2005). The uptake of 3'-deoxy-3'-[18F]fluorothymidine into L5178Y tumours in vivo is dependent on thymidine kinase 1 protein levels. Eur J Nucl Med Mol Imaging, 32(3), 257-263.

Basundra, R., Kumar, A., Amrane, S., Verma, A., Phan, A. T., & Chowdhury, S. (2010). A novel G-quadruplex motif modulates promoter activity of human thymidine kinase 1. FEBS J, 277(20), 4254-4264.

Benz, M. R., Czernin, J., Allen-Auerbach, M. S., Dry, S. M., Sutthiruangwong, P., Spick, C., . . . Eilber, F. C. (2012). 3'-deoxy-3'-[(18) F]fluorothymidine positron emission tomography for response assessment in soft tissue sarcoma: A *pilot study to correlate imaging findings with tissue thymidine kinase 1 and Ki-67 activity and histopathologic response. Cancer, 118(12), 3135-3144.*

Birringer, M. S., Claus, M. T., Folkers, G., Kloer, D. P., Schulz, G. E., & Scapozza, L. (2005). Structure of a type II thymidine kinase with bound dTTP. FEBS Lett, 579(6), 1376-1382.

Birringer, M. S., Perozzo, R., Kut, E., Stillhart, C., Surber, W., Scapozza, L., & Folkers, G. (2006). High-level expression and purification of human thymidine kinase 1: quaternary structure, stability, and kinetics. Protein Expr Purif, 47(2), 506-515.

Bohman, C., & Eriksson, S. (1988). Deoxycytidine kinase from human leukemic spleen: preparation and characteristics of homogeneous enzyme. Biochemistry, 27(12), 4258-4265.

Bradshaw, H. D., Jr., & Deininger, P. L. (1984). Human thymidine kinase gene: molecular cloning and nucleotide sequence of a cDNA expressible in mammalian cells. Mol Cell Biol, 4(11), 2316-2320.

Bristow, H., O'Neill, K., Hannigan, B. M., & McKenna, P. G. (1988). Leakage of Thymidine Kinase from proliferating cells Biochemical Society Transactions, 16(1), 55-56.

Brockenbrough, J. S., Morihara, J. K., Hawes, S. E., Stern, J. E., Rasey, J. S., Wiens, L. W., . . . Vesselle, H. (2009). Thymidine kinase 1 and thymidine phosphorylase expression in non-small-cell lung carcinoma in relation to angiogenesis and proliferation. J Histochem Cytochem, 57(11), 1087-1097.

Brockenbrough, J. S., Souquet, T., Morihara, J. K., Stern, J. E., Hawes, S. E., Rasey, J. S., . . . Vesselle, H. (2011). Tumor 3'-deoxy-3'-(18)F-fluorothymidine ((18)F-FLT) uptake by PET correlates with thymidine kinase 1 expression: static and kinetic analysis of (18)F-FLT PET studies in lung tumors. J Nucl Med, 52(8), 1181-1188.

Broet, P., Romain, S., Daver, A., Ricolleau, G., Quillien, V., Rallet, A., . . . Lu, G. O. F. N. C. (2001). Thymidine kinase as a proliferative marker: Clinical relevance in 1,692 primary breast cancer patients. Journal of Clinical Oncology, 19(11), 2778-2787.

Carlsson, L., Larsson, A., & Lindman, H. (2009). Elevated levels of thymidine kinase 1 peptide in serum from patients with breast cancer. Ups J Med Sci, 114(2), 116-120.

Catalano, L., Frigeri, F., De Rosa, G., Camera, A., & Rotoli, B. (1989). Serum thymidine kinase peaks early during AML induction therapy. Leukemia, 3(5), 396.

Chang, Z. F., Huang, D. Y., & Chi, L. M. (1998). Serine 13 is the site of mitotic phosphorylation of human thymidine kinase. J Biol Chem, 273(20), 12095-12100.

Chang, Z. F., Huang, D. Y., & Hsue, N. C. (1994). Differential phosphorylation of human thymidine kinase in proliferating and M phase-arrested human cells. J Biol Chem, 269(33), 21249-21254.

Chang, Z. F., Huang, D. Y., & Hu, S. F. (1999). NF-Y-mediated trans-activation of the human thymidine kinase promoter is closely linked to activation of cyclin-dependent kinase. J Cell Biochem, 75(2), 300-309.

Chang, Z. F., & Liu, C. J. (1994). Human thymidine kinase CCAAT-binding protein is NF-Y, whose A subunit expression is serum-dependent in human IMR-90 diploid fibroblasts. J Biol Chem, 269(27), 17893-17898.

Chen, Eriksson, S., & Chang, Z. F. (2010). Regulation and functional contribution of thymidine kinase 1 in repair of DNA damage. Journal of Biological Chemistry, 285(35), 27327-27335.

Chen, Huang, S. Q., Wang, Y. D., Yang, A. Z., Wen, J., Xu, X. H., . . . Skog, S. (2011). Serological Thymidine Kinase 1 is a Biomarker for Early Detection of Tumours-A Health Screening Study on 35,365 People, Using a Sensitive Chemiluminescent Dot Blot Assay. Sensors, 11(12), 11064-11080.

Chen, Ying, M. G., Chen, Y. S., Hu, M. H., Lin, Y. Y., Chen, D. D., . . . Skog, S. (2010). Serum thymidine kinase 1 correlates to clinical stages and clinical reactions and monitors the outcome of therapy of 1,247 cancer patients in routine clinical settings. International Journal of Clinical Oncology, 15(4), 359-368.

Chen, Zhou, H., Li, S. L., He, E., Hu, J. Y., Zhou, J., & Skog, S. (2008). Serological Thymidine Kinase 1 (STK1) Indicates an Elevated Risk for the Development of Malignant Tumours. Anticancer Research, 28(6B), 3897-3907.

Chevinsky, A. H. (1991). CEA in tumors of other than colorectal origin. Semin Surg Oncol, 7(3), 162-166.

Chou, W. L., & Chang, Z. F. (2001). Cap-independent translation conferred by the 5'-untranslated region of human thymidine kinase mRNA. Biochim Biophys Acta, 1519(3), 209-215.

De Blasio, F., Alonzo, M., Zofra, S., De Colle, R., Romano, L., & Pezza, A. (1990). [Thymidine kinase as a biological marker in neoplasms of the lung and mediastinum]. Arch Monaldi Mal Torace, 45(1), 39-48.

Demeter, A., Abonyi, M., Look, K. Y., Keszler, G., Staub, M., & Weber, G. (2001). Differences in thermostability of thymidine kinase isoenzymes in normal ovary and ovarian carcinoma. Anticancer Research, 21(1A), 353-358.

Di Cresce, C., Figueredo, R., Ferguson, P. J., Vincent, M. D., & Koropatnick, J. (2011). Combining Small Interfering RNAs Targeting Thymidylate Synthase and Thymidine Kinase 1 or 2 Sensitizes Human Tumor Cells to 5-Fluorodeoxyuridine and Pemetrexed. Journal of Pharmacology and Experimental Therapeutics, 338(3), 952-963.

Di Raimondo, F., Giustolisi, R., Lerner, S., Cacciola, E., O'Brien, S., Kantarjian, H., & Keating, M. J. (2001). Retrospective study of the prognostic role of serum thymidine kinase level in CLL patients with active disease treated with fludarabine. Ann Oncol, 12(5), 621-625.

Dobrovolsky, V. N., Bucci, T., Heflich, R. H., Desjardins, J., & Richardson, F. C. (2003). Mice deficient for cytosolic thymidine kinase gene develop fatal kidney disease. Mol Genet Metab, 78(1), 1-10.

Dou, Q. P., Fridovich-Keil, J. L., & Pardee, A. B. (1991). Inducible proteins binding to the murine thymidine kinase promoter in late G1/S phase. Proc Natl Acad Sci U S A, 88(4), 1157-1161.

Dowsett, M., Nielsen, T. O., A'Hern, R., Bartlett, J., Coombes, R. C., Cuzick, J., . . . Hayes, D. F. (2011). Assessment of Ki67 in breast cancer: recommendations from the International Ki67 in Breast Cancer working group. J Natl Cancer Inst, 103(22), 1656-1664.

Elfagieh, M., Abdalla, F., Gliwan, A., Boder, J., Nichols, W., & Buhmeida, A. (2012). Serum tumour markers as a diagnostic and prognostic tool in Libyan breast cancer. Tumour Biol, 33(6), 2371-2377.

Eriksson, S., Kierdaszuk, B., Munch-Petersen, B., Oberg, B., & Johansson, N. G. (1991). Comparison of the substrate specificities of human thymidine kinase 1 and 2 and deoxycytidine kinase toward antiviral and cytostatic nucleoside analogs. Biochem Biophys Res Commun, 176(2), 586-592.

Eriksson, S., Munch-Petersen, B., Johansson, K., & Eklund, H. (2002). Structure and function of cellular deoxyribonucleoside kinases. Cell Mol Life Sci, 59(8), 1327-1346.

Euler, v., & Eriksson, S. (2011). Comparative aspects of the proliferation marker thymidine kinase 1 in human and canine tumour diseases. Vet Comp Oncol, 9(1), 1-15.

Euler, V., Rivera, P., Aronsson, A. C., Bengtsson, C., Hansson, L. O., & Eriksson, S. K. (2009). Monitoring therapy in canine malignant lymphoma and leukemia with serum thymidine kinase 1 activity--evaluation of a new, fully automated non-radiometric assay. Int J Oncol, 34(2), 505-510.

Fanciullino, R., Evrard, A., Cuq, P., Giacometti, S., Peillard, L., Mercier, C., . . . Ciccolini, J. (2006). Genetic and biochemical modulation of 5-fluorouracil through the overexpression of thymidine kinase: an in-vitro study. Anticancer Drugs, 17(4), 463-470.

Faria, M., Halquist, M. S., Kindt, E., Li, W., Karnes, H. T., & O'Brien, P. J. (2012). Liquid chromatography-tandem mass spectrometry method for quantification of thymidine kinase activity in human serum by monitoring the conversion of 3'-deoxy-3'-fluorothymidine to 3'-deoxy-3'-fluorothymidine monophosphate. J Chromatogr B Analyt Technol Biomed Life Sci, 907, 13-20.

Fernandez-Fernandez, L., Tejero, E., Tieso, A., Rabadan, L., Munoz, M., & Santos, I. (1996). Receiver operating characteristic (ROC) curve analysis of the tumor markers CEA, CA 19-9 and CA 72-4 in gastric cancer. Int Surg, 81(4), 400-402.

Foekens, J. A., Romain, S., Look, M. P., Martin, P. M., & Klijn, J. G. (2001). Thymidine kinase and thymidylate synthase in advanced breast cancer: response to tamoxifen and chemotherapy. Cancer Res, 61(4), 1421-1425.

Fujiwaki, R., Hata, K., Moriyama, M., Iwanari, O., Katabuchi, H., Okamura, H., & Miyazaki, K. (2001). Clinical value of thymidine kinase in patients with cervical carcinoma. Oncology, 61(1), 47-54.

Gakis, G., Hennenlotter, J., Scharpf, M., Hevler, J., Schilling, D., Kuehs, U., . . . Schwentner, C. (2011). XPA-210: a new proliferation marker to characterize tumor biology and progression of renal cell carcinoma. World J Urol, 29(6), 801-806.

Gasparri, F., Wang, N., Skog, S., Galvani, A., & Eriksson, S. (2009). Thymidine kinase 1 expression defines an activated G1 state of the cell cycle as revealed with site-specific antibodies and ArrayScan assays. Eur J Cell Biol, 88(12), 779-785.

Good, L., Chen, J., & Chen, K. Y. (1995). Analysis of sequence-specific binding activity of cis-elements in human thymidine kinase gene promoter during G1/S phase transition. J Cell Physiol, 163(3), 636-644.

Guan, H., Sun, Y., Zan, Q., Xu, M., Li, Y., Zhou, J., . . . Skog, S. (2009). Thymidine kinase 1 expression in atypical ductal hyperplasia significantly differs from usual ductal hyperplasia and ductal carcinoma in situ: A useful tool in tumor therapy management. Mol Med Report, 2(6), 923-929.

Hallek, M., Langenmayer, I., Nerl, C., Knauf, W., Dietzfelbinger, H., Adorf, D., . . . Emmerich, B. (1999). Elevated serum thymidine kinase levels identify a subgroup at high risk of disease progression in early, nonsmoldering chronic lymphocytic leukemia. Blood, 93(5), 1732-1737.

Harper, J. W. (2002). A phosphorylation-driven ubiquitination switch for cell-cycle control. Trends Cell Biol, 12(3), 104-107.

Haveman, J., Sigmond, J., van Bree, C., Franken, N. A., Koedooder, C., & Peters, G. J. (2006). Time course of enhanced activity of deoxycytidine kinase and thymidine kinase 1 and 2 in cultured human squamous lung carcinoma cells, SW-1573, induced by gamma-irradiation. Oncol Rep, 16(4), 901-905.

He, Fornander, T., Johansson, H., Johansson, U., Hu, G. Z., Rutqvist, L. E., & Skog, S. (2006). Thymidine kinase 1 in serum predicts increased risk of distant or loco-regional recurrence following surgery in patients with early breast cancer. Anticancer Research, 26(6C), 4753-4759.

He, Mao, Y., Wu, J., Decker, C., Merza, M., Wang, N., . . . Skog, S. (2004). Cytosolic thymidine kinase is a specific histopathologic tumour marker for breast carcinomas. Int J Oncol, 25(4), 945-953.

He, Skog, S., & Tribukait, B. (1991). Cell cycle related studies on thymidine kinase and its isoenzymes in Ehrlich ascites tumours. Cell Prolif, 24(1), 3-14.

He, Skog, S., Wu, C. J., Johansson, A., & Tribukait, B. (1996). Existence of phosphorylated and dephosphorylated forms of cytosolic thymidine kinase (TK1). Biochimica Et Biophysica Acta-General Subjects, 1289(1), 25-30.

He, Xu, X. H., Guan, H., Chen, Y., Chen, Z. H., Pan, Z. L., . . . Skog, S. (2010). Thymidine Kinase 1 is a Potential Marker for Prognosis and Monitoring the Response to Treatment of Patients with Breast, Lung, and Esophageal Cancer and Non-Hodgkin's Lymphoma. Nucleosides Nucleotides & Nucleic Acids, 29(4-6), 352-358.

He, Zhang, P. G., Zou, L., Li, H. X., Wang, X. Q., Zhou, S., . . . Skog, S. (2005). Concentration of thymidine kinase 1 in serum (S-TK1) is a more sensitive proliferation marker in human solid tumors than its activity. Oncology Reports, 14(4), 1013-1019.

He, Zou, L., Zhang, P. A., Lui, J. X., Skog, S., & Fornander, T. (2000). The clinical significance of thymidine kinase 1 measurement in serum of breast cancer patients using anti-TK1 antibody. Int J Biol Markers, 15(2), 139-146.

He, Q., Skog, S., Welander, I., & Tribukait, B. (2002). X-irradiation effects on thymidine kinase (TK): II. The significance of deoxythymidine triphosphate for inhibition of TK1 activity. Cell Prolif, 35(2), 83-92.

Hengstschlager, M., Knofler, M., Mullner, E. W., Ogris, E., Wintersberger, E., & Wawra, E. (1994). Different regulation of thymidine kinase during the cell cycle of normal versus DNA tumor virus-transformed cells. J Biol Chem, 269(19), 13836-13842.

Huang, & Chang, Z. F. (2001). Interaction of human thymidine kinase 1 with p21(Waf1). Biochem J, 356(Pt 3), 829-834.

Huang, Lin, J., Guo, N., Zhang, M., Yun, X., Liu, S., . . . Skog, S. (2011). *Elevated serum thymidine kinase 1 predicts risk of pre/early cancerous progression. Asian Pac J Cancer Prev, 12(2), 497-505.*

Huang, Tian, X. S., Li, R., Wang, X. M., Wen, W., Guan, H., & Yang, Y. J. (2012). *Elevated thymidine kinase 1 in serum following neoadjuvant chemotherapy predicts poor outcome for patients with locally advanced breast cancer. Experimental and Therapeutic Medicine, 3(2), 331-335.*

Ishikawa, Y., Kudo, H., Suzuki, S., Nemoto, N., Sassa, S., & Sakamoto, S. (2008). *Down regulation by a low-zinc diet in gene expression of rat prostatic thymidylate synthase and thymidine kinase. Nutr Metab (Lond), 5, 12.*

Jeong, M. H., Jin, Y. H., Kang, E. Y., Jo, W. S., Park, H. T., Lee, J. D., . . . Jeong, S. J. (2004). *The modulation of radiation-induced cell death by genistein in K562 cells: activation of thymidine kinase 1. Cell Res, 14(4), 295-302.*

Kameyama, R., Yamamoto, Y., Izuishi, K., Sano, T., & Nishiyama, Y. (2011). *Correlation of F-18-FLT uptake with equilibrative nucleoside transporter-1 and thymidine kinase-1 expressions in gastrointestinal cancer. Nuclear Medicine Communications, 32(6), 460-465.*

Karbownik, M., Brzezianska, E., Zasada, K., & Lewinski, A. (2003). *Expression of genes for certain enzymes of pyrimidine and purine salvage pathway in peripheral blood leukocytes collected from patients with Graves' or Hashimoto's disease. Journal of Cellular Biochemistry, 89(3), 550-555.*

Karlstrom, A. R., Neumuller M., Gronowitz J.S., Kallander C.F.R. (1990). *Molecular forms in human serum of enzymes synthesizing DNA precursors and DNA. Molecular and Cellular Biochemistry, 92, 23-35.*

Katz, S. I., Zhou, L., Ferrara, T. A., Wang, W., Mayes, P. A., Smith, C. D., & El-Deiry, W. S. (2011). *FLT-PET may not be a reliable indicator of therapeutic response in p53-null malignancy. Int J Oncol, 39(1), 91-100.*

Kauffman, M. G., & Kelly, T. J. (1991). *Cell cycle regulation of thymidine kinase: residues near the carboxyl terminus are essential for the specific degradation of the enzyme at mitosis. Mol Cell Biol, 11(5), 2538-2546.*

Ke, P. Y., & Chang, Z. F. (2004). *Mitotic degradation of human thymidine kinase 1 is dependent on the anaphase-promoting complex/cyclosome-CDH1-mediated pathway. Mol Cell Biol, 24(2), 514-526.*

Ke, P. Y., Hu, C. M., Chang, Y. C., & Chang, Z. F. (2007). *Hiding human thymidine kinase 1 from APC/C-mediated destruction by thymidine binding. FASEB J, 21(4), 1276-1284.*

Ke, P. Y., Yang, C. C., Tsai, I. C., & Chang, Z. F. (2003). *Degradation of human thymidine kinase is dependent on serine-13 phosphorylation: involvement of the SCF-mediated pathway. Biochem J, 370(Pt 1), 265-273.*

Kim, & Lee. (1992). *Identification of a protein-binding site in the promoter of the human thymidine kinase gene required for the G1-S-regulated transcription. J Biol Chem, 267(4), 2723-2727.*

Kim, & Lee, A. S. (1991). *Identification of a 70-base-pair cell cycle regulatory unit within the promoter of the human thymidine kinase gene and its interaction with cellular factors. Mol Cell Biol, 11(4), 2296-2302.*

Kim, Rawlings, S. L., Li, L. J., Roy, B., & Lee, A. S. (1996). *Identification of a set of protein species approximately 40 kDa as high-affinity DNA binding factor(s) to the cell cycle regulatory region of the human thymidine kinase promoter. Cell Growth Differ, 7(12), 1741-1749.*

Kim, Y. K., Wells, S., Lau, Y. F., & Lee, A. S. (1988). *Sequences contained within the promoter of the human thymidine kinase gene can direct cell-cycle regulation of heterologous fusion genes. Proc Natl Acad Sci U S A, 85(16), 5894-5898.*

Konoplev, S. N., Fritsche, H. A., O'Brien, S., Wierda, W. G., Keating, M. J., Garnet, T. G., . . . Bueso-Ramos, C. E. (2010). *High Serum Thymidine Kinase 1 Level Predicts Poorer Survival in Patients With Chronic Lymphocytic Leukemia. American Journal of Clinical Pathology, 134(3), 472-477.*

Korkmaz, T., Seber, S., Okutur, K., Basaran, G., Yumuk, F., Dane, F., . . . Turhal, N. S. (2013). *Serum thymidine kinase 1 levels correlates with FDG uptake and prognosis in patients with non small cell lung cancer. Biomarkers, 18(1), 88-94.*

Kreder, N. C., van Bree, C., Peters, G. J., Loves, W. J., & Haveman, J. (2002). Enhanced levels of deoxycytidine kinase and thymidine kinase 1 and 2 after pulsed low dose rate irradiation as an adaptive response to radiation. Oncol Rep, 9(1), 141-144.

Kristensen, T., Jensen, H. K., & Munch-Petersen, B. (1994). Overexpression of human thymidine kinase mRNA without corresponding enzymatic activity in patients with chronic lymphatic leukemia. Leuk Res, 18(11), 861-866.

Kruck, S., Hennenlotter, J., Vogel, U., Schilling, D., Gakis, G., Hevler, J., . . . Schwentner, C. (2012). Exposed proliferation antigen 210 (XPA-210) in renal cell carcinoma (RCC) and oncocytoma: clinical utility and biological implications. BJU Int, 109(4), 634-638.

Kuroiwa, N., Yusa, T., Nakamura, Y., Sakiyama, S., Hiwasa, T., Lin, L., . . . Fujimura, S. (2000). Regulation of the activity and polymerization status of recombinant human cytosolic thymidine kinase by thiols and ATP. Int J Oncol, 16(2), 305-313.

Lee, S. J., Lee, H. J., & Moon, D. H. (2011). Quantitative Analysis of Thymidine Kinase 1 and 5 '(3 ')-Deoxyribonucleotidase mRNA Expression: The Role of Fluorothymidine Uptake. Anticancer Research, 31(6), 2135-2139.

Li, Lei, D. S., Wang, X. Q., Skog, S., & He, Q. (2005). Serum thymidine kinase 1 is a prognostic and monitoring factor in patients with non-small cell lung cancer. Oncol Rep, 13(1), 145-149.

Li, Lu, C. Y., Ke, P. Y., & Chang, Z. F. (2004). Perturbation of ATP-induced tetramerization of human cytosolic thymidine kinase by substitution of serine-13 with aspartic acid at the mitotic phosphorylation site. Biochem Biophys Res Commun, 313(3), 587-593.

Li, Naeve, G. S., & Lee, A. S. (1993). Temporal regulation of cyclin A-p107 and p33cdk2 complexes binding to a human thymidine kinase promoter element important for G1-S phase transcriptional regulation. Proc Natl Acad Sci U S A, 90(8), 3554-3558.

Li, Wang, Y., He, J., Ma, J., Zhao, L., Chen, H., . . . Skog, S. (2010). Serological thymidine kinase 1 is a prognostic factor in oesophageal, cardial and lung carcinomas. Eur J Cancer Prev, 19(4), 313-318.

Lin, L., Kuroiwa, N., Moriyama, Y., & Fujimura, S. (2003). Continuous increase in phosphorylation of cytosolic thymidine kinase during proliferation of rat hepatoma JB1 cells. Oncol Rep, 10(3), 665-669.

Lipson, K. E., Liang, G., Xia, L., Gai, X., Prystowsky, M. B., & Mao, X. (1995). Protein that binds to the distal, but not to the proximal, CCAAT of the human thymidine kinase gene promoter. J Cell Biochem, 57(4), 711-723.

Liu, Y. P., Ling, Y., Qi, Q. F., Tang, Y. X., Xu, J. Z., Zhou, T., . . . Pan, Y. D. (2011). Changes in serum thymidine kinase 1 levels during chemotherapy correlate with objective response in patients with advanced gastric cancer. Experimental and Therapeutic Medicine, 2(6), 1177-1181.

Luo, P., He, E., Eriksson, S., Zhou, J., Hu, G., Zhang, J., & Skog, S. (2009). Thymidine kinase activity in serum of renal cell carcinoma patients is a useful prognostic marker. Eur J Cancer Prev, 18(3), 220-224.

Luo, P., Wang, N., He, E., Eriksson, S., Zhou, J., Hu, G., . . . Skog, S. (2010). The proliferation marker thymidine kinase 1 level is high in normal kidney tubule cells compared to other normal and malignant renal cells. Pathol Oncol Res, 16(2), 277-283.

Madec, A., Javre, J. L., Haras, D., Samperez, S., & Jouan, P. (1988). Some characteristics of fetal and adult isoenzymes of thymidine kinase in human breast cancers. Bull Cancer, 75(2), 187-194.

Mao, Wu, J., Skog, S., Eriksson, S., Zhao, Y., Zhou, J., & He, Q. (2005). Expression of cell proliferating genes in patients with non-small cell lung cancer by immunohistochemistry and cDNA profiling. Oncol Rep, 13(5), 837-846.

Mao, Wu, J., Wang, N., He, L., Wu, C., He, Q., & Skog, S. (2002). A comparative study: immunohistochemical detection of cytosolic thymidine kinase and proliferating cell nuclear antigen in breast cancer. Cancer Invest, 20(7-8), 922-931.

Mao, X., Xia, L., Liang, G., Gai, X., Huang, D. Y., Prystowsky, M. B., & Lipson, K. E. (1995). CCAAT-box contributions to human thymidine kinase mRNA expression. J Cell Biochem, 57(4), 701-710.

McKenna, P. G., O'Neill, K. L., Abram, W. P., & Hannigan, B. M. (1988). Thymidine kinase activities in mononuclear leukocytes and serum from breast cancer patients. Br J Cancer, 57(6), 619-622.

McKenna, P. G., Yasseen, A. A., & McKelvey, V. J. (1985). Evidence for indirect involvement of thymidine kinase in excision repair processes in mouse cell lines. Somat Cell Mol Genet, 11(3), 239-246.

McKinley, E. T., Ayers, G. D., Smith, R. A., Saleh, S. A., Zhao, P., Washington, M. K., . . . Manning, H. C. (2013). Limits of [(18)F]-FLT PET as a Biomarker of Proliferation in Oncology. PLoS One, 8(3), e58938.

Mizutani, Y., Wada, H., Yoshida, O., Fukushima, M., Kamoi, K., & Miki, T. (2002). Prognostic significance of thymidine kinase activity in bladder carcinoma. Cancer, 95(10), 2120-2125.

Mizutani, Y., Wada, H., Yoshida, O., Fukushima, M., Nakao, M., & Miki, T. (2003). Significance of thymidine kinase activity in renal cell carcinoma. J Urol, 169(2), 706-709.

Munch-Petersen, B. (1990). Thymidine kinase in human leukemia--expression of three isoenzyme variants in six patients with chronic myelocytic leukemia. Leuk Res, 14(1), 39-45.

Munch-Petersen, B. (2009). Reversible tetramerization of human TK1 to the high catalytic efficient form is induced by pyrophosphate, in addition to tripolyphosphates, or high enzyme concentration. FEBS J, 276(2), 571-580.

Munch-Petersen, B. (2010). Enzymatic regulation of cytosolic thymidine kinase 1 and mitochondrial thymidine kinase 2: a mini review. Nucleosides Nucleotides Nucleic Acids, 29(4-6), 363-369.

Munch-Petersen, B., Cloos, L., Jensen, H. K., & Tyrsted, G. (1995). Human thymidine kinase 1. Regulation in normal and malignant cells. Adv Enzyme Regul, 35, 69-89.

Munch-Petersen, B., Cloos, L., Tyrsted, G., & Eriksson, S. (1991). Diverging substrate specificity of pure human thymidine kinases 1 and 2 against antiviral dideoxynucleosides. J Biol Chem, 266(14), 9032-9038.

Munch-Petersen, B., Tyrsted, G., & Cloos, L. (1993). Reversible ATP-dependent transition between two forms of human cytosolic thymidine kinase with different enzymatic properties. J Biol Chem, 268(21), 15621-15625.

Musto, P., Bodenizza, C., Falcone, A., D'Arena, G., Scalzulli, P., Perla, G., . . . Carotenuto, M. (1995). Prognostic relevance of serum thymidine kinase in primary myelodysplastic syndromes: relationship to development of acute myeloid leukaemia. Br J Haematol, 90(1), 125-130.

Musto, P., Cascavilla, N., Ladogana, S., Longo, S., Modoni, S., Ficola, U., & Carotenuto, M. (1989). Cerebro-spinal fluid thymidine kinase in acute leukemia. Leukemia, 3(9), 679-680.

Mutahir, Z., Clausen, A. R., Andersson, K. M., Wisen, S. M., Munch-Petersen, B., & Piskur, J. (2013). Thymidine kinase 1 regulatory fine-tuning through tetramer formation. Febs Journal, 280(6), 1531-1541.

Nisman, B., Allweis, T., Kadouri, L., Mali, B., Hamburger, T., Baras, M., . . . Peretz, T. (2013). Comparison of diagnostic and prognostic performance of two assays measuring thymidine kinase 1 activity in serum of breast cancer patients. Clinical Chemistry and Laboratory Medicine, 51(2), 439-447.

Nisman, B., Allweis, T., Kaduri, L., Maly, B., Gronowitz, S., Hamburger, T., & Peretz, T. (2010). Serum thymidine kinase 1 activity in breast cancer. Cancer Biomarkers, 7(2), 65-72.

Nisman, B., Yutkin, V., Nechushtan, H., Gofrit, O. N., Peretz, T., Gronowitz, S., & Pode, D. (2010). Circulating tumor M2 pyruvate kinase and thymidine kinase 1 are potential predictors for disease recurrence in renal cell carcinoma after nephrectomy. Urology, 76(2), 513 e511-516.

O'Neill, Abram, P., Hannigan, B., & McKenna, G. (1987). Elevated serum and mononuclear leukocyte thymidine kinase activities in patients with cancer. Ir Med J, 80(9), 264-265.

O'Neill, Buckwalter, M. R., & Murray, B. K. (2001). Thymidine kinase: diagnostic and prognostic potential. Expert Rev Mol Diagn, 1(4), 428-433.

O'Neill, Zhang, F., Li, H., Fuja, D. G., & Murray, B. K. (2007). Thymidine kinase 1--a prognostic and diagnostic indicator in ALL and AML patients. Leukemia, 21(3), 560-563.

O'Neill, K. L., Abram, W. P., & McKenna, P. G. (1986). Serum thymidine kinase levels in cancer patients. Ir J Med Sci, 155(8), 272-274.

O'Neill, K. L., Hoper, M., & Odling-Smee, G. W. (1992). Can thymidine kinase levels in breast tumors predict disease recurrence? J Natl Cancer Inst, 84(23), 1825-1828.

O'Neill, K. L., McKelvey, V. J., Hoper, M., Monteverde, H., Odling-Smee, G. W., Logan, H., . . . McKenna, P. G. (1992). Breast tumour thymidine kinase levels and disease recurrence. Med Lab Sci, 49(4), 244-247.

Oh, J. Y., Park, M. Y., Kim, D. R., Lee, J. H., Shim, S. H., Chung, J. H., . . . Lee, C. T. (2010). Combination gene therapy of lung cancer with conditionally replicating adenovirus and adenovirus-herpes simplex virus thymidine kinase. International Journal of Molecular Medicine, 25(3), 369-376.

Ohrvik, A., Lindh, M., Einarsson, R., Grassi, J., & Eriksson, S. (2004). Sensitive nonradiometric method for determining thymidine kinase 1 activity. Clin Chem, 50(9), 1597-1606.

Pan, Z.-L., Ji, X.-Y., Shi, Y.-M., Zhou, J., He, E., & Skog, S. (2010). Serum thymidine kinase 1 concentration as a prognostic factor of chemotherapy-treated non-Hodgkin's lymphoma patients. Journal of Cancer Research and Clinical Oncology, 136(8), 1193-1199.

Pang, J. H., & Chen, K. Y. (1993). A specific CCAAT-binding protein, CBP/tk, may be involved in the regulation of thymidine kinase gene expression in human IMR-90 diploid fibroblasts during senescence. J Biol Chem, 268(4), 2909-2916.

Posch, M., Hauser, C., & Seiser, C. (2000). Substrate binding is a prerequisite for stabilisation of mouse thymidine kinase in proliferating fibroblasts. J Mol Biol, 300(3), 493-502.

Priego, E. M., Karlsson, A., Gago, F., Camarasa, M. J., Balzarini, J., & Perez-Perez, M. J. (2012). Recent advances in thymidine kinase 2 (TK2) inhibitors and new perspectives for potential applications. Curr Pharm Des, 18(20), 2981-2994.

Prochazka, V., Faber, E., Raida, L., Langova, K., Indrak, K., & Papajik, T. (2012). High baseline serum thymidine kinase 1 level predicts unfavorable outcome in patients with follicular lymphoma. Leuk Lymphoma, 53(7), 1306-1310.

Radivoyevitch, T., Saunthararajah, Y., Pink, J., Ferris, G., Lent, I., Jackson, M., . . . Kunos, C. A. (2012). dNTP Supply Gene Expression Patterns after P53 Loss. Cancers (Basel), 4(4), 1212-1224.

Rasey, J. S., Grierson, J. R., Wiens, L. W., Kolb, P. D., & Schwartz, J. L. (2002). Validation of FLT uptake as a measure of thymidine kinase-1 activity in A549 carcinoma cells. J Nucl Med, 43(9), 1210-1217.

Reichard, P. (1988). Interactions between deoxyribonucleotide and DNA synthesis. Annu Rev Biochem, 57, 349-374.

Rhea, J. M., & Molinaro, R. J. (2011). Cancer biomarkers: surviving the journey from bench to bedside. MLO Med Lab Obs, 43(3), 10-12, 16, 18; quiz 20, 22.

Robertson, J. F., O'Neill, K. L., Thomas, M. W., McKenna, P. G., & Blamey, R. W. (1990). Thymidine kinase in breast cancer. Br J Cancer, 62(4), 663-667.

Romain, S., Bendahl, P. O., Guirou, O., Malmstrom, P., Martin, P. M., & Ferno, M. (2001). DNA-synthesizing enzymes in breast cancer (thymidine kinase, thymidylate synthase and thymidylate kinase): association with flow cytometric S-phase fraction and relative prognostic importance in node-negative premenopausal patients. Int J Cancer, 95(1), 56-61.

Romain, S., Spyratos, F., Descotes, F., Daver, A., Rostaing-Puissant, B., Bougnoux, P., . . . Martin, P. M. (2000). Prognostic of DNA-synthesizing enzyme activities (thymidine kinase and thymidylate synthase) in 908 T1-T2, N0-N1, M0 breast cancers: a retrospective multicenter study. Int J Cancer, 87(6), 860-868.

Saada, A., Shaag, A., Mandel, H., Nevo, Y., Eriksson, S., & Elpeleg, O. (2001). Mutant mitochondrial thymidine kinase in mitochondrial DNA depletion myopathy. Nat Genet, 29(3), 342-344.

Sarup, J. C., & Fridland, A. (1987). Identification of purine deoxyribonucleoside kinases from human leukemia cells: substrate activation by purine and pyrimidine deoxyribonucleosides. Biochemistry, 26(2), 590-597.

Schwartz, J. L., Tamura, Y., Jordan, R., Grierson, J. R., & Krohn, K. A. (2004). *Effect of p53 activation on cell growth, thymidine kinase-1 activity, and 3'-deoxy-3'fluorothymidine uptake. Nucl Med Biol, 31(4), 419-423.*

Segura-Pena, D., Lichter, J., Trani, M., Konrad, M., Lavie, A., & Lutz, S. (2007). *Quaternary structure change as a mechanism for the regulation of thymidine kinase 1-like enzymes. Structure, 15(12), 1555-1566.*

Segura-Pena, D., Lutz, S., Monnerjahn, C., Konrad, M., & Lavie, A. (2007). *Binding of ATP to TK1-like enzymes is associated with a conformational change in the quaternary structure. J Mol Biol, 369(1), 129-141.*

Sharif, H., Kiran Kumar, J., Wang, L., He, E., & Eriksson, S. (2012). *Quaternary structures of recombinant, cellular, and serum forms of Thymidine Kinase 1 from dogs and humans. BMC Biochem, 13(1), 12.*

Sharif, H., von Euler, H., Westberg, S., He, E., Wang, L., & Eriksson, S. (2012). *A sensitive and kinetically defined radiochemical assay for canine and human serum thymidine kinase 1 (TK1) to monitor canine malignant lymphoma. Veterinary Journal, 194(1), 40-47.*

Sherley, J. L., & Kelly, T. J. (1988). *Regulation of human thymidine kinase during the cell cycle. J Biol Chem, 263(17), 8350-8358.*

Shields, A. F. (2012). *PET imaging of tumor growth: not as easy as it looks. Clin Cancer Res, 18(5), 1189-1191.*

Shinomiya, A., Kawai, N., Okada, M., Miyake, K., Nakamura, T., Kushida, Y., . . . Tamiya, T. (2013). *Evaluation of 3'-deoxy-3'- F-18 -fluorothymidine (F-18-FLT) kinetics correlated with thymidine kinase-1 expression and cell proliferation in newly diagnosed gliomas. European Journal of Nuclear Medicine and Molecular Imaging, 40(2), 175-185.*

Siegel, R., Naishadham, D., & Jemal, A. (2013). *Cancer statistics, 2013. CA: A Cancer Journal for Clinicians, 63(1), 11-30.*

Span, P., Heuvel, J., Romain, S., Piffanelli, A., Martin, P. M., Geurts-Moespot, A., & Sweep, F. (2000). *EORTC receptor and biomarker study group report analytical and technical evaluation of a thymidine kinase radio-enzymatic assay in breast cancer cytosols. Anticancer Research, 20(2A), 681-687.*

Stalhandske, P., Wang, L., Westberg, S., von Euler, H., Groth, E., Gustafsson, S. A., . . . Lennerstrand, J. (2013). *Homogeneous assay for real-time and simultaneous detection of thymidine kinase 1 and deoxycytidine kinase activities. Anal Biochem, 432(2), 155-164.*

Struthers, H., Viertl, D., Kosinski, M., Spingler, B., Buchegger, F., & Schibli, R. (2010). *Charge dependent substrate activity of C3' and N3 functionalized, organometallic technetium and rhenium-labeled thymidine derivatives toward human thymidine kinase 1. Bioconjug Chem, 21(4), 622-634.*

Svobodova, S., Topolcan, O., Holubec, L., Treska, V., Sutnar, A., Rupert, K., . . . Finek, J. (2007). *Prognostic importance of thymidine kinase in colorectal and breast cancer. Anticancer Research, 27(4A), 1907-1909.*

Thamm, D. H., Kamstock, D. A., Sharp, C. R., Johnson, S. I., Mazzaferro, E., Herold, L. V., . . . Selting, K. A. (2012). *Elevated serum thymidine kinase activity in canine splenic hemangiosarcoma*. Vet Comp Oncol, 10(4), 292-302.*

Thomas, W. M., Robertson, J. F., McKenna, P. G., O'Neill, K. L., Robinson, M. H., & Hardcastle, J. D. (1995). *Serum thymidine kinase in colorectal neoplasia. Eur J Surg Oncol, 21(6), 632-634.*

Topolcan, & Holubec, L. (2008). *The role of thymidine kinase in cancer diseases. Expert Opinion on Medical Diagnostics, 2(2), 129-141.*

Topolcan, Holubec, L., Jr., Finek, J., Stieber, P., Holdenrieder, S., Lamerz, R., . . . Lipska, L. (2005). *Changes of thymidine kinase (TK) during adjuvant and palliative chemotherapy. Anticancer Research, 25(3A), 1831-1833.*

Tzeng, H. F., & Hung, H. P. (2005). *Simultaneous determination of thymidylate and thymidine diphosphate by capillary electrophoresis as a rapid monitoring tool for thymidine kinase and thymidylate kinase activities. Electrophoresis, 26(11), 2225-2230.*

von Euler, H. P., Ohrvik, A. B., & Eriksson, S. K. (2006). *A non-radiometric method for measuring serum thymidine kinase activity in malignant lymphoma in dogs. Res Vet Sci, 80(1), 17-24.*

Votava, T., Topolcan, O., Holubec, L., Jr., Cerna, Z., Sasek, L., Finek, J., & Kormunda, S. (2007). Changes of serum thymidine kinase in children with acute leukemia. Anticancer Research, 27(4A), 1925-1928.

Wakazono, Y., Kubota, M., Furusho, K., Liu, L., & Gerson, S. L. (1996). Thymidine kinase deficient cells with decreased TTP pools are hypersensitive to DNA alkylating agents. Mutat Res, 362(1), 119-125.

Wang, & Eriksson, S. (2000). Cloning and characterization of full-length mouse thymidine kinase 2: the N-terminal sequence directs import of the precursor protein into mitochondria. Biochem J, 351 Pt 2, 469-476.

Wang, He, Q., Skog, S., Eriksson, S., & Tribukait, B. (2001). Investigation on cell proliferation with a new antibody against thymidine kinase 1. Anal Cell Pathol, 23(1), 11-19.

Weber, G., Ichikawa, S., Nagai, M., & Natsumeda, Y. (1990). Azidothymidine inhibition of thymidine kinase and synergistic cytotoxicity with methotrexate and 5-fluorouracil in rat hepatoma and human colon cancer cells. Cancer Commun, 2(4), 129-133.

Welin, M., Kosinska, U., Mikkelsen, N. E., Carnrot, C., Zhu, C., Wang, L., . . . Eklund, H. (2004). Structures of thymidine kinase 1 of human and mycoplasmic origin. Proc Natl Acad Sci U S A, 101(52), 17970-17975.

Wu, Li, W. P., Qian, C., Ding, W., Zhou, Z. W., & Jiang, H. (2013). Increased serum level of thymidine kinase 1 correlates with metastatic site in patients with malignant melanoma. Tumour Biol, 34(2), 643-648.

Wu, Mao, Y., He, L., Wang, N., Wu, C., He, Q., & Skog, S. (2000). A new cell proliferating marker: cytosolic thymidine kinase as compared to proliferating cell nuclear antigen in patients with colorectal carcinoma. Anticancer Research, 20(6C), 4815-4820.

Wu, Yang, R., Zhou, J., Bao, S., Zou, L., Zhang, P., . . . He, Q. (2003). Production and characterisation of a novel chicken IgY antibody raised against C-terminal peptide from human thymidine kinase 1. J Immunol Methods, 277(1-2), 157-169.

Xu, Shi, Q. L., Ma, H. H., Zhou, H. B., Lu, Z. F., Yu, B., . . . Skog, S. (2012). High thymidine kinase 1 (TK1) expression is a predictor of poor survival in patients with pT1 of lung adenocarcinoma. Tumor Biology, 33(2), 475-483.

Xu, Zhang, Y. M., Shu, X. H., Shan, L. H., Wang, Z. W., Zhou, Y. L., . . . Skog, S. (2008). Serum thymidine kinase 1 reflects the progression of pre-malignant and malignant tumors during therapy. Mol Med Report, 1(5), 705-711.

Xu, W., Cao, X., Miao, K.-R., Qiao, C., Wu, Y.-J., Liu, Q., . . . Li, J.-Y. (2009). Serum thymidine kinase 1 concentration in Chinese patients with chronic lymphocytic leukemia and its correlation with other prognostic factors. International Journal of Hematology, 90(2), 205-211.

Zacchetti, A., van Garderen, E., Teske, E., Nederbragt, H., Dierendonck, J. H., & Rutteman, G. R. (2003). Validation of the use of proliferation markers in canine neoplastic and non-neoplastic tissues: comparison of KI-67 and proliferating cell nuclear antigen (PCNA) expression versus in vivo bromodeoxyuridine labelling by immunohistochemistry. Apmis, 111(3), 430-438.

Zaharevitz, D. W., Anderson, L. W., Malinowski, N. M., Hyman, R., Strong, J. M., & Cysyk, R. L. (1992). Contribution of de-novo and salvage synthesis to the uracil nucleotide pool in mouse tissues and tumors in vivo. Eur J Biochem, 210(1), 293-296.

Zhang, Jia, Q., Zou, S., Zhang, P., Zhang, X., Skog, S., . . . He, Q. (2006). Thymidine kinase 1: a proliferation marker for determining prognosis and monitoring the surgical outcome of primary bladder carcinoma patients. Oncol Rep, 15(2), 455-461.

Zhang, Kang, C. S., Shi, L., Zhao, P., Liu, N., & You, Y. P. (2010). Use of thymidine kinase gene-modified endothelial progenitor cells as a vector targeting angiogenesis in glioma gene therapy. Oncology, 78(2), 94-102.

Zhang, Shao, X., Li, H., Robison, J. G., Murray, B. K., & O'Neill, K. L. (2001). A monoclonal antibody specific for human thymidine kinase 1. Hybridoma, 20(1), 25-34.

Zhang, C. C., Yan, Z., Li, W., Kuszpit, K., Painter, C. L., Zhang, Q., . . . Christensen, J. G. (2012). [(18)F]FLT-PET imaging does not always "light up" proliferating tumor cells. Clin Cancer Res, 18(5), 1303-1312.

Zhu, C., Harlow, L. S., Berenstein, D., Munch-Petersen, S., & Munch-Petersen, B. (2006). *Effect of C-terminal of human cytosolic thymidine kinase (TK1) on in vitro stability and enzymatic properties. Nucleosides Nucleotides Nucleic Acids, 25(9-11), 1185-1188.*

Zou, L., Zhang, P. G., Zou, S., Li, Y., & He, Q. (2002). *The half-life of thymidine kinase 1 in serum measured by ECL dot blot: a potential marker for monitoring the response to surgery of patients with gastric cancer. Int J Biol Markers, 17(2), 135-140.*

Diagnosis of Primary Gastrointestinal Lymphomas and Mimics

Mingyi Chen

Department of Pathology and Laboratory Medicine
University of California at Davis Medical Center, Sacramento, CA, USA

Thomas J. Semrad

Department of Internal Medicine, Division of Hematology and Oncology
University of California at Davis Medical Center, Sacramento, CA, USA

Jun Wang

Department of Pathology and Laboratory Medicine
Loma Linda University Medical Center, Loma Linda, CA, USA

1   Introduction

Primary gastrointestinal (GI) lymphomas typically refer to a lymphoma that predominantly involves any section of the GI tract from the oropharynx to the rectum (Bautista-Quach, Ake, Chen, & Wang, 2012).While the disease often involves a single primary site, multiple sites within the GI tract may be involved, as can local and distant lymph nodes. Primary GI tract lymphomas are uncommon, while secondary involvement of the GI tract by lymphoma is relatively frequent (Lewin, Ranchod, & Dorfman, 1978). Nonetheless, primary lymphomas of the GI tract are important since their evaluation, diagnosis, management and prognosis are distinct from that of lymphoma at other sites and other cancers of the GI tract (Dawson, Cornes, & Morson, 1961).

1.1   Background

The amount and nature of GI tract associated lymphoid tissue varies greatly within the GI tract, thus influencing the type of lymphomas developing in each location (Radic-Kristo *et al.*, 2010). The character of these lymphoid tissues is determined by innate genetic factors and acquired immune stimulation, often directed by exposure to the innumerable dietary and microbial antigens and inflammatory responses. The normal esophagus essentially has no lymphoid tissue associated with the mucosa. Likewise, B-lymphocytes, plasma cells, and granulocytes are almost completely absent in the normal stomach (Cardona, Layne, & Lagoo, 2012). A few CD8+ T-cells are present in intraepithelial locations and CD4+ T-cells are localized mainly in the lamina propria of stomach, accompanied by macrophages and very few CD1-positive Langerhans' cells (Brenchley *et al.*, 2004; Cardona *et al.*, 2012). In contrast, the intestines contain a large amount of lymphoid tissue, concentrated in the mucosa and submucosa, which is collectively referred to as mucosa associated lymphoid tissue or MALT (Isaacson PG, 2008).

Intestinal MALT is the primary site for eliciting adaptive immune responses towards mucosal antigens and can be divided into three components including Peyer's patches, isolated lymphoid follicules, and efferent lymphatics. Most well-known among these are the organized lymphoid aggregates called Peyer's patches, which first appear during 19th week of gestation on the antimesenteric border of the entire small intestine starting at the upper jejunum. Their numbers appear to be predetermined but their size steadily increases until puberty, followed by gradual involution in old age. They resemble miniature lymph nodes and contain both B- and T-cells, segregated in the follicles and interfollicular areas, respectively. The luminal antigens are carried to the Peyer's patches through specialized epithelial cells called M cells, present in the intestinal lining covering the dome region of the patch, and presented to the dendritic cells (Burke, 2011). Structures closely related to Peyer's patches but containing only an isolated lymphoid follicle develop after exposure to intestinal commensals and are particularly numerous in the colon, which lacks Peyer's patches. Efferent lymphatics from the Peyer's patches carry memory B-cells and plasma cells to mesenteric lymph nodes and hematogenous lymphocytes traffic through MALT by virtue of specific adhesion molecules (Isaacson PG, 2008).

Gastrointestinal lymphomas comprise a group of distinctive clinicopathological entities of B- or T-cell type, with primary gastrointestinal Hodgkin's disease being extremely uncommon (Devaney & Jaffe, 1991). Most low-grade B-cell gastrointestinal lymphomas are MALT type, so called because they recapitulate the features of MALT rather than those of lymph nodes. Paradoxically, however, most MALT lymphomas arise in the stomach, which normally contains no organized lymphoid tissue. The gastrointestinal (GI) tract is the predominant site of extranodal marginal zone lymphoma of mucosa-associated lymphoid tissue (MALT lymphoma), accounting for 30–40% of cases of all extranodal lymphomas (Isaacson PG, 2008). Although B-cell lymphomas are by far the most frequent type found in this location, gastrointestinal lymphomas are a diverse group of neoplasms, many of which are characterized by distinctive clinicopathologic settings. Diffuse large B-cell lymphoma (DLBCL) and MALT lymphoma are commonly encountered, but other less common entities can pose diagnostic challenges, mimicking both benign, reactive conditions and each other (Bautista-Quach et al., 2012).

Primary GI lymphomas are derived from lymphoid tissue of the MALT and lymph nodes of the intestine (including Peyer's patches). In western countries, the estimated frequency of GI lymphomas based on the site are stomach (48%) > small bowel (26%) > colon (12%) > pancreas (2%) > esophagus (rare). In the Middle East and Mediterranean basin, small bowel lymphoma is most common, and accounts for up to 75 percent of primary GI lymphomas. The incidence of Burkitt lymphoma (BL) in Africa is approximately 50-fold higher than it is in the US, and its classic GI presentation is that of an obstructing lesion in the terminal ileum (Koch et al., 2001).

1.2   Predisposing Conditions

The conditions that predispose to GI lymphoma include (Andrews et al., 2008; Isaacson PG, 2008):

- Helicobacter pylori infection — H. pylori infection is highly associated with the development of MALT lymphoma of the stomach (Suzuki, Saito, & Hibi, 2009).

- Autoimmune diseases — A variety of autoimmune diseases, including rheumatoid arthritis, Sjögren's syndrome, systemic lupus erythematosus and granulomatosis with polyangiitis (previously Wegener's granulomatosis), have been associated with an increased risk of lymphoma. Immunosuppression, rather than the disease itself, is thought to be responsible for the increased risk.

- Immunodeficiency and immunosuppression — Congenital immunodeficiency syndromes (eg, Wiskott-Aldrich syndrome, severe combined immunodeficiency syndrome, ataxia-telangiectasia, X-linked agammaglobulinemia) and acquired immunodeficiency (eg, HIV infection, iatrogenic immunosuppression) are associated with an increased incidence of B cell lymphoma. Lymphomas occurring in this setting tend to be aggressive and widespread at the time of diagnosis (Jamieson, Thiru, Calne, & Evans, 1981; Sandler & Kaplan, 1996).

- Celiac disease — Patients with gluten-sensitive enteropathy (celiac disease) are at increased risk of developing enteropathy-associated T cell lymphoma (EATL) (Smedby et al., 2005).

- Inflammatory bowel disease — An association between inflammatory bowel disease (IBD) and lymphoma has been described, as has been a possible association between tumor necrosis factor-alpha inhibitors and hepatic gamma delta T-cell lymphoma (Aithal & Mansfield, 2001; Kandiel, Fraser, Korelitz, Brensinger, & Lewis, 2005; Thayu et al., 2005).

- Nodular lymphoid hyperplasia — Nodular lymphoid hyperplasia, also known as follicular lymphoid hyperplasia, is a benign condition that has been implicated as a possible risk factor for primary lymphomas of the small intestine (Burke, 2011).

1.3   Clinical Presentation

The clinical signs and symptoms of GI lymphomas are typically nonspecific, attributable to the site of involvement:

Gastric lymphoma is the most common site of GI lymphoma and typically presents with nonspecific symptoms such as epigastric pain or discomfort, anorexia, weight loss, nausea and/or vomiting, occult GI bleeding, and/or early satiety. The diagnosis is usually established during upper endoscopy with biopsy. The vast majority (greater than 90 percent) of gastric lymphomas is approximately equally divided between extranodal marginal zone B cell lymphoma of gut-mucosa (gut)-associated lymphoid tissue (MALT) type (referred to as MALT lymphoma in this chapter) and diffuse large B cell lymphoma.

Lymphoma of the small intestine is the second most common site and the clinical presentation varies depending upon whether the tumor is associated with immunoproliferative small intestinal disease (IPSID), celiac disease (enteropathy-associated T cell lymphoma, EATL), or neither. The diagnosis may be suggested on computed tomography (CT) and/or contrast radiography, but requires a biopsy for confirmation.

Colorectal lymphoma is an uncommon form of GI lymphoma and may present with abdominal pain, overt or occult bleeding, diarrhea, intussusception, or rarely, bowel obstruction. Colonoscopy with biopsy is the principal diagnostic modality for colorectal lymphomas. The most common histologic types include diffuse large B cell lymphoma, mantle cell lymphoma, and Burkitt lymphoma.

Esophagus is perhaps the most uncommon site for primary GI lymphoma, which appears to more commonly involve the distal esophagus. Most patients are asymptomatic or present with complaints of dysphagia or odynophagia. There is a diverse appearance on imaging and the diagnosis is made by endoscopic biopsy in most cases.

1.4 Staging

Lymphoma of the GI tract is staged using the Ann Arbor System, with the GI tract being considered an extranodal site (Boot, 2010):

- I-Single nodal or extranodal site

- II-More than one nodal group on same side of diaphragm or single extranodal group with adjacent lymph nodes

- III- Multiple nodal sites on both sides of diaphragm

- IV-Bone, central nerve system (CNS), diffuse visceral involvement

2   Lymphomas by Anatomic Location

2.1 Gastric Lymphoma

The stomach is the most common extranodal site of lymphoma. Primary gastric lymphoma accounts for 3 percent of gastric neoplasms and 10 percent of lymphomas (Isaacson PG, 2008; Lewin *et al.*, 1978). Stomach is the most common site of GI tract involved by lymphoma, accounting for 68 to 75 percent of GI lymphomas (Koch *et al.*, 2001). Gastric lymphoma reaches its peak incidence between the ages of 50 to 60 years. There is a slight male predominance.

Gastric lymphoma is clinically heterogeneous. While the vast majority of cases occur in individuals infected with Helicobacter pylori, the cases can show a range of histologies and can follow diverse natural histories. Tumors may comprise mainly small cells, contain predominantly large cells with a small-cell component, or consist entirely of large cells, similar to diffuse large B-cell lymphomas occurring in nodes or other extranodal tissues (Cardona *et al.*, 2012; Starostik *et al.*, 2002). The disease originates on inflammatory background brought about by a chronic Helicobacter pylori infection that initiates buildup of MALT in originally lymphoid follicle-free stomach. Further development of lymphoma out of the MALT is the result of continuous antigen-dependent growth of B lymphocytes in the early phase that then progresses into a stage of autonomous proliferation of a true low-grade lymphoma. That lymphoma can and in some cases does develop into a high-grade lymphoma (Starostik *et al.*, 2002).

The diagnosis of gastric lymphoma is usually established during upper endoscopy with biopsy. The vast majority (greater than 90 percent) of gastric lymphomas are approximately equally divided into two histologic subtypes, gastric extranodal marginal zone B cell lymphoma of MALT type (MALT lymphoma), and DLBCL (Isaacson PG, 2008; Koch *et al.*, 2001; Lewin *et al.*, 1978). The remaining cases of gastric lymphoma may represent any histology including mantle cell lymphoma (1 percent), follicular lymphoma, and peripheral T cell lymphoma.

2.2 Lymphoma of the Small Intestine

Small intestine has abundant mucosal lymphoid tissue which contains both B- and T-cells and lymphomas of both cell types occur in this location. Reactive lymphohistiocytic infiltrate due to infections can occur and mimic Hodgkin lymphoma in immunocompromised patients. The most common lymphoma in adults is DLBCL, but in children Burkitt lymphoma is more common (Matuchansky *et al.*, 1985). Some lymphomas are rather unique to the small intestine or have unique features when they occur in this GI tract site.

These lymphomas may be broadly categorized into three main groups, 1) Immunoproliferative small intestinal disease (IPSID, also called alpha heavy chain disease, Mediterranean lymphoma, or Seligmann disease). This lymphoma is a variant of MALT lymphoma which secretes alpha heavy chains, 2) Enteropathy-associated T cell lymphoma (EATL), also called intestinal T cell lymphoma, is a tumor that is highly associated with gluten-sensitive enteropathy (celiac disease), and 3) Other western-type non-IPSID lymphomas, including diffuse large B cell lymphoma, mantle cell lymphoma, Burkitt lymphoma, follicular lymphoma (Mori *et al.*, 2010). In the Middle East and Mediterranean basin, primary small intestinal lymphoma, usually of the IPSID type, accounts for up to 75 percent of primary GI lymphomas (Salem *et al.*, 1987). Although uncommon, enteropathy-associated T cell lymphoma (EATL) is most common in areas with a high incidence of gluten-sensitive enteropathy (celiac disease), such as the Western part of Ireland and Northern Europe (Verbeek *et al.*, 2008).

IPSID-associated lymphomas generally appear as a diffuse infiltrating lesion of the proximal small intestine, sometimes resembling cobblestoning. The presence of multiple polyps of varying size within the bowel (lymphomatous polyposis) is particularly common in mantle cell lymphoma. Patients with enteropathy-associated T cell lymphoma of the jejunum typically demonstrate large circumferential ulcers without overt tumor masses. Biopsies of the involved mucosa demonstrate lymphoma, while biopsies of the normal appearing mucosa usually show villous atrophy characteristic of celiac disease (Salem *et al.*, 1987).

Patients with mantle cell lymphoma may demonstrate typical small nodular or polypoid tumors (2 mm to more than 2 cm in size), with or without normal intervening mucosa referred to as "lymphomatous polyposis" (Bautista-Quach *et al.*, 2012).

Patients with primary intestinal follicular lymphoma most often (commonly) present with multiple small (1 to 5 mm) polypoid lesions in the descending part of the duodenum. The lesions are solitary in approximately 15 percent of cases and may grossly resemble adenomas (Iwamuro *et al.*, 2013).

2.3   Colorectal Lymphoma

Colorectal lymphomas are uncommon, accounting for approximately 3 percent of the GI lymphomas and 0.3 percent of large intestinal malignancies (Koch *et al.*, 2001; Lewin *et al.*, 1978). There is a male predominance, twice as often in males compared with females (Aledavood *et al.*, 2012). The diagnosis of colorectal lymphoma is dependent upon the histologic evaluation of an adequate biopsy specimen. The most common lymphomas seen in this region include: DLBCL, mantle cell lymphoma, Burkitt lymphoma, and follicular lymphoma. Almost all primary colorectal lymphomas reported from the West have B-cell lineage, but rare T-cell lymphomas are reported in the East. While MALT lymphomas are relatively uncommon in large intestine, DLBCLs may show a low grade component in a minority of cases. In immunocompetent patients the cecum is involved most often but in immunodeficient patients, the rectum (and anal canal) is more likely to be involved (Koch *et al.*, 2001). The difference could be due to the viral infectious etiology (Hyder & Mackeigan, 1988).

2.4   Esophageal Lymphoma

Primary esophageal lymphoma is very rare, accounting for less than 1 percent of primary GI lymphomas. More commonly, lymphoma may involve the esophagus as an extension of mediastinal or gastric involvement. Only case reports and series of primary esophageal lymphoma have been reported in the literature (Kalogeropoulos *et al.*, 2009). Primary esophageal lymphoma appears to more commonly involve the distal esophagus. Most patients are asymptomatic or present with complaints of dysphagia or odynophagia. There is a diverse appearance on imaging and the diagnosis is made by endoscopic biopsy in most cases (Ghai, Pattison, O'Malley, Khalili, & Stephens, 2007).

3   Morphologic Classification

In this section, the characteristic pathological, immunophenotypic, and genetic features of different GI lymphomas categorized according to World Health Organization (WHO) classification are discussed. The epidemiological, clinical, and pathological features of lymphomas occurring in each part of the GI tract are summarized and the key points regarding lymphomas at each site are emphasized.

3.1   Overview

The current lymphoma classification is based on morphological, immunophenotypic, genetic, and clinical features (Isaacson PG, 2008). In addition to characteristic cell morphology, most GI lymphomas also demonstrate fairly typical architectural features which are useful in diagnosis. Specific cytogenetic abnormalities are seen in many lymphomas and appear to influence their clinical behavior to a great extent. Making the correct diagnosis, according to the WHO classification, is critical because treatments can vary widely from a simple "wait and watch" approach to local radiation or surgery to high dose chemotherapy with or without stem cell transplantation. No separate classification for gastrointestinal lymphomas is offered by the World Health Organization (WHO), although extranodal marginal zone lymphoma of MALT (including immunoproliferative small-intestinal disorder) and enteropathy-associated T-cell lymphoma form 2 distinct categories among the mature B-, T- and natural killer (NK)–cell neoplasms. The distinguishing clinicopathological features of the major types of lymphomas occurring in the GI tract are summarized in Table 1.

Hodgkin Lymphoma	T-cell lymphomas
Non-Hodgkin Lymphoma	type II (non–enteropathy associated)
B-cell lymphomas	NK/T, nasal type
Extranodal marginal zone lymphoma, MALT type	Gamma-Delta type
IPSID (heavy chain disease)	Anaplastic large cell lymphoma
Mantle cell (lymphomatous polyposis)	Peripheral T-cell lymphoma, not otherwise specified
Follicular lymphoma	Angioimmunoblastic T-cell lymphoma
Diffuse large B-cell lymphoma	Adult T-cell lymphoma
Burkitt lymphoma	Precursor T-lymphoblastic lymphoma
Small lymphocytic lymphoma	Others
Precursor B-lymphoblastic lymphoma	
Plasmacytoma	
Plasmablastic lymphoma	
Others	

Table 1: Classification of Primary Gastrointestinal Lymphomas Histologic Type.

3.2   B-Cell Lymphomas

I. Extranodal marginal zone mucosa associated lymphoid tissue (MALT) lymphoma

MALT lymphomas comprise over 50% of primary gastric non-Hodgkin lymphomas, occurring predominately in patients older than 50 years, with a noted peak in the seventh decade and a male: female ratio of about 1.5:1 (Psyrri, Papageorgiou, & Economopoulos, 2008). Patients commonly present with nonspecific gastritis and/or a peptic ulcer. Endoscopy commonly demonstrates erythematous and slightly thickened rugae with superficial spreading of lesions without formation of a distinct mass. The gastric lesions commonly are multifocal, and most patients have stage I or II disease (Isaacson PG, 2008; Nakamura *et al.*, 2008). Cases of MALT transformation to DLBCL have also been recognized (Isaacson PG, 2008; Nakamura *et al.*, 2008).

Pathogenesis

A strong association between chronic *H. pylori* infection and gastric MALT lymphoma has been demonstrated in 80 to 90% of cases, and it is widely accepted that the bacterial infection plays a crucial role in the pathogenesis of this tumor (Isaacson PG, 2008; Nakamura *et al.*, 2000; Psyrri *et al.*, 2008). Chronic *H. pylori* infection provides the antigenic stimulus, resulting in the clonal expansion of lymphoid cells leading to the evolution of MALT lymphoma. According to the study by Arnold and colleagues, *H. pylori* strains expressing the cytotoxin-associated gene A *(CagA)* protein carry the major histocompatibility complex (MHC) class II T cell epitope. Therefore, infection with this specific strain induces activation of CD4+ T cells which has been postulated to instigate neoplasia (Arnold *et al.*, 2011; Mills, Kurjanczyk, & Penner, 1992).

On the other hand, lymphomagenesis has also been hypothesized to evolve independent of *H. pylori* infection (Farinha & Gascoyne, 2005; Isaacson PG, 2008), particularly in the setting of translocation (11;18)(q21;q21) positive cases (Nakamura *et al.*, 2000). This aberration is further described under *molecular abnormalities*. Transformation to DLBCL has been documented in cases independent of *H. pylori* infection, as well as in cases harboring genomic alterations of the MYC, p53, p15, p16, and retinoblastoma (Rb) genes (Farinha & Gascoyne, 2005).

Morphology and immunophenotype

Gastric MALT lymphomas are characterized by lymphoepithelial lesions (LEL) (Figure 1) with glandular invasion by neoplastic centrocyte-like cells or small lymphoid cells with irregular nuclear contour, nuclear clefting, hyperchromasia, and with scant to fair amount of cytoplasm. Occasional atypical plasmacytoid/plasmacytic lymphocytes and/or plasma cells may also be observed. Nevertheless, care must be taken to avoid over-interpretation of LELs as these lesions may also appear in benign settings including reactive lymphoid infiltrates. Lymphoepithelial lesions are not reliable in distinguishing chronic active H. Pylori gastritis from MALT-lymphoma since they can occur in both (Aledavood *et al.*, 2012).

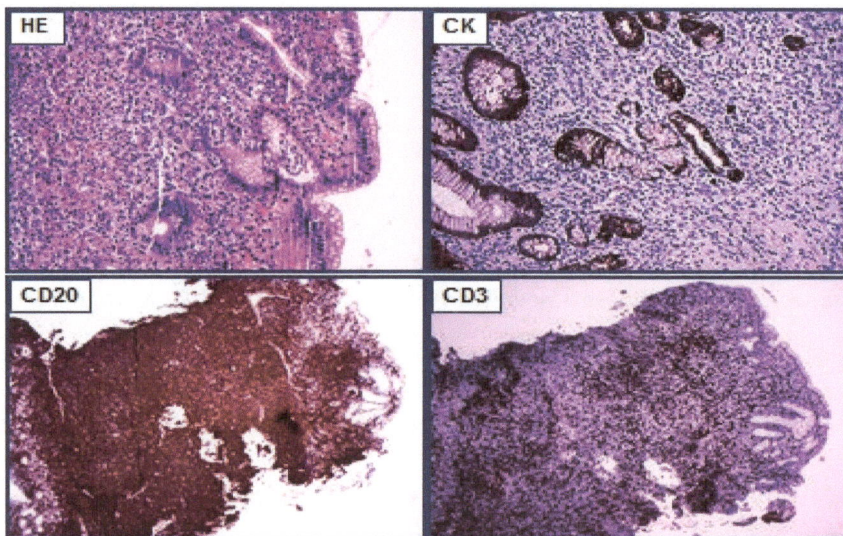

Figure 1: H&E stained section of extranodal marginal zone lymphoma, MALT type lymphoma of stomach. The dense atypical lymphoid infiltrate in MALT lymphoma extends deeper into the lamina propria. Immunohistochemistry for CD20 highlights sheets of B-cells and lymphoepithelial lesions. Cytokeratin (CK) stain shows the glandular epithelial cells. CD3 stain is positive in the reactive non-neoplastic T-cells.

The distinction between reactive LEL and neoplastic LEL may be very difficult. A large infiltrate, a relatively monotonous lymphoid population, cytologic atypia and numerous Dutcher bodies are supportive of a malignant diagnosis. The presence of halos around LEL's and broad interconnecting bands of atypical lymphoid cells (centrocyte-like or monocytoid B cells) are features supporting the diagnosis of lymphoma. With progression, the LEL's are destroyed, reactive follicles are infiltrated and replaced and the process extends outside the gland (Bautista-Quach *et al.*, 2012; Isaacson PG, 2008). Reactive germinal centers, common in the deeper mucosa associated with *H. pylori* gastritis, may be colonized by lymphoma cells, with obliteration of mantle zone and the appearance of so-called "naked" follicles. The atypical lymphoid infiltrate usually expands the lamina propria or submucosa. Muscularis mucosae infiltration and disruption can be a useful clue to the diagnosis in small biopsy specimens. In more extensive cases, the lymphoma can create mucosal ulcers and can infiltrate through the muscularis propria.

While MALT lymphoma does not show a specific immunohistochemical profile, there is usually an overabundance of neoplastic B cells as highlighted by CD20 immunostain. Large series have demonstrated that up to 50% of the cases may also aberrantly co-express CD43 and/or BCL2 by these neoplastic B cells (Isaacson PG, 2008; Psyrri *et al.*, 2008). The tumor cells show variable surface and cytoplasmic immunoglobulin reactivity, with most cases expressing IgM, and a few cases showing IgA or IgG reactivity, whereas IgD expression is rare. The neoplastic B cells are negative for CD10, CD23, and cyclin D1, and typically do not co-express CD5, although rare cases of CD5-positive MALT lymphomas have been documented (Terada, 2012). In cases with extensive or nearly complete plasmacytic differentiation, immunostains for kappa and lambda light chains can be extremely useful in highlighting possible monotypic plasma cell population (Bautista-Quach *et al.*, 2012).

Molecular abnormalities

For MALT lymphomas in general, the genetic abnormalities encompass trisomies 3, 12 and 18, as well as balanced translocations, specifically t(11;18)(q21;q21), t(14;18)(q32;q21), t(1;14)(p22;q32) and t(3;14)(p14;q32). The most common translocation in gastric MALT lymphoma, arising in approximately 20-30% of cases (although lower in North America) is t(11;18)(q21;q21), in which the t(11;18) fuses the amino terminal of the apoptosis inhibitor *API2* at 11q21 to the carboxyl terminal of *MALT1* at 18q21 leading to a chimeric fusion protein (Sugano, 1998). *MALT1* is involved in antigen receptor-mediated nuclear factor kB (NF-kB) activation (32,33). However, t(11;18)(q21;q21) is usually not associated with *H. pylori* gastritis; hence, such cases are believed to show resistance to antibiotic therapy (Nakamura *et al.*, 2000).

All aforementioned translocations induce activation of the nuclear factor kB (NF-kB) oncogenic pathway (Psyrri *et al.*, 2008). It has been postulated that chronic inflammation leads to activation of NF-kB pathway via the antigen receptor signaling in MALT lymphoma cells. Antigen stimulation and CD40 triggering synergize NF-kB activation through formation of *CARMA1–BCL10–MALT1* ternary complex. In addition, the continuous and sustained antiapoptotic stimuli driven by *API2-MALT1* are most likely to play key roles in the pathogenesis of MALT lymphomas (Farinha & Gascoyne, 2005; Sagaert, De Wolf-Peeters, Noels, & Baens, 2007).

Prognosis

The response of low grade MALT lymphoma to *H. pylori* eradication is predicted by stage. Complete regression of low-grade, early stage MALT lymphoma following successful *H. pylori* eradication has been confirmed in about 75-80% of cases (Chiang, Wang, Cheng, Lin, & Su, 1996; Isaacson PG, 2008). Studies have documented that complete response has been achieved in nearly all patients where disease is limited to the gastric mucosa or submucosa. Complete response rates have decreased in cases where disease extended to the muscularis propria or serosa (Freeman, Berg, & Cutler, 1972). Furthermore, it has been shown that no patients with nodal disease achieved complete response with *H. pylori* eradication alone (Nakamura *et al.*, 2008).

It is important to note, however, that approximately 10% of gastric MALT lymphomas have the t(11;18)(q21;q21) translocation and are resistant to *H. pylori* antibiotic therapy, suggesting importance of strict follow up, and if clinically indicated, a trial of chemotherapy, immunotherapy (i.e., Rituximab), and/or radiotherapy for localized disease, may be pursued (Isaacson PG, 2008; Nakamura *et al.*, 2008). Studies suggest that medical therapy alone is superior to surgery, although surgical intervention may be appropriate in specific circumstances such as in cases with gastric outlet obstruction and/or other complications (Yoon, Coit, Portlock, & Karpeh, 2004).

Diagnosis of gastric MALT lymphoma

It should be emphasized that essentially not all of the above described histopathologic features are seen in every case of low-grade gastric MALT lymphoma, and virtually everyone can be seen in other neoplasms or even benign reactive conditions. Even prominent lymphoepithelial lesions, often regarded as among the features most suggestive of MALT lymphoma, can be seen in florid follicular gastritis as well as non-MALT lymphomas. Thus, the histologic diagnosis of gastric MALT lymphoma is based on analysis of the gestalt of features present, rather than on the presence of any individual feature. These difficulties are magnified in small mucosal biopsies, where limited sampling and crush artifact can further limit assessment.

In general, it has been suggested that an unequivocal diagnosis of low grade MALT lymphoma be made on the basis of histologic analysis of small gastric mucosal biopsies only if all three of the following features are present in full flower: 1) a dense, extensive, interfollicular lymphoid infiltrate (sometimes defined as occupying at least half of a low-power field using a 4X objective), 2) the predominance within the infiltrate of atypical centrocyte-like cells, with or without clear cytoplasm, and 3) prominent lymphoepithelial lesions, generally associated with expansion and distortion of glandular structures, and eosinophilic degeneration of the epithelial cytoplasm. Specimens showing lesser degrees of atypia should be termed "suspicious lymphoid infiltrates"; in such cases repeat biopsies to provide material for immunophenotyping and lymphoid antigen receptor gene rearrangement studies could be helpful if warranted clinically. The histologic scoring system initially described by Wotherspoon *et al.* (1993) for assessment of post-therapy biopsies (but equally applicable to initial diagnostic specimens) is reproduced here (Table 2), and can be useful in categorizing suspicious lymphoid infiltrates (Copie-Bergman *et al.*, 2003).

Grade	Description	Histological Features
0	Normal	Scattered plasma cells in LP. No LFs
1	Chronic active gastritis	Small clusters of lymphocytes in LP. No LFs. No LELs.
2	Chronic active gastritis with florid LF formation	Prominent LFs with surrounding MZ and plasma cells. No LELs.
3	Suspicious lymphoid infiltrate in LP, probably reactive	LFs surrounded by small lymphocytes that infiltrate diffusely in LP and occasionally into epithelium
4	Suspicious lymphoid infiltrate in LP, probably lymphoma	LFs surrounded by CCL cells that infiltrate diffusely in LP and into epithelium in small groups
5	Low-grade B-cell lymphoma of MALT	Presence of dense diffuse infiltrate of CCL cells in LP with prominent LELs

LP = Lamina propria, LF = lymphoid follicle, LEL = lymphoepithelial lesion, MZ = mantle zone
CCL = centrocyte-like, MALT = mucosa associated lymphoid tissue

Table 2: Histologic grading system for gastric MALT lymphoma.

Although less common than gastric primaries, MALT lymphomas also not infrequently present in the intestines. Most involve the small intestine; colorectal tumors are rare. The most common form of intestinal MALT lymphoma histopathologically and immunophenotypically resembles gastric MALT lymphoma, and is diagnosed in the same manner. It apparently shows a somewhat less favorable prognosis than gastric primaries, however. Despite its occurrence throughout the world, this form is termed the "Western type" of intestinal MALT lymphoma, largely to distinguish it from a form endemic in the Mediterranean and Middle East, previously referred to a "Mediterranean lymphoma", but now more commonly referred to as immunoproliferative small intestinal disease (IPSID)(Salem *et al.*, 1987). This latter entity is the subject of the next section.

II. Immunoproliferative Small Intestinal Disease (IPSID)

IPSID is a variant form of MALT lymphoma arising in the small intestine that has also been described as alpha heavy chain disease (alpha-HCD). The neoplastic cells of IPSID show a characteristic production of alpha immunoglobulin heavy chains without light chain, which occurs as a paraprotein in the serum, leading this alternate designation. IPSID or alpha-HCD is the most common form of the heavy chain diseases (HCD). It accounts for about one-third of all GI lymphomas in the Middle-East areas. IPSID occurs in a younger age population, with most patients presenting at the age of 20 to 30 years. Molecular and immunohistochemical studies demonstrated an association with epidemiology of Campylobacter jejuni (Salem *et al.*, 1987). The typical presentation in young adults is as a malabsorption syndrome. Pathologically, it can be thought of a low grade B-cell MALT lymphoma with marked plasma cell differentiation, showing a dense lymphoplasmacytic infiltrate which expands and blunts the intestinal villi.

Pathogenesis

As in cases of *H. pylori* associated MALT lymphoma, an infectious etiology has been suspected in cases of IPSID. Studies have mirrored the efficacy of antimicrobial therapy in disease regression. Lecuit, et al demonstrated *C. jejuni* as a possible stimulus for this proliferation (Lecuit *et al.*, 2004). C. *jejuni* has been shown to persist in Peyer's patches and mesenteric lymph nodes, and is capable of eliciting strong IgA mucosal response. Persistent infection may lead to sustained stimulation of B cells eventually resulting in the production of monotypic IgA such as that seen in IPSID (Peterson, 2004).

Morphology and immunophenotype

IPSID is morphologically characterized by small bowel infiltration by a monotypic lymphoplasmacytic cells, and is associated with a variety of histopathological changes which range from small to medium atypical lymphoid propagation to DLBCL. The centrocyte-like lymphocytes are CD20 positive, and both atypical lymphocytic and plasmacytic populations will stain strongly with IgA heavy chain, with absence of light chain staining (7).

Molecular abnormality

Much like *H. pylori* associated MALT lymphoma, IPSID appears to arise from monoclonal overgrowth secondary to chronic immune stimulation by an infectious organism in this case by *C. jejuni* (7). Deletions of alpha heavy chain gene are observed which lead to expression of a faulty heavy chain that precludes binding of light chain to form an intact immunoglobulin molecule (7, 41).

Prognosis

The disease follows a variable clinical course, but in its early phases may respond to broad spectrum antibiotics, again suggesting the possibility of an infectious etiology, possibly *C. jejuni*. Nonetheless, transformation to DLBCL is not uncommon (7). The diagnosis is made in a manner similar to other forms of MALT lymphoma.

III. Diffuse large B cell lymphoma (DLBCL)

Diffuse large B-cell lymphoma is the 2nd most common lymphoma of the stomach after MALT lymphoma. About 75% of all cases arise *de novo* whereas the rest are transformations of MALT lymphoma and other low grade lymphomas (Koch *et al.*, 2001). The normal architecture is replaced by a diffuse proliferation of large lymphoid cells. The tumors may form large gastric mass or an ulcer with perforation. DLBCL of the gastrointestinal tract, either *de novo* or transformed from another low grade type, is an aggressive lymphoma, more commonly affecting males with a median age range of 50 to 60 years (Aledavood *et al.*, 2012; Isaacson PG, 2008; Zhang, Shen, Shen, & Ni, 2012).

Pathogenesis

MALTomas may transform into a diffuse large B-cell lymphoma. There is usually nothing specific appearance or immunophenotype of the large cell lymphoma itself to suggest MALT origin, but rather the existence of a prior or coexistent low grade MALT lymphoma which permits the inference that a particular large B-cell lymphoma is derived from MALT. Since many gastrointestinal large B-cell lymphomas are discovered without any known previous or coexistent low grade MALT lymphoma, this raises the interesting question of whether all gastrointestinal diffuse large B-cell lymphomas are of MALT origin (discussed further below). Current research suggests that the transformation from low grade to high grade MALT lymphoma may involve decreased expression of *bcl*-2 and acquisition of increased p53 abnormalities resulting in overexpression of the p53 protein product (Psyrri *et al.*, 2008; Zhang *et al.*, 2012). No definite risk factors for gastric DLBCL have been identified, although some evidences suggest that this neoplasm may arise in a background of atrophic gastritis, particularly in the setting of immuno-deficiency.

Large Cells in Gastric B-cell Lymphomas

Primary gastric DLBCL is a heterogeneous disease entity that includes patients with and without detectable MALT lymphoma components. Foci of DLBCL may be found in MALT lymphomas, ranging from small number of transformed cells to predominant large cell population with minimal residual MALT lymphoma (2). Distinction of the latter from DLBCL can be difficult, and may require correlation of identical rearranged immunoglobulin (Ig) genes with co-existent low-grade MALT lymphoma (Isaacson PG, 2008). A case can be made that most are of MALT origin given a common pattern of oncogene expression in gastric low grade MALT lymphomas and large cell lymphomas compared with node-based tumors.

It is generally accepted that DLBCL can be diagnosed when large lymphoid cells with distinct nu-cleoli are present in compact clusters, confluent aggregates, or sheets (not counting large cells confined to apparent colonized follicles), although if the high grade tumor is a minor component within a larger low grade MALT lymphoma, it should be so noted. If the tumor is predominantly of large cell type, there is no significant difference in behavior if a low grade component can be identified, although again it is suggested that the presence of the minor component be noted. Shrinkage artifact in poorly fixed specimens can sometimes obscure the recognition of large cells, which may be difficult to tell from the surrounding centrocyte-like cells, which may have somewhat open chromatin and small nucleoli. It has been suggested that large cells be counted as such only if they show distinct nucleoli and a rim of amphophilic cytoplasm (Burke, 2011). Given the heterogenecity of the large cell component in some tumors, failure to detect a high grade large cell component in mucosal biopsies does not exclude the possibility of transformation, and a re-biopsy should be suggested in cases where the clinical suspicion is high (e.g., a significant clinical mass lesion, or failure to respond to antibiotic therapy)(Isaacson PG, 2008).

In hematopathology, a large lymphoid cell is by definition larger than the nucleus of a histiocyte. This "internal yardstick" is helpful to avoid incorrect assessment due to swelling of cells(Cardona *et al.*, 2012). MALT lymphomas typically contain a mixture of large and small lymphoid cells, but presence of up to 10% large cells dispersed throughout does not change the outcome. The WHO classification does not recommend categorization as "high grade MALT lymphoma" for cases with higher number of large cells mixed with small cells. However, when large cells are present in confluent sheets or clusters with other areas showing typical MALT lymphoma morphology, the diagnosis should be "DLBCL associated with MALT lymphoma in stage I or II gastric lymphomas." DLBCL with associated low grade MALT component appear to have a better outcome than DLBCL without associated MALT component, prolonging the event free survival but not necessarily the overall survival. *De novo* DLBCL is also not uncommon in the stomach (Aledavood *et al.*, 2012; Psyrri *et al.*, 2008).

Morphology and immunophenotype

DLBCL is characterized by large lymphoid cells (Figure 2), with nuclei greater than twice the size of a small lymphocyte, and frequently larger than nuclei of tissue macrophage (Stein, 2008). The tumor cells are medium to large sized cells and contain round, oval, or slightly irregular nuclei with vesicular nuclear chromatin, prominent nucleoli, and moderate to ample amount of basophilic cytoplasm, and show a moderate to high proliferation index marker Ki-67 (usually >40%). In most cases, the predominant cells resemble either large centroblasts or immunoblasts; nonetheless, a mixture of these two cell types is also commonly encountered. Histologically, there is an intense cellular infiltration of the lamina propria (Boot, 2010).

Transformed MALT lymphomas may be distinguished from de novo germinal center DLBCL by immunophenotype. Both transformed MALT lymphomas and DLBCLs show BCL6 positivity; however, DLBCLs with a germinal center-like phenotype are frequently CD10 and BCL2 positive, whereas transformed MALT lymphomas are CD10 and BCL2 negative (Burke, 2011).

Molecular abnormalities

A number of genetic variability in DLBCLs has been documented. Studies continue to subdivide these processes into separate disease entities with associated overall clinical circumstances. However, approximately 30% of DLBCL has been demonstrated to show BCL6 abnormalities. BCL2 translocation has been documented in about 25%, and presence of c-MYC rearrangements have been postulated to occur at an average of about 10% of patients (42, 47).

Prognosis

Several factors affect the prognosis of gastrointestinal DLBCL. Age, stage of disease, lactate dehydro-genase (LDH) level, and use of chemotherapy are independently and significantly associated with survival. A more aggressive clinical course has been reported in patients with more extensive disease,

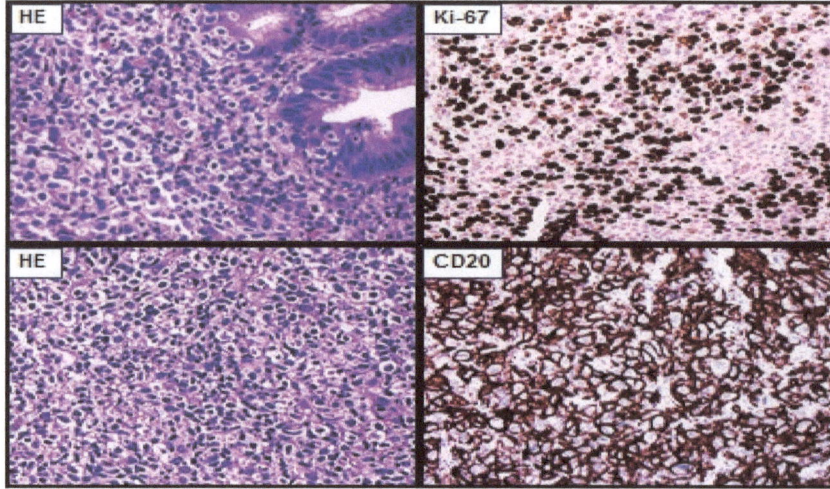

Figure 2: Gastric diffuse Large B-cell Lymphoma arising MALT lymphoma. The H&E stained sections show confluent collections sheets of large atypical lymphoid cells and high cell proliferation index marker Ki-67 (>40%). Evidence of an underlying MALT lymphoma is seen in this case as lymphoepithelial lesions and presence of a polymorphous infiltrate including plasma cell. CD20 stain is positive in the sheets of B-cell infiltrate.

such as presence of systemic symptoms, bulky lymphadenopathy, and elevated serum LDH levels. Interestingly, patients with CD10-positive disease showed a significantly higher survival rate compared to patients with CD10-negative lymphomas. The prognostic and diagnostic roles of some molecular variables, like microsatellite instability, allelic imbalance and chromosomal trisomies, are matters of continued investigation (Akaza *et al.*, 1995; Boot, 2010).

IV. Burkitt lymphoma (BL)

Burkitt lymphoma is a substantially much more aggressive mature B cell neoplasm mainly in children and young adults. This entity has three recognized clinical variants: endemic form which is usually associated with EBV infection, sporadic variant where only about 30% of the cases are related to EBV infection, and immunodeficiency-associated BL (Howell *et al.*, 2012; Lewin *et al.*, 1978; Sugano, 1998). Extranodal disease is frequently observed but GI tract involvement varies among the three clinical subtypes, with the sporadic variant usually presenting as an abdominal mass, commonly in the terminal ileum. Rare cases of gastric and cecal BL have also been described (Faltas & Kramer, 2009; Sugano, 1998).

Pathogenesis

All three variants harbor chromosomal rearrangement of c-MYC oncogene which modifies cell cycle regulation, cellular metabolism, adhesion, differentiation and apoptosis ultimately leading to tumor formation. Baumgaertner and colleagues reported a case of *H. pylori*-associated Burkitt lymphoma with complete disease remission after *H. pylori* eradication therapy. This occurrence may imply probable role of *H. pylori* in some cases of BL (Faltas & Kramer, 2009; Grewal *et al.*, 2008).

Morphology and immunophenotype

BL displays a diffuse, monotonous infiltrate of medium-sized neoplastic lymphoid cells with round nuclei showing finely clumped and dispersed chromatin, with multiple basophilic nucleoli (Figure 3). The profoundly basophilic cytoplasm generally encloses multiple lipid vacuoles on Wright-Giemsa or Diff-Quick stained smears. Frequent mitotic figures and apoptotic bodies are encountered; the apoptotic body-containing scattered tingible body macrophages impart the characteristic "starry sky" pattern.

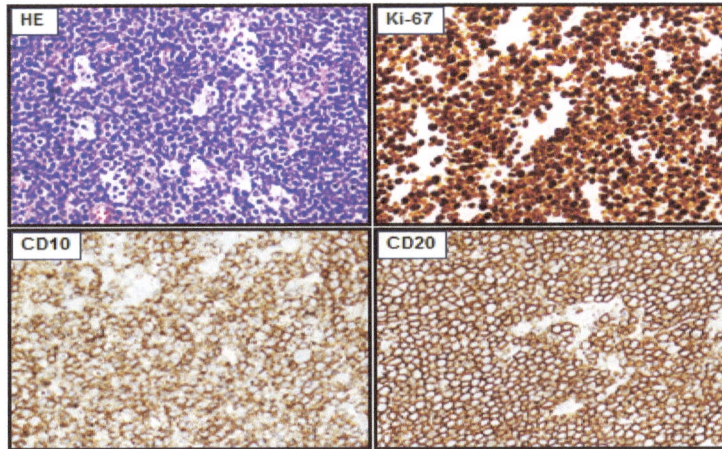

Figure 3: Burkitt lymphoma of colon. The lymphoma cells are medium sized with round nuclei, coarse chromatin, multiple nucleoli, and frequent mitoses. Numerous tingible-body macrophages create a starry sky pattern. By immunohistochemistry, the tumor cells are diffusely positive for B-cell marker CD20 with co-expression of CD10 and very high cell proliferation index marker Ki-67 (nearly 100%).

The tumor cells co-express pan B-cell markers such as CD19, CD20, as well as CD10, BCL6, and demonstrate light chain restriction, but are generally negative for BCL2 and TdT. In rare cases, Bcl-2 can be weakly positive. The neoplastic cells show an extremely high proliferation index with nearly 100% of Ki-67 reactivity (Bautista-Quach *et al.*, 2012; Burke, 2011).

Currently Burkitt's lymphoma can be divided into three main clinical variants: the endemic, the sporadic and the immunodeficiency-associated variants. The endemic variant occurs in equatorial Africa. It is the most common malignancy of children in this area. The sporadic type of Burkitt lymphoma (also known as "non-African") is found outside of Africa. Sporadic lymphomas are rarely associated with the Epstein-Barr virus. Immunodeficiency-associated Burkitt lymphoma is usually associated with HIV infection or occurs in the setting of post-transplant patients who are taking immunosuppressive drugs (Bellan *et al.*, 2003).

Molecular abnormalities

As previously mentioned, all three subtypes of BL typically demonstrate any of three c-MYC translocations at band 8q24; the most common of which is with immunoglobulin heavy (IgH) chain gene at 14q32, and infrequently with Ig kappa (IgK) at 2p12 or Ig lambda (IgL) at 22q11. However, c-MYC rearrangement is not specific for BL (Sugano, 1998). The WHO criteria for Burkitt lymphoma include demonstration of a translocation involving *MYC* oncogene on chromosome 8 with one of the immunoglobulin genes, involving kappa, IgH, and lambda, respectively) in small to medium, uniform B-cells which express CD10 and BCL6 and surface immunoglobulin but lack expression of BCL2 and TdT (Sugano, 1998). The proliferation fraction, as measured by Ki67 immunostaining, is 99% or higher (Cogliatti *et al.*, 2006). The characteristic morphology (diffuse proliferation of uniform, small non-cleaved cells with cytoplasmic vacuoles and a starry sky appearance) must be accompanied by the translocation involving MYC and immunoglobulin gene for a diagnosis of BL.

Prognosis

BL is chemosensitive and the advent of high intensity, multi-agent chemotherapeutic regimen has led to an astoundingly high remission rate. Because BL specific aggressive chemotherapy protocols offer a chance of cure, whereas routine chemotherapy such as CHOP used for DLBCL is usually associated with suboptimal response, every effort should be made to provide the accurate diagnosis (Burke, 2011). In one case, a BL patient with concomitant *H. pylori* infection benefitted from *H. pylori* eradication (44).

V. Gray zone lymphoma

Approximately 28-50% of GI tract, *de novo* DLBCLs, and DLBCL, unclassifiable, with features intermediate between DLBCL and BL (DLBCL/BL) show c-MYC translocation with a non-Ig gene partner, complex karyotype, and simultaneous BCL2, BCL6 and/or PAX5 translocations. These are referred to as "double or triple hit" lymphoma. The 2008 WHO classification resurrects the concept of a high-grade B-cell lymphoma occupying a gray zone between BL and DLBCL in a new category with the ungainly title of "B-cell lymphoma, unclassifiable, with features intermediate between DLBCL and BL," which is commonly abbreviated DLBCL/BL (Hasserjian *et al.*, 2009). DLBCL/BL is one of the two officially sanctioned "gray zone" lymphomas in the updated 2008 WHO classification. Morphological overlap exists between BL and high-grade DLBCL and/or DLBCL/BL; therefore, it is imperative to differentiate BL from DLBCL and DLBCL/BL, particularly since the latter two entities are more resistant to chemotherapy and carry a poorer prognosis overall (47). Currently, the category of previous Burkitt-like lymphoma is usually defined as a lymphoma with features intermediate between Burkitt lymphoma and diffuse large B-cell lymphoma. The immunophenotype is similar to Burkitt lymphoma, but some cases are BCL2 positive and the cell morphology is less uniform and resembles DLBCL. Furthermore, the cytogenetic abnormalities may involve both MYC and BCL2 or BCL6 genes (Hasserjian *et al.*, 2009).

VI. Mantle cell lymphoma

Small cell lymphomas other than low grade MALT lymphomas can involve the GI tract, including CLL/SLL, follicular lymphoma, and, most notably mantle cell lymphoma. Mantle cell lymphoma may involve virtually any portion of the gastrointestinal tract, which is the most common site of extranodal involvement by this tumor (Akaza *et al.*, 1995; Boot, 2010; Burke, 2011). Overall, between 20% and 30% of mantle cell lymphoma cases involve the GI tract, not uncommonly as the primary site of involvement. A particularly characteristic form of GI tract involvement is the presence of multiple polypoid lesions, most commonly in the ileocecal region (where regional lymph nodes are also frequently involved), a condition termed lymphomatous polyposis (Figure 4). Lymphomatous polyposis has been regarded as synonymous with mantle cell lymphoma in the past, but it is now clear that other forms of non-Hodgkin's lymphoma, especially follicular lymphoma, may on occasion present in an identical fashion, so attention to pertinent diagnostic cytoarchitectural features is important (Howell *et al.*, 2012). In other cases, GI mantle cell lymphomas may present clinically as discrete masses, ulcers, and mucosal thickenings which may more closely mimic other lymphomas (Howell *et al.*, 2012).

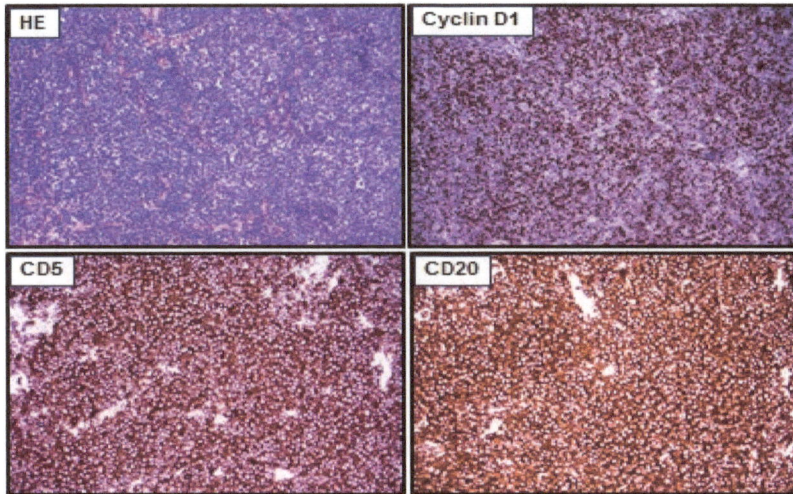

Figure 4: Mantle Cell Lymphoma involvement GI tract can be multifocal, known as "lymphomatoid polyposis". The lymphoma cells are monomorphic small to medium sized with co-expression of CD5 and CD20. Nuclear staining of variable intensity with Cyclin D1 is characteristic.

Because of its worse prognosis (median survival 2-3 years) compared with other small cell lymphomas, it is important to distinguish mantle cell lymphoma of the GI tract from its histologic mimics, particularly the much more indolent low grade MALT lymphomas. The histologic features of mantle cell lymphoma include a monomorphic population of small lymphocytes, typically resembling small cleaved cells, but with nuclei which may range from round to frankly convoluted. In contrast to MALT lymphoma, there is a paucity of other admixed cell types such as large non-cleaved lymphocytes. The tumor cells are usually present in diffuse sheets, although a mantle zone pattern, with tumor cells surrounding naked germinal centers, may provide a clue in some cases. A nodular pattern has also been reported on occasion. An increased mitotic rate may be seen, particularly in the blastic variant. Unlike low grade MALT lymphomas, lymphoepithelial lesions are uncommon.

Mantle cell lymphoma shows a variety of immunophenotypic characteristics which can be quite useful in arriving at the correct diagnosis. By frozen section or flow immunophenotyping, the cells appear as B-cells with immunoglobulin light chain restriction which are CD5+ and CD23-, an immunophenotype virtually diagnostic of mantle cell lymphoma, given that the only other common CD5+ small cell lymphoma, CLL/SLL, is characteristically CD23+. Even if only paraffin-embedded material is available, immunophenotyping is still helpful, as CD43 coexpression is usually seen, which, though not specific for mantle cell lymphoma, does suggest a B-cell neoplasm. In addition, cyclin D1 overexpression can be detected by antibodies which work well in paraffin sections. This overexpression, which represents activation of the PRAD1/CCND1 gene at the *bcl*-1 locus at 11q13 by the characteristic t(11;14) translocation found in most mantle cell lymphomas, appears to date to be quite specific for mantle cell lymphoma.

VII. Intestinal Follicular Lymphoma

Primary FL of the GI tract is a predominantly female lymphoma that most frequently involves the small intestine with a predilection to the ileum (Damaj *et al.*, 2003). This entity is recognized as a variant of follicular lymphoma in the 2008 edition of WHO classification (Figure 5).

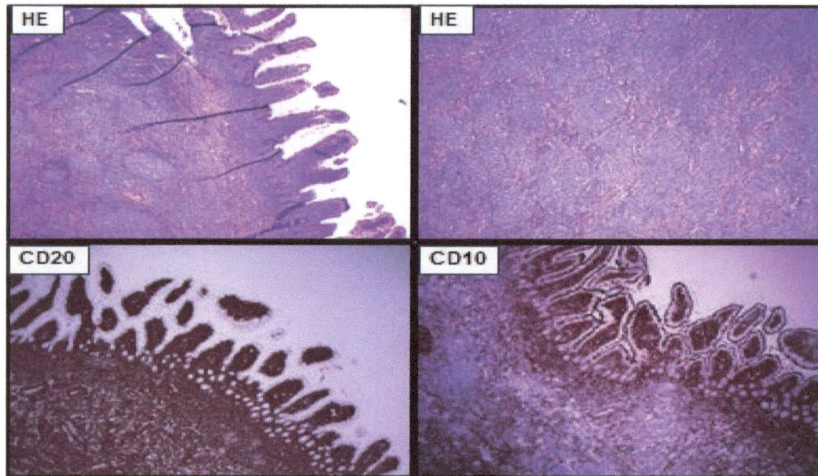

Figure 5: Follicular lymphoma in the duodenum which is the usual site of involvement by follicular lymphoma, but may occur anywhere along the GI tract. The follicular architecture is variably prominent on H & E staining. Immunohistochemical stains show the atypical follicle centers are positive for CD20 and CD10 which confirm the follicular center origin of the lymphoma. In addition BCL2 positive staining (not shown) confirms the malignant nature of the follicles.

Since the endoscopic and clinical presentation may not be different from seconday GI involvement by a nodal follicular lymphoma or lymphomatous polyposis, which is often associated with mantle cell origin of tumor cells, it is mandatory to perform an immunohistological and, if possible, a molecular analysis of GI lymphoma. A comprehensive recent review show that this lymphoma is similar to node based follicular lymphoma with regard to morphology and immunophenotype (CD10+, BCL6+, BCL2+), but has a superior prognosis compared to nodal disease (Damaj *et al.*, 2003). It is often detected as an incidental polyp or plaque in the duodenum or terminal ileum during endoscopy, but more advanced techniques such as double balloon endoscopy or capsule endoscopy shows multifocal involvement of the entire small intestine in many cases. The course of the disease is indolent and does not differ from nodal FL. Thus, therapy may not be required unless significant clinical symptoms are present or until disease progression. Nevertheless, a majority of patients may not require specific treatment (Boot, 2010; Burke, 2011).

VIII. AIDS-Related lymphomas

Non-Hodgkin's lymphomas represent the most common malignancy in AIDS patients after Kaposi's sarcoma, and unlike KS, occur with increased frequency in all AIDS risk groups. About 30% of AIDS-related non-Hodgkin's lymphomas involve the GI tract at presentation (Sandler & Kaplan, 1996; Wotherspoon *et al.*, 1996), with the stomach and small intestine representing the most common sites of involvement. Pain, ulceration with bleeding, obstruction, and constitutional symptoms are all seen as presenting complaints. The vast majority of AIDS-related lymphomas have been reported to correspond to one of three "diffuse aggressive". Frequently, it is difficult to precisely sub-classify AIDS-related lymphomas, as many display histopathologic features which vary significantly within the tumor (Imrie *et al.*, 1995). Precise histologic sub-classification may be of largely semantic interest, however, since in

AIDS patients, essentially all of these lymphomas behave in an aggressive, high-grade fashion, with reported median survivals of 5 to 11 months in most series (Imrie *et al.*, 1995; Simcock *et al.*, 2007). Histologically, all tend to show a high mitotic rate with significant necrosis. Virtually all are B-cell lymphomas, and are generally thought to develop secondary to the impaired immunosurveillance which occurs in AIDS. Many cases (including a majority of the immunoblastic lymphomas) show evidence of EBV infection, and most show evidence of c-MYC proto-oncogene activation which may be etiologic. High grade Burkitt's and Burkitt's-like lymphomas also commonly involve the GI tract in non-AIDS patients, particularly among pediatric and young adult patients.

Some uncommon variants of large B-cell lymphoma are seen in this population. Their diagnosis may be challenging due to their atypical morphology and immunophenotype. Plasmablastic lymphomas and extra-cavitary variant of primary effusion lymphoma deserve special mention (Sarode, Zarkar, Desai, Sabane, & Kulkarni, 2009). The former is most commonly seen in the oral cavity of chronically HIV infected patients but can occur in other parts of the GI tract including the anorectal region and a majority of cases are associated with EBV (Figure 6).

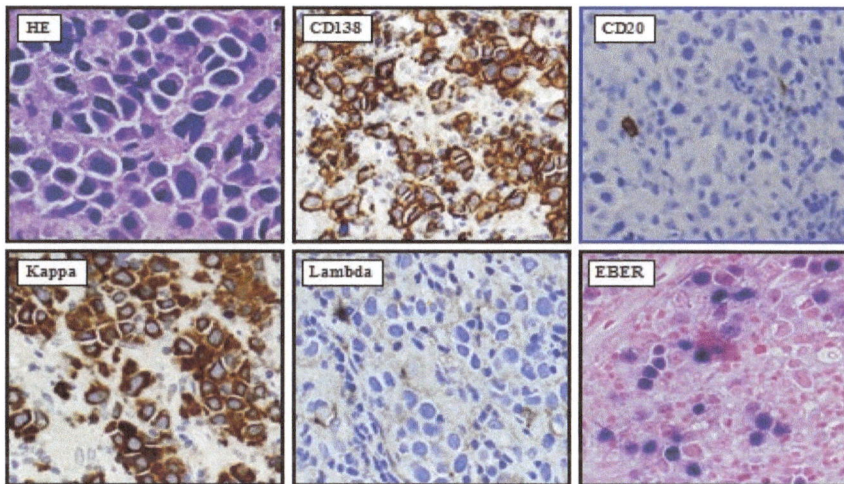

Figure 6: Plasmablastic Lymphoma usually occurs in the oral cavity of HIV positive patients. Anorectal location has been noted, but other parts of the GI tract such as the small intestine, esophagus, as in this case, can be involved. The lymphoma cells do not express CD45 or CD20 (not shown), but are CD138+, and restrictive kappa cytoplasmic light chain+. In situ hybridization shows EBV early RNA (EBER) expression.

On the other hand, primary effusion lymphoma is associated with HHV8 (or Kaposi Sarcoma herpes virus, KSHV) and often presents as pleural effusions but can occur as a solid tumor. KSHV may be seen in a relatively high proportion of aggressive B-cell lymphomas in HIV patients and all morphological and immunophenotypic characteristics should be considered for appropriate diagnosis. A plasmacytoid morphology or an immunophenotype that is closer to plasma cells than to B-cells is observed in these lymphomas as both lymphomas often lack expression of pan B-cell antigen CD20 and PAX5, but often express CD79a and always express MUM1, CD38 and CD138. Distinction of these lymphomas from plasmablastic myeloma may be difficult as they share nearly identical immunophenotypic profiles, but is important for correct treatment (Cardona *et al.*, 2012; Vega *et al.*, 2005). The only significant difference between plasmablastic lymphoma and plasma cell myeloma was the presence of EBV-encoded RNA, which was positive in all plasmablastic lymphoma cases tested and negative in all plasma cell myelomas (Vega *et al.*, 2005). Marked reactive lymphoid hyperplasia may produce localized masses referred to as "Anorectal Tonsils", which must be distinguished from low grade lymphomas (Burke, 2011).

IX. Post-transplant lymphoproliferative disorders (PTLDs)

Transplant patients receiving immunosuppressive drugs constitute the other major class of immunocompromised hosts to experience high rates of non-Hodgkin's lymphomas (Semakula, Rittenbach, & Wang, 2006). As in AIDS, most are EBV-driven B-cell proliferations, but in contrast to AIDS, these proliferations are a heterogeneous group which range from benign hyperplasias to frankly malignant high grade lymphomas. Most patients with PTLDs have extranodal involvement, with the GI tract being the principal site of clinical presentation. Most of these GI involving cases are of B-lymphocyte origin and are associated with Epstein-Barr virus infection. Overall, the GI tract is involved in about 35% of PTLD cases, with the small bowel being the most common site. In many cases, it is difficult to determine from routine histopathologic examination whether the lesions are benign or malignant, leading to use of the more general term PTLD (Lai *et al.*, 2006; Nalesnik, 1990). A variety of classification schemes for PTLDs have been proposed over the years. The 2008 World Health Organization (WHO) classification system recognizes 4 major histopathologic subtypes of PTLD: (1) early hyperplastic lesions, (2) polymorphic lesions (which may be polyclonal or monoclonal), (3) monomorphic lesions, and (4) classic Hodgkin-type lymphomas (Glotz *et al.*, 2012; Pitman *et al.*, 2006).

3.3   T-Cell Lymphomas

I. Enteropathy-associated T-cell lymphoma (EATL)

Two components of intestinal MALT are present more diffusely in the mucosa. Firstly, lamina propria immune cells are a heterogeneous collection of antigen presenting macrophages and dendritic cells, antibody producing plasma cells and helper T-cells. Few eosinophils and mast cells are also present, particularly in the small intestine. Secondly, intra-epithelial lymphocytes are predominantly cytotoxic T-cells, present diffusely in low numbers throughout the intestines, with somewhat higher proportions in small intestines. Distinct types of lymphomas arise from the three components of intestinal MALT and recapitulate the structure and function of the cells of origin to a variable degree.

While virtually any T-cell lymphoma can affect the GI tract, EATL is perhaps the most distinctive one. Most cases occur in elderly individuals, many of whom have histories of malabsorption syndromes, particularly celiac disease. Clinically, the jejunum is most frequently involved, often as multiple well-circumscribed ulcers without a clinical mass lesion (Chan *et al.*, 2011; Smedby *et al.*, 2005). Biopsies or resection specimens show lymphoid infiltrates which typically resemble a large cell lymphoma, but which may vary considerably, even within a given patient, with other areas resembling small cell lymphomas or even Hodgkin's disease. Tumor cells commonly invade the overlying epithelium, sometimes in aggregates resembling lymphoepithelial lesions (Figure 7). The presence of numerous associated eosinophils, and other inflammatory cells related to the ulceration, together with the often polymorphous nature of the infiltrate, may mask the neoplastic nature of this disorder, which should nonetheless be suspected in this clinical setting. Most cases previously described in the literature as "ulcerative jejunitis" are now suspected of being EATLs, given some studies which have found clonal T-cell receptor gene rearrangements by PCR (Chan *et al.*, 2011; Smedby *et al.*, 2005). Most cases (classical

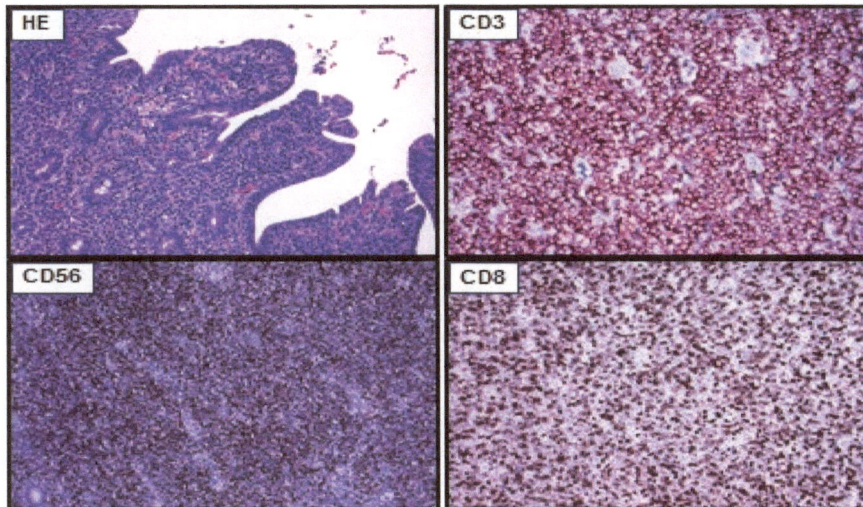

Figure 7: Enteropathy associated T-cell Lymphoma (EATL) type II in the small intestine: The Uniform small cells in this lymphoma closely mimic cells of mantle cell lymphoma. Immunohistochemistry shows the lymphoma cells are positive for CD3, CD8, and CD56, as well as TIA-1 and Granzyme B (not shown).

type I EATL) have a characteristic CD3+, CD7+, CD4-, and CD8- immunophenotype. As this is also the typical immunophenotype for intestinal intraepithelial T-cells, and an origin from native intraepithelial T-cells has been proposed. The tumor tends to follow an aggressive clinical course, with frequent dissemination to multiple body sites (Andrews *et al.*, 2008). Type II EATL develops sporadically and is independent of celiac disease (Yang, Batth, Chen, Borys, & Phan, 2012), and it comprises 10 to 20% of EATL cases. It is a distinct aggressive T-cell lymphoma with frequent gamma-delta ($\gamma\delta$) T-cell receptor expression (Chan *et al.*, 2011; Smedby *et al.*, 2005). This type of EATL is mainly composed of medium-sized cells, which are positive for CD3, CD7, CD8, and CD56. Recent studies suggest to separate type II EATL from the EATL category as a distinct form of lymphoma, for which it was proposed the designation of "monomorphic intestinal T-cell lymphoma" (Burke, 2011; Chan *et al.*, 2011).

II. Hepatosplenic T-cell lymphoma

Hepatosplenic T-cell lymphoma presents with marked hepatosplenomegaly in the absence of lymphadenopathy. The great majority of cases are of $\gamma\delta$ T-cell origin. Most patients are male, with a peak incidence in young adults. There is an association with iatrogenic immunosuppression, both in solid organ transplant recipients and in patients with Crohn's disease receiving immunosuppressive agents, in particular purine analogs and infliximab, an inhibitor of tumor necrosis factor. Although patients may respond initially to chemotherapy, relapse has been seen in the majority of cases, and the median survival is <3 years. Allogeneic hematopoietic cell transplantation has led to long-term disease-free survival in some cases.

The cells of hepatosplenic T-cell lymphoma are usually moderate in size, with a rim of pale cytoplasm (Figure 8). The nuclear chromatin is dispersed, with small inconspicuous nucleoli. The pattern of infiltration mimics the homing pattern of $\gamma\delta$ T cells with marked sinusoidal infiltration in liver and spleen. Abnormal cells are usually present in the sinusoids of the bone marrow but may be difficult to identify

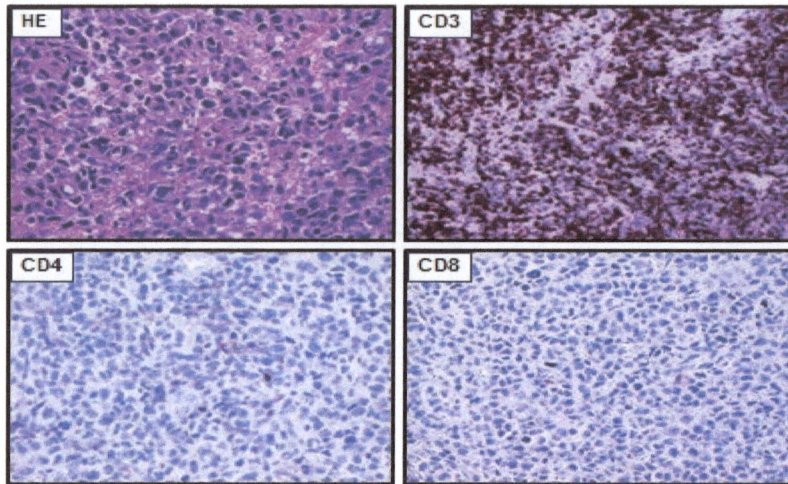

Figure 8: Gamma-delta T-cell lymphoma of the liver. Malignant T cells are small to intermediate in size with regular oval or folded nuclei; occasional cells may be larger with highly atypical nuclei. The lymphoma cells are diffuse positive for T-cell marker CD3, but are double negative for CD4 and CD8.

without immunohistochemical stains. The neoplastic cells also have a phenotype that resembles that of normal resting $\gamma\delta$ T cells. They are often negative for both CD4 and CD8, although CD8 may be expressed in some cases. CD56 is typically positive. The neoplastic cells express markers associated with cytotoxic T cells, such as TIA-1. However, perforin and granzyme B are usually negative, suggesting that these cells are not activated. Isochromosome 7q is a consistent cytogenetic abnormality, and is often seen in association with trisomy 8 (Thayu *et al.*, 2005). Cases of $\alpha\beta$ T-cell derivation have similar immuno-phenotypic and genetic features, but are more common in females, with an older age distribution. Interestingly, they have a gene expression profile very similar to tumors of $\gamma\delta$ T-cell derivation (Burke, 2011).

III. Extranodal NK/T cell lymphoma, nasal type (ENKTL)

This aggressive entity primarily occurs in the nasal cavity, nasopharynx and paranasal sinuses but also involves a number of extranasal locations including the GI tract where it may present as ulceration or perforation (Bautista-Quach *et al.*, 2012). The disease is more commonly seen in Asians, Mexicans and natives of Central and South America, and more frequently affects males than females. Virtually all cases of ENKTL are associated with EBV infection (Burke, 2011).

The infiltrate often effaces the mucosal architecture and consists of varying sizes of pleomorphic neoplastic lymphoid cells with irregular, convoluted nuclear contour with indistinct nucleoli (Figure 9). The larger lymphoid cells show irregular nuclei with vesicular chromatin. The moderate to abundant cytoplasm is usually clear or faint. In particular, the neoplastic lymphoid infiltrates characteristically show an angiocentric and angiodestructive pattern where they aggregate around and infiltrate blood vessel wall. Admixed inflammatory cells consisting of histiocytes, plasma cells and small lymphocytes, ulceration of the overlying mucosa and geographic necrosis are frequently observed (Sun, Lu, Yang, & Chen, 2011). The tumor cells are distinctively CD2, CD56, cytoplasmic CD3 positive and express

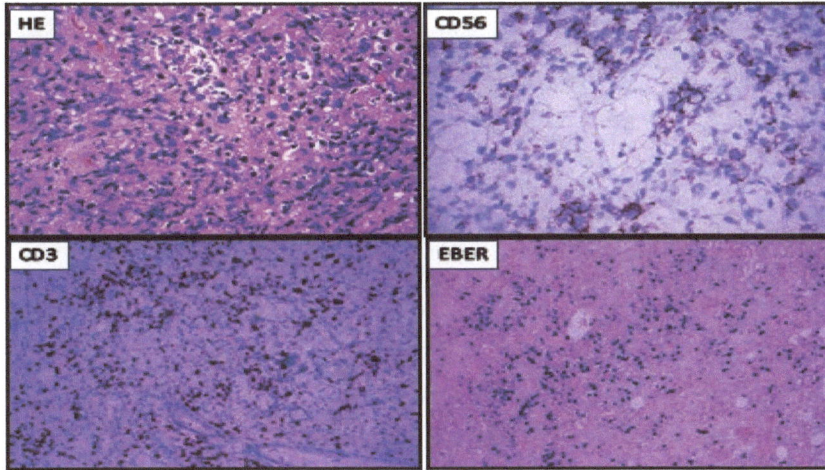

Figure 9: Extranodal NK/T cell lymphoma, nasal type in the esophagus. The neoplastic lymphoid cells are invading and destroying the wall of a blood vessel. The neoplastic cells are positive for CD56, and CD3 as well as EBV by EBER in situ hybridization.

cytotoxic molecules (Granzyme B, TIA-1 and/or perforin) but are negative for surface CD3 and other T or NK cell markers such as CD4, CD5, CD8, TCR delta, beta F1, CD16 and CD57. Some cases demonstrate reactivity for CD7 or CD30 (Burke, 2011).

3.4 Other Rare Type of Primary Gastrointestinal Lymphomas

The primary GI tract Hodgkin lymphoma, myeloid sarcoma, histiocytic sarcoma, dendtric cell sarcoma, extramedullary plasmacytoma or other rare types of primary GI tract B-cells lymphomas (T-cell histiocytes rich large B-cell lymphoma, B lymphoblastic lymphoma, lymphomatoid granulomatosis etc) or T-cells lymphomas (anaplastic large cell lymphoma, peripheral T-cell lymphoma and T-lymphoblastic lymphoma etc) should also be considered if unusual morphologic and immunophenotypical features are present. A complete morphologic immunophenotypical and molecular study analysis is required for the differential diagnosis.

3.5 Mimics of Gastrointestinal Lymphomas

1. Distinguishing between reactive lymphoid hyperplasia and MALT lymphoma

This has been discussed in the section on low grade MALT lymphoma above. While reactive lymphoid follicles can be present in virtual any gastrointestinal biopsy, the presence of an extensive dense interfollicular lymphoid infiltrate, a predominance of centrocyte-like cells (which may include monocytoid cells) in the infiltrate, deep extension of the infiltrate into the wall, and prominent destructive lymphoepithelial lesions should alert one to the possibility of a low grade MALT lymphoma (Figure 10).

The suspicious of MALT lymphoma is relied on histology in combination with immunohistochemistry and ancillary studies if available, but diagnose unequivocally only if most or all of the above features are present. A monomorphous dense lymphoid infiltrate should raise suspicion of a non-MALT lymphoma, such as mantle cell lymphoma, follicular lymphoma, or small lymphocytic lymphoma. Ancillary studies are recommended to support the diagnosis.

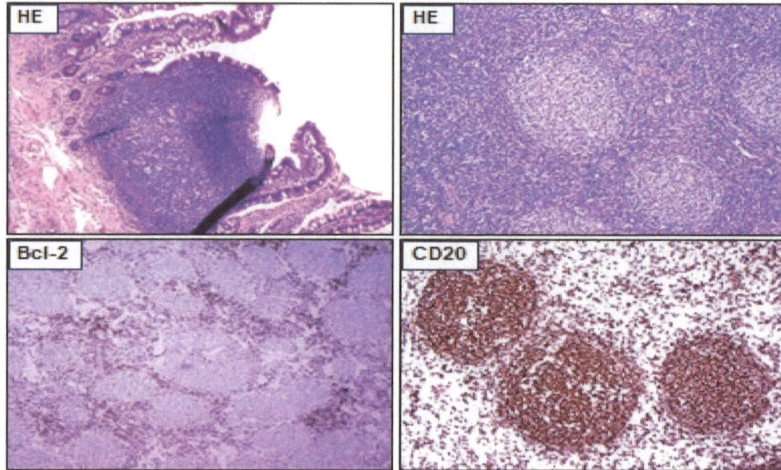

Figure 10: Reactive lymphoid aggregates in the cecum. Reactive follicles are composed follicular B-cells (CD20 positive) and perifollicular/intrafollicular T-cells (Bcl-2 positive) and with normal compartmentalization. The follicles, particularly the reactive germinal centers are negative for BCL2.

2. Inflammatory pesudotumor (IPT) and lymphomas

Inflammatory pseudotumor (inflammatory myofibroblastic tumor) is a benign, chronic inflammatory disorder of unknown cause that manifests as a solid mesenteric mass, indistinguishable from malignancy. IPT can be differentiated from lymphoma because IPT has both T and B cells, in contradistinction to lymphoma, in which a clonal population of T or B cells is present (Figure 11) (Burke, 2011). Some pseudotumors are thought to be secondary to infection. Various organisms have been implicated in pathologic specimens, including mycoplasmata and nocardiae in lung pseudotumors, actinomycetes in liver pseudotumors, Epstein-Barr virus in splenic and nodal pseudotumors, and mycobacteria in spindle cell tumors. Histologically, the lesions were characterized by a fibrous/inflammatory process that showed marked heterogeneity associated with both acute and chronic inflammation, including lymphocytes and plasma cells, myofibroblastic spindle cells, and collagen (a fibrous reaction). IPT of lymph node represents an evolving, dynamic process that may adopt different morphological appearances depending on its stage of evolution (Makhlouf & Sobin, 2002).

Some IPTs have been found to be associated with IgG4-related sclerosing disease, a systemic disease in which there is extensive IgG4-positive plasma cell and T-cell infiltration of various tissues. This condition manifests itself as autoimmune pancreatitis, sclerosing cholangitis, cholecystitis, sialadenitis, retroperitoneal fibrosis, tubulointerstitial nephritis, interstitial pneumonia, prostatitis, IPT, and lymphadenopathy. IgG4-related IPTs have been found in patients with and those without autoimmune pancreatitis (Cheuk & Chan, 2010).

3. NK-cell enteropathy or lymphomatoid gastropathy

Recently, benign, indolent NK-cell enteropathy or lymphomatoid gastropathy have been described, and therefore should be differentiated from the aggressive ENKTL. Mansoor and associates documented eight cases of atypical NK-cell proliferation limited to the GI tract (stomach, duodenum and colon) (Mansoor *et al.*, 2011). The atypical cells express NK cell markers such as CD56, cytoplasmic CD3, CD7, TIA-1 and/or Granzyme B, but are non-reactive for CD4, CD8, CD5, CD10, CD20, CD30, CD68, or CD138.

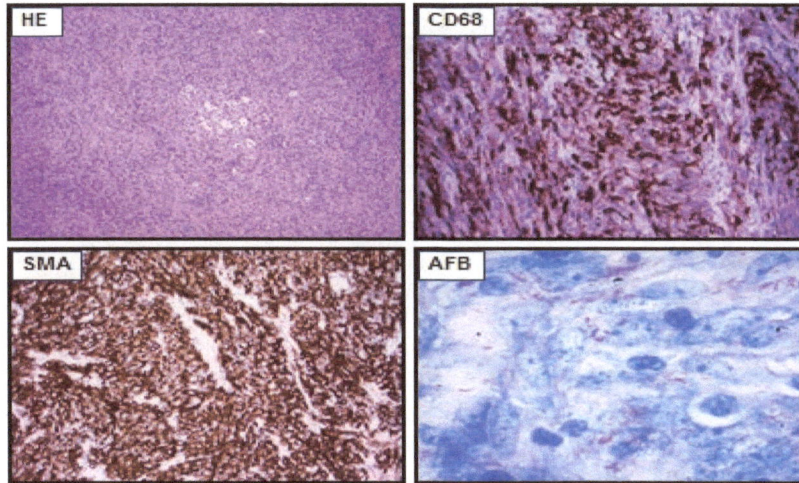

Figure 11: Inflammatory pseudotumor of mesentery lymph node from a patient with AIDS. The smooth muscle and histiocytic proliferations are positive for SMA and CD68 respectively. Acid Fast stain highlights the microorganisms.

The proliferative index marker Ki-67 nuclear staining is usually low. Furthermore, in contrast to ENKTL, NK-cell enteropathy or lymphomatoid gastropathy is not typically associated with EBV infection. This lesion clinically behaves in a benign and an indolent manner. Disease persistence was observed in 67% to 75% of the patients, with recurrence in one patient two years after spontaneous regression of the disease. Moreover, none of the patients showed evidence of disease progression, and there was no reported mortality (Mansoor *et al.*, 2011). It is therefore essential to distinguishing this entity from the more aggressive NK/T-cell lymphomas in order to avoid unnecessary therapy and its associated risks.

4. Non-lymphoid disease

Non-hematolymphoid lesions such as poorly differentiated carcinoma or melnoma morphologically can mimic GI tract lymphoma (Burke, 2011). In addition, many system diseases have GI tact involvement; therefore the clinical and radiological correlation is required for differential diagnosis. A complete immunohistochemistry work up is helpful in order to figure out the origin or the disease processes. For example, systemic mastocytosis and Langerhans' histiocytosis can be distinguished with CD117 and CD1a immunostains, respectively (Bautista-Quach, *et al*, 2012).

4   Diagnostic Approach for Suspected GI Lymphomas

In every case of GI tract lymphoma, the goal is to provide a diagnosis according to the WHO classification so that the correct treatment can be given. Detailed algorithms or practical guide to diagnosis with relatively modest ancillary techniques have been published but must be adopted for the individual practice situation. A judicious use of immunohistochemistry can provide a great deal of information with relatively low cost. Generous sampling during endoscopy, prompt fixation, and optimal processing are required to produce consistently high quality H&E sections, which must form the basis for decisions about additional ancillary testing. In general, diffuse large B-cell lymphomas, which form the largest single type of GI lymphomas, are unlikely to be mistaken for a benign process but may mimic non lymphoma entities. Immunohistochemical staining for CD20 may be sufficient to arrive at the correct diagnosis in most of these cases. Staining with CD45, CD138, pancytokeratin and S-100 antibodies is robust and usually reliable in cases of acute leukemia, plasma cell neoplasm, poorly differentiated carcinoma and melanoma, respectively (Burke, 2011; Cardona *et al.*, 2012). The infiltrates composed of small or mixed lymphoid cells prove most challenging as do the presence of lymphoid follicles. The pathologist should be familiar with the characteristics of reactive follicles (presence of zonation, tingible body macrophages, and complete mantle zones), but BCL2 immunohistochemistry may be required to make the distinction between reactive and neoplastic follicles and follicular colonization by mantle zone or marginal zone lymphoma cells. The pathologist should also remember that benign reactive lymphoid follicles may co-exist with extranodal marginal zone lymphoma involving GI tract.

The clinical context is extremely important in deciding which ancillary tests are required. Because most chronic gastritis and gastric MALT lymphoma patients are initially treated with antibiotics, the exact distinction may not be necessary. Demonstrating the proportion of B-cells with one or two immunostains may be adequate. However, distinction between mantle cell lymphoma, EATL type II and other reactive small lymphocytic infiltrates is crucial and Cyclin D1 staining should be included in any GI tract lymphoma composed of small cells. Clinical correlation is essential in every case of suspected lymphoma and GI tract lymphomas have no exception. In particular, the distinction between primary GI tract lymphoma and secondary involvement of GI tract by lymphoma cannot be performed on the basis of pathological examination alone. The prognosis for primary and secondary GI tract lymphoma of the same WHO type may be entirely different, supposed to be due to the low clinical stage of the primary lesions. The presence of HIV infection or other causes of immunodeficiency (for example, post-transplant status) should be noted because of the possibility of unusual types of lymphomas and the vastly inferior prognosis to the usual types.

In summary, GI lymphomas are common extranodal lymphomas occurring in all age groups. Accurate diagnosis of the types of lymphoma is vitally important for correct treatment and determining prognosis. The close connection between chronic inflammation in GI tract and lymphoma has shed much light on the growth and natural history of the lymphomas.

References

Aithal, G. P., & Mansfield, J. C. (2001). Review article: the risk of lymphoma associated with inflammatory bowel disease and immunosuppressive treatment. [Case Reports Review]. Aliment Pharmacol Ther, 15(8), 1101-1108.

Akaza, K., Motoori, T., Nakamura, S., Koshikawa, T., Kitoh, K., Futamura, N., . . . et al. (1995). Clinicopathologic study of primary gastric lymphoma of B cell phenotype with special reference to low-grade B cell lymphoma of mucosa-associated lymphoid tissue among the Japanese. [Research Support, Non-U.S. Gov't]. Pathol Int, 45(11), 832-845.

Aledavood, A., Nasiri, M. R., Memar, B., Shahidsales, S., Raziee, H. R., Ghafarzadegan, K., & Mohtashami, S. (2012). Primary gastrointestinal lymphoma. J Res Med Sci, 17(5), 487-490.

Andrews, C. N., John Gill, M., Urbanski, S. J., Stewart, D., Perini, R., & Beck, P. (2008). Changing epidemiology and risk factors for gastrointestinal non-Hodgkin's lymphoma in a North American population: population-based study. Am J Gastroenterol, 103(7), 1762-1769. doi: 10.1111/j.1572-0241.2008.01794.x

Arnold, I. C., Hitzler, I., Engler, D., Oertli, M., Agger, E. M., & Muller, A. (2011). The C-terminally encoded, MHC class II-restricted T cell antigenicity of the Helicobacter pylori virulence factor CagA promotes gastric preneoplasia. [Research Support, Non-U.S. Gov't]. J Immunol, 186(11), 6165-6172. doi: 10.4049/jimmunol.1003472.

Bautista-Quach, M. A., Ake, C. D., Chen, M., & Wang, J. (2012). Gastrointestinal lymphomas: Morphology, immunophenotype and molecular features. J Gastrointest Oncol, 3(3), 209-225. doi: 10.3978/j.issn.2078-6891.2012.024.

Bellan, C., Lazzi, S., De Falco, G., Nyongo, A., Giordano, A., & Leoncini, L. (2003). Burkitt's lymphoma: new insights into molecular pathogenesis. J Clin Pathol, 56(3), 188-192. doi: Doi 10.1136/Jcp.56.3.188.

Boot, H. (2010). Diagnosis and staging in gastrointestinal lymphoma. [Review]. Best Pract Res Clin Gastroenterol, 24(1), 3-12. doi: 10.1016/j.bpg.2009.12.003.

Brenchley, J. M., Schacker, T. W., Ruff, L. E., Price, D. A., Taylor, J. H., Beilman, G. J., . . . Douek, D. C. (2004). CD4+ T cell depletion during all stages of HIV disease occurs predominantly in the gastrointestinal tract. [Research Support, U.S. Gov't, P.H.S.]. J Exp Med, 200(6), 749-759. doi: 10.1084/jem.20040874.

Burke, J. S. (2011). Lymphoproliferative disorders of the gastrointestinal tract: a review and pragmatic guide to diagnosis. [Review]. Arch Pathol Lab Med, 135(10), 1283-1297. doi: 10.5858/arpa.2011-0145-RA

Cardona, D. M., Layne, A., & Lagoo, A. S. (2012). Lymphomas of the gastro-intestinal tract - pathophysiology, pathology, and differential diagnosis. [Review]. Indian J Pathol Microbiol, 55(1), 1-16. doi: 10.4103/0377-4929.94847.

Chan, J. K., Chan, A. C., Cheuk, W., Wan, S. K., Lee, W. K., Lui, Y. H., & Chan, W. K. (2011). Type II enteropathy-associated T-cell lymphoma: a distinct aggressive lymphoma with frequent gammadelta T-cell receptor expression. Am J Surg Pathol, 35(10), 1557-1569. doi: 10.1097/PAS.0b013e318222dfcd.

Cheuk, W., & Chan, J. K. (2010). IgG4-related sclerosing disease: a critical appraisal of an evolving clinicopathologic entity. [Review]. Adv Anat Pathol, 17(5), 303-332. doi: 10.1097/PAP.0b013e3181ee63ce.

Chiang, I. P., Wang, H. H., Cheng, A. L., Lin, J. T., & Su, I. J. (1996). Low-grade gastric B-cell lymphoma of mucosa-associated lymphoid tissue: clinicopathologic analysis of 19 cases. J Formos Med Assoc, 95(11), 857-865.

Cogliatti, S. B., Novak, U., Henz, S., Schmid, U., Moller, P., & Barth, T. F. (2006). Diagnosis of Burkitt lymphoma in due time: a practical approach. [Research Support, Non-U.S. Gov't]. Br J Haematol, 134(3), 294-301. doi: 10.1111/j.1365-2141.2006.06194.x

Copie-Bergman, C., Gaulard, P., Lavergne-Slove, A., Brousse, N., Flejou, J. F., Dordonne, K., . . . Wotherspoon, A. C. (2003). Proposal for a new histological grading system for post-treatment evaluation of gastric MALT lymphoma. [Letter]. Gut, 52(11), 1656.

Damaj, G., Verkarre, V., Delmer, A., Solal-Celigny, P., Yakoub-Agha, I., Cellier, C., . . . Adulte, G. E. L. (2003). Primary follicular lymphoma of the gastrointestinal tract: a study of 25 cases and a literature review. Annals of Oncology, 14(4), 623-629. doi: DOI 10.1093/annonc/mdg168.

Dawson, I. M., Cornes, J. S., & Morson, B. C. (1961). Primary malignant lymphoid tumours of the intestinal tract. Report of 37 cases with a study of factors influencing prognosis. Br J Surg, 49, 80-89.

Devaney, K., & Jaffe, E. S. (1991). The surgical pathology of gastrointestinal Hodgkin's disease. Am J Clin Pathol, 95(6), 794-801.

Faltas, B., & Kramer, Z. B. (2009). Gastric Burkitt lymphoma associated with Efalizumab and Helicobacter pylori. [Case Reports Letter]. Leuk Lymphoma, 50(9), 1538-1539. doi: 10.1080/10428190903085969.

Farinha, P., & Gascoyne, R. D. (2005). Molecular pathogenesis of mucosa-associated lymphoid tissue lymphoma. [Comparative Study Research Support, Non-U.S. Gov't Review]. J Clin Oncol, 23(26), 6370-6378. doi: 10.1200/JCO.2005.05.011.

Freeman, C., Berg, J. W., & Cutler, S. J. (1972). Occurrence and prognosis of extranodal lymphomas. Cancer, 29(1), 252-260.

Ghai, S., Pattison, J., O'Malley, M. E., Khalili, K., & Stephens, M. (2007). Primary gastrointestinal lymphoma: spectrum of imaging findings with pathologic correlation. [Review]. Radiographics, 27(5), 1371-1388. doi: 10.1148/rg.275065151.

Glotz, D., Chapman, J. R., Dharnidharka, V. R., Hanto, D. W., Castro, M. C. R., Hirsch, H. H., . . . Gross, T. G. (2012). The Seville Expert Workshop for Progress in Posttransplant Lymphoproliferative Disorders. Transplantation, 94(8), 784-793. doi: Doi 10.1097/Tp.0b013e318269e64f.

Grewal, S. S., Hunt, J. P., O'Connor, S. C., Gianturco, L. E., Richardson, M. W., & Lehmann, L. E. (2008). Helicobacter pylori associated gastric Burkitt lymphoma. [Case Reports]. Pediatr Blood Cancer, 50(4), 888-890. doi: 10.1002/pbc.21201.

Hasserjian, R. P., Ott, G., Elenitoba-Johnson, K. S., Balague-Ponz, O., de Jong, D., & de Leval, L. (2009). Commentary on the WHO classification of tumors of lymphoid tissues (2008): "Gray zone" lymphomas overlapping with Burkitt lymphoma or classical Hodgkin lymphoma. J Hematop, 2(2), 89-95. doi: 10.1007/s12308-009-0039-7.

Howell, J. M., Auer-Grzesiak, I., Zhang, J., Andrews, C. N., Stewart, D., & Urbanski, S. J. (2012). Increasing incidence rates, distribution and histological characteristics of primary gastrointestinal non-Hodgkin lymphoma in a North American population. Can J Gastroenterol, 26(7), 452-456.

Hyder, J. W., & Mackeigan, J. M. (1988). Anorectal and Colonic Disease and the Immunocompromised Host. Diseases of the Colon & Rectum, 31(12), 971-976. doi: Doi 10.1007/Bf02554899.

Imrie, K. R., Sawka, C. A., Kutas, G., Brandwein, J., Warner, E., Burkes, R., . . . Shepherd, F. A. (1995). HIV-associated lymphoma of the gastrointestinal tract: the University of Toronto AIDS-Lymphoma Study Group experience. [Case Reports]. Leuk Lymphoma, 16(3-4), 343-349. doi: 10.3109/10428199509049774.

Isaacson PG, C. A., Nakamura S, et al. . (2008). Extranodal marginal zone lymphoma of mucosa-associated lymphoid tissue (MALT lymphoma). In C. E. Swerdlow SH, Harris NL, Jaffe ES, et al, eds (Ed.), World Health Organization Classification of Tumours of Haematopoietic and Lymphoid Tissues (4th edition ed., pp. 214-217). Lyon, France: IARC Press.

Iwamuro, M., Kawai, Y., Takata, K., Kawano, S., Yoshino, T., Okada, H., & Yamamoto, K. (2013). Primary intestinal follicular lymphoma: How to identify follicular lymphoma by routine endoscopy. World J Gastrointest Endosc, 5(1), 34-38. doi: 10.4253/wjge.v5.i1.34.

Jamieson, N. V., Thiru, S., Calne, R. Y., & Evans, D. B. (1981). Gastric lymphomas arising in two patients with renal allografts. [Case Reports]. Transplantation, 31(3), 224-225.

Kalogeropoulos, I. V., Chalazonitis, A. N., Tsolaki, S., Laspas, F., Ptohis, N., Neofytou, I., & Rontogianni, D. (2009). A case of primary isolated non-Hodgkin's lymphoma of the esophagus in an immunocompetent patient. [Case Reports]. World J Gastroenterol, 15(15), 1901-1903.

Kandiel, A., Fraser, A. G., Korelitz, B. I., Brensinger, C., & Lewis, J. D. (2005). Increased risk of lymphoma among inflammatory bowel disease patients treated with azathioprine and 6-mercaptopurine. [Meta-Analysis Research Support, N.I.H., Extramural Research Support, U.S. Gov't, P.H.S.]. Gut, 54(8), 1121-1125. doi: 10.1136/gut.2004.049460.

Koch, P., del Valle, F., Berdel, W. E., Willich, N. A., Reers, B., Hiddemann, W., . . . Tiemann, M. (2001). Primary gastrointestinal non-Hodgkin's lymphoma: I. Anatomic and histologic distribution, clinical features, and survival data of 371 patients registered in the German Multicenter Study GIT NHL 01/92. [Comparative Study Research Support, Non-U.S. Gov't]. J Clin Oncol, 19(18), 3861-3873.

Lai, Y. C., Ni, Y. H., Jou, S. T., Ho, M. C., Wu, J. F., Chen, H. L., . . . Lee, P. H. (2006). Post-transplantation lymphoproliferative disorders localizing to the gastrointestinal tract after liver transplantation: report of five pediatric cases. [Case Reports]. Pediatr Transplant, 10(3), 390-394. doi: 10.1111/j.1399-3046.2005.00457.x

Lecuit, M., Abachin, E., Martin, A., Poyart, C., Pochart, P., Suarez, F., . . . Lortholary, O. (2004). Immunoproliferative small intestinal disease associated with Campylobacter jejuni. [Case Reports Research Support, Non-U.S. Gov't]. N Engl J Med, 350(3), 239-248. doi: 10.1056/NEJMoa031887.

Lewin, K. J., Ranchod, M., & Dorfman, R. F. (1978). Lymphomas of the gastrointestinal tract: a study of 117 cases presenting with gastrointestinal disease. [Comparative Study Review]. Cancer, 42(2), 693-707.

Makhlouf, H. R., & Sobin, L. H. (2002). Inflammatory myofibroblastic tumors (inflammatory pseudotumors) of the gastrointestinal tract: how closely are they related to inflammatory fibroid polyps? Hum Pathol, 33(3), 307-315.

Mansoor, A., Pittaluga, S., Beck, P. L., Wilson, W. H., Ferry, J. A., & Jaffe, E. S. (2011). NK-cell enteropathy: a benign NK-cell lymphoproliferative disease mimicking intestinal lymphoma: clinicopathologic features and follow-up in a unique case series. [Research Support, N.I.H., Intramural]. Blood, 117(5), 1447-1452. doi: 10.1182/blood-2010-08-302737.

Matuchansky, C., Touchard, G., Lemaire, M., Babin, P., Demeocq, F., Fonck, Y., . . . Preud'Homme, J. L. (1985). Malignant lymphoma of the small bowel associated with diffuse nodular lymphoid hyperplasia. [Case Reports]. N Engl J Med, 313(3), 166-171. doi: 10.1056/NEJM198507183130307.

Mills, S. D., Kurjanczyk, L. A., & Penner, J. L. (1992). Antigenicity of Helicobacter pylori lipopolysaccharides. [Research Support, U.S. Gov't, P.H.S.]. J Clin Microbiol, 30(12), 3175-3180.

Mori, M., Kobayashi, Y., Maeshima, A. M., Gotoda, T., Oda, I., Kagami, Y., . . . Tobinai, K. (2010). The indolent course and high incidence of t(14;18) in primary duodenal follicular lymphoma. [Research Support, Non-U.S. Gov't]. Ann Oncol, 21(7), 1500-1505. doi: 10.1093/annonc/mdp557.

Nakamura, T., Nakamura, S., Yonezumi, M., Suzuki, T., Matsuura, A., Yatabe, Y., . . . Seto, M. (2000). Helicobacter pylori and the t(11;18)(q21;q21) translocation in gastric low-grade B-cell lymphoma of mucosa-associated lymphoid tissue type. [Research Support, Non-U.S. Gov't]. Jpn J Cancer Res, 91(3), 301-309.

Nakamura, T., Seto, M., Tajika, M., Kawai, H., Yokoi, T., Yatabe, Y., & Nakamura, S. (2008). Clinical features and prognosis of gastric MALT lymphoma with special reference to responsiveness to H. pylori eradication and API2-MALT1 status. [Comparative Study Research Support, Non-U.S. Gov't]. Am J Gastroenterol, 103(1), 62-70. doi: 10.1111/j.1572-0241.2007.01521.x.

Nalesnik, M. A. (1990). Involvement of the gastrointestinal tract by Epstein-Barr virus--associated posttransplant lymphoproliferative disorders. [Case Reports Research Support, Non-U.S. Gov't]. Am J Surg Pathol, 14 Suppl 1, 92-100.

Peterson, M. C. (2004). Immunoproliferative small intestinal disease associated with Campylobacter jejuni. [Comment Letter]. N Engl J Med, 350(16), 1685-1686; author reply 1685-1686. doi: 10.1056/NEJM200404153501619.

Pitman, S. D., Huang, Q., Zuppan, C. W., Rowsell, E. H., Cao, J. D., Berdeja, J. G., . . . Wang, J. (2006). Hodgkin lymphoma-like posttransplant lymphoproliferative disorder (HL-like PTLD) simulates monomorphic B-cell PTLD both clinically and pathologically. Am J Surg Pathol, 30(4), 470-476.

Psyrri, A., Papageorgiou, S., & Economopoulos, T. (2008). Primary extranodal lymphomas of stomach: clinical presentation, diagnostic pitfalls and management. [Review]. Ann Oncol, 19(12), 1992-1999. doi: 10.1093/annonc/mdn525.

Radic-Kristo, D., Planinc-Peraica, A., Ostojic, S., Vrhovac, R., Kardum-Skelin, I., & Jaksic, B. (2010). Primary gastrointestinal non-Hodgkin lymphoma in adults: clinicopathologic and survival characteristics. Coll Antropol, 34(2), 413-417.

Sagaert, X., De Wolf-Peeters, C., Noels, H., & Baens, M. (2007). The pathogenesis of MALT lymphomas: where do we stand? [Review]. Leukemia, 21(3), 389-396. doi: 10.1038/sj.leu.2404517.

Salem, P., el-Hashimi, L., Anaissie, E., Geha, S., Habboubi, N., Ibrahim, N., . . . Allam, C. (1987). Primary small intestinal lymphoma in adults. A comparative study of IPSID versus non-IPSID in the Middle East. [Research Support, Non-U.S. Gov't]. Cancer, 59(9), 1670-1676.

Sandler, A. S., & Kaplan, L. D. (1996). Diagnosis and management of systemic non-Hodgkin's lymphoma in HIV disease. [Review]. Hematol Oncol Clin North Am, 10(5), 1111-1124.

Sarode, S. C., Zarkar, G. A., Desai, R. S., Sabane, V. S., & Kulkarni, M. A. (2009). Plasmablastic lymphoma of the oral cavity in an HIV-positive patient: a case report and review of literature. [Case Reports Review]. Int J Oral Maxillofac Surg, 38(9), 993-999. doi: 10.1016/j.ijom.2009.03.720.

Semakula, B., Rittenbach, J. V., & Wang, J. (2006). Hodgkin lymphoma-like posttransplantation lymphoproliferative disorder. [Review]. Arch Pathol Lab Med, 130(4), 558-560. doi: 10.1043/1543-2165(2006)130[558:HLPLD]2.0.CO;2.

Simcock, M., Blasko, M., Karrer, U., Bertisch, B., Pless, M., Blumer, L., . . . Koller, M. T. (2007). Treatment and prognosis of AIDS-related lymphoma in the era of highly active antiretroviral therapy: findings from the Swiss HIV Cohort Study. [Research Support, Non-U.S. Gov't]. Antivir Ther, 12(6), 931-939.

Smedby, K. E., Akerman, M., Hildebrand, H., Glimelius, B., Ekbom, A., & Askling, J. (2005). Malignant lymphomas in coeliac disease: evidence of increased risks for lymphoma types other than enteropathy-type T cell lymphoma. [Multicenter Study Research Support, Non-U.S. Gov't]. Gut, 54(1), 54-59. doi: 10.1136/gut.2003.032094.

Starostik, P., Patzner, J., Greiner, A., Schwarz, S., Kalla, J., Ott, G., & Muller-Hermelink, H. K. (2002). Gastric marginal zone B-cell lymphomas of MALT type develop along 2 distinct pathogenetic pathways. Blood, 99(1), 3-9. doi: DOI 10.1182/blood.V99.1.3.

Stein, H. W., RA; Chan, WC et al. (2008). Diffuse large B-cell lymphoma, not otherwise specified. . In C. E. Swerdlow SH, Harris NL, Jaffe ES, et al, eds (Ed.), World Health Organization Classification of Tumours of Haematopoietic and Lymphoid Tissues (4th edition ed., pp. 233-237). Lyon, France: IARC Press.

Sugano, K. (1998). Molecular and cytogenetic diagnosis of lymphoproliferative disorders of the gastrointestinal tract. [Comment Editorial]. J Gastroenterol, 33(5), 782-783.

Sun, J., Lu, Z., Yang, D., & Chen, J. (2011). Primary intestinal T-cell and NK-cell lymphomas: a clinicopathological and molecular study from China focused on type II enteropathy-associated T-cell lymphoma and primary intestinal NK-cell lymphoma. Mod Pathol, 24(7), 983-992. doi: 10.1038/modpathol.2011.45.

Suzuki, H., Saito, Y., & Hibi, T. (2009). Helicobacter pylori and Gastric Mucosa-associated Lymphoid Tissue (MALT) Lymphoma: Updated Review of Clinical Outcomes and the Molecular Pathogenesis. Gut Liver, 3(2), 81-87. doi: 10.5009/gnl.2009.3.2.81.

Terada, T. (2012). CD5-positive marginal zone B-cell lymphoma of the mucosa-associated lymphoid tissue (MALT) of the lung. [Case Reports]. Diagn Pathol, 7, 16. doi: 10.1186/1746-1596-7-16.

Thayu, M., Markowitz, J. E., Mamula, P., Russo, P. A., Muinos, W. I., & Baldassano, R. N. (2005). Hepatosplenic T-cell lymphoma in an adolescent patient after immunomodulator and biologic therapy for Crohn disease. [Case Reports]. J Pediatr Gastroenterol Nutr, 40(2), 220-222.

Vega, F., Chang, C. C., Medeiros, L. J., Udden, M. M., Cho-Vega, J. H., Lau, C. C., . . . Jorgensen, J. L. (2005). Plasmablastic lymphomas and plasmablastic plasma cell myelomas have nearly identical immunophenotypic profiles. Modern Pathology, 18(6), 806-815. doi: DOI 10.1038/modpathol.3800355.

Verbeek, W. H., Van De Water, J. M., Al-Toma, A., Oudejans, J. J., Mulder, C. J., & Coupe, V. M. (2008). Incidence of enteropathy--associated T-cell lymphoma: a nation-wide study of a population-based registry in The Netherlands. [Research Support, Non-U.S. Gov't]. Scand J Gastroenterol, 43(11), 1322-1328. doi: 10.1080/00365520802240222.

Wotherspoon, A. C., Diss, T. C., Pan, L., Singh, N., Whelan, J., & Isaacson, P. G. (1996). Low grade gastric B-cell lymphoma of mucosa associated lymphoid tissue in immunocompromised patients. [Case Reports]. Histopathology, 28(2), 129-134.

Yang, Y. F., Batth, S. S., Chen, M. Y., Borys, D., & Phan, H. (2012). Enteropathy-Associated T Cell Lymphoma Presenting with Acute Abdominal Syndrome: a Case Report and Review of Literature. Journal of Gastrointestinal Surgery, 16(7), 1446-1449. doi: DOI 10.1007/s11605-012-1878-6.

Yoon, S. S., Coit, D. G., Portlock, C. S., & Karpeh, M. S. (2004). The diminishing role of surgery in the treatment of gastric lymphoma. [Review]. Ann Surg, 240(1), 28-37.

Zhang, Z., Shen, Y., Shen, D., & Ni, X. (2012). Immunophenotype classification and therapeutic outcomes of Chinese primary gastrointestinal diffuse large B-cell lymphoma. BMC Gastroenterol, 12, 77. doi: 10.1186/1471-230X-12-77.

The Complex Role of Chemokines in Cancer: The Case of the CX3CL1/CX3CR1 Axis

Manuel Tardáguila

Department of Immunology and Oncology
Centro Nacional de Biotecnología (CNB/CSIC), Madrid, Spain

Santos Mañes

Department of Immunology and Oncology
Centro Nacional de Biotecnología (CNB/CSIC), Madrid, Spain

1   Introduction

Cancer is a miscellany of diseases that involves uncontrolled growth and proliferation of neoplastic cells; they originate from normal cells that undergo genetic and epigenetic alterations that affect proto-oncogenes and tumor suppressor genes. These genomic modifications allow tumor cells to escape the strict constraints of the multicellular structure, unleashing their replicative potential and the capacity to colonize distant tissues, which finally leads to the death of the organism. The hallmarks of cancer include self-sufficiency in growth signals, insensitivity to anti-growth signals, evasion of apoptosis, sustained angiogenesis, acquisition of limitless replicative potential, and the ability to invade and metastasize (Hanahan & Weinberg, 2000). Two additional characteristics of cancer have recently been suggested, reprogramming of energy metabolism and evasion of immune destruction (Hanahan & Weinberg, 2011).

The role of the immune system in tumor progression was traditionally defined as a counter-force to tumor growth to destroy neoplastic lesions that arise naturally through somatic mutation (Bissell & Hines, 2011). When tumor cells reach a critical number of alterations, the relationship between the two forces enters equilibrium; in this phase, the immune system precludes tumor expansion but does not eradicate the lesion (Murphy *et al.*, 2008; Pardoll, 2003). This equilibrium phase involves immunoediting of the tumor; the immune system eliminates highly immunogenic clones, effectively selecting for those with low immunogenicity. The immune system is eventually unable to cope with the tumor, which reaches the escape phase (Murphy *et al.*, 2008; Pardoll, 2003). It is now thought that the immune system has a more complex role in cancer progression; the types of immune cells and molecular mediators involved in the response are central to its outcome, and effectively curb tumor growth or, paradoxically, promote it (DeNardo & Coussens, 2007).

The cells of the immune system, the leukocytes, are divided into myeloid and lymphoid lineages. Myeloid cells compose the innate immune system, which includes monocytes, neutrophils, granulocytes, mastocytes, dendritic cells, natural killer (NK) cells and macrophages. With the complement system, the innate immune system forms the body's first line of defense against pathogens and tumors. Lymphoid cells constitute the adaptive immune system. These cells are comprised of B lymphocytes, which origi-nate in the bone marrow, and CD4 and CD8 T lymphocytes, both of which arise in the thymus; there is also an NK cell population (NK-T cells) of thymic origin (Ballas & Rasmussen, 1990). Once antigens are presented to them by professional antigen-presenting cells (APC) of the innate immune system, the lym-phoid cells can elicit an antigen-specific response.

In the context of tumor inflammation, cell types in charge of maintaining tissue homeostasis, such as mastocytes and macrophages, secrete soluble mediators in the tissue. Among these are the chemokines, low molecular weight proteins that recruit immune cells to the neoplastic lesion (Allavena *et al.*, 2011; Balkwill, 2012; González-Martín *et al.*, 2012). Depending on the leukocyte type recruited and the tumor microenvironment, an acute or a chronic inflammatory response is evoked (DeNardo & Coussens, 2007). Tumor progression can be stemmed by acute inflammatory responses, characterized by the presence of CD4 helper type 1 T cells (Th1), CD8 cytolytic T cells (CTL), NK cells, Th1 cytokines (IFN-g and IL-1) and antibodies secreted by B cells (DeNardo & Coussens, 2007; Mosser & Edwards, 2008). In chronic immune responses to tumors, CD4 helper type 2 T cells (Th2) and regulatory T cells (Treg) suppress the cytotoxic activity of CTL (Gu *et al.*, 2000; Viola *et al.*, 2006) and polarize innate immune cells towards phenotypes that enhance tumor progression (Bailey *et al.*, 2007; Fridlender *et al.*, 2009). Chronically activated B cells further enhance the accumulation of these cells in tumors (DeNardo & Coussens, 2007).

Tumors are thus selected for genetic programs that skew immune responses towards chronicity (Allavena *et al.*, 2008; Balkwill & Mantovani, 2001).

Chemokines are among the many factors in the tumor milieu that might function as chemotactic factors; they are a family of small soluble molecules that direct leukocyte trafficking in homeostasis and inflammation (Baggiolini *et al.*, 1997; Mellado *et al.*, 2001). Some chemokines are costimulatory molecules for T cell activation and anti-tumor responses (Contento *et al.*, 2008; González-Martín *et al.*, 2011; Molon *et al.*, 2005). The role of the chemokine ligand-receptor system in cancer is nonetheless complex, as these molecules not only act as cues for leukocyte recruitment to the tumor, but also influence neoplastic cell biology in many ways (Allavena *et al.*, 2011; Balkwill, 2012; Viola *et al.*, 2012). We will provide an overview of the chemokine system in homeostasis and cancer, and focus on the CX3CL1/CX3CR1 axis to illustrate the complex interplay between the chemokines and other molecules that shape a tumor's microenvironment and its progression.

2   Chemokines and Chemokine Receptors

2.1   Chemokine Structure and Classification

The chemokine superfamily comprises 44 members in humans (45 in mice), divided into four groups (Figure 1) based on the position of two conserved N-terminal cysteine residues (Zlotnik & Yoshie, 2000). For the CXC chemokines, also termed a-chemokines (CXCL1-CXCL17), the two cysteine residues are separated by one amino acid; for the CC or b-chemokines (CCL1-CCL28; CCL6, CCL9/10 and CCL12 are exclusively murine), the cysteines are adjacent (Baggiolini *et al.*, 1994, 1997). The XC or g-chemokines (XCL1-2) have lost one of the conserved cysteines (Kelner *et al.*, 1994), and in the CX3C or d-chemokines (with a single known member, CX3CL1), the cysteines are separated by three amino acids (Bazan *et al.*, 1997). The CXC chemokines are in turn subdivided as ELR^+ and ELR^-, based on a glutamic acid-leucine-arginine (ELR) motif adjacent to the first conserved cysteine at the N terminus (Clark-Lewis *et al.*, 1991). This motif has important functional consequences, since ELR^+ chemokines (including CXCL1-3, CXCL8 and CXCL12) attract neutrophils and promote angiogenesis (Gupta *et al.*, 1998; Smith *et al.*, 1994; Strieter *et al.*, 1995; Zlotnik *et al.*, 2006), whereas ELR^- chemokines (including CXCL4, CXCL9 and CXCL10) recruit different types of lymphocytes and have angiostatic properties (Angiolillo *et al.*, 1995; Arenberg *et al.*, 1997; Strieter *et al.*, 1995; Zlotnik *et al.*, 2006).

Chemokines are low molecular weight proteins (8-10 kDa) secreted to the extracellular medium (except CXCL16 and CX3CL1, which are synthesized as transmembrane proteins and can subsequently be cleaved); they form gradients that allow receptor-expressing cells to migrate towards higher concentrations of the chemokine (Bazan *et al.*, 1997; Handel *et al.*, 2005; Matloubian *et al.*, 2000; Mellado *et al.*, 2001; Pan *et al.*, 1997). Chemokine binding to glycosaminoglycans (GAG) of the extracellular matrix stabilizes these gradients, and this interaction is a central attribute of the *in vivo* chemoattractant function of chemokines (Bonecchi *et al.*, 2011).

Chemokines signal by binding to G protein-coupled receptors (GPCR), which activate heterotrimeric G proteins of the inhibitory subclass (G_i). These receptors share a common structure (except PIT-PNM3/Nir1) (Murphy, 1994), with seven transmembrane domains connected by intra- and extracellular loops. They are classified according to the chemokines they bind (Figure 1) as CXC (CXCR1-10), CC (CCR1-6), XC (XCR1) and CX3C (CX3CR1) receptors (de Brevern *et al.*, 2005; Premack & Schall, 1996). The two atypical receptors, D6 and Duffy, bind chemokines without triggering an intracellular

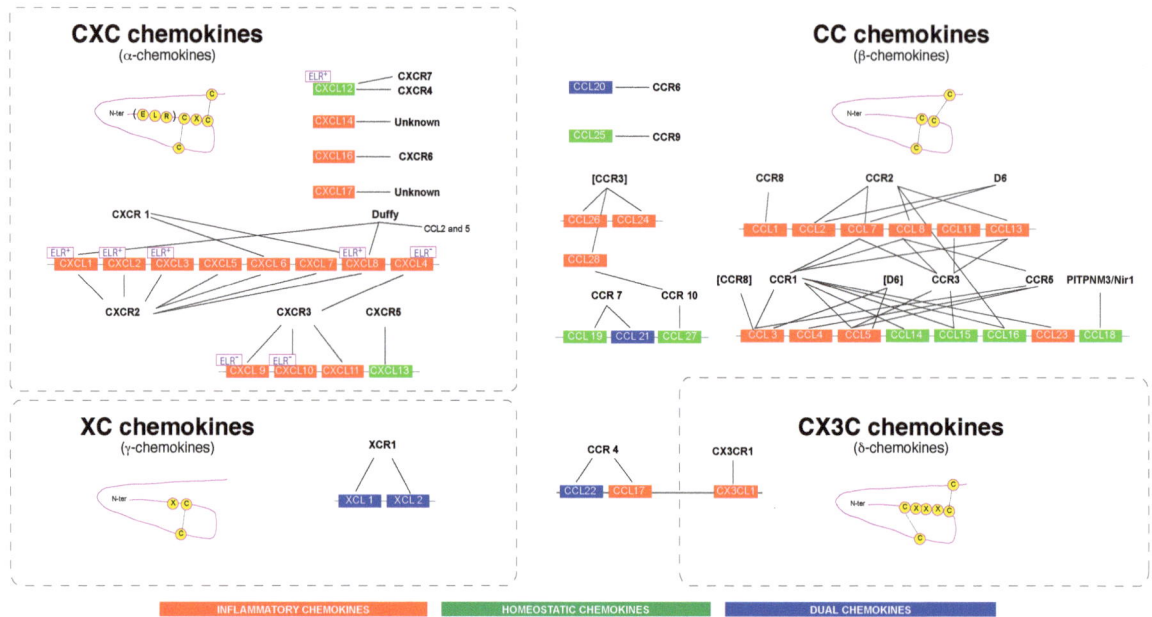

Figure 1: Chemokines and chemokine receptors. Chemokines are grouped in clusters, as they appear in the genome, or shown separately when they do not cluster (Zlotnik *et al.*, 2006). The position of the conserved cysteine residues is detailed for each family, as is the ELR motif in CXC chemokines. The functional classification of chemokines is also shown; inflammatory chemokines are in red, homeostatic in green and dual in blue. When necessary, chemokine receptors that bind chemokines in different clusters are duplicated and included in brackets.

signal, and are hypothesized to function as decoy receptors (Allavena *et al.*, 2011; Hansell *et al.*, 2006). Signaling routes activated by chemokine binding include calcium mobilization, as well as survival and proliferation pathways (Balkwill, 2012).

Chemokines and their receptors can be further categorized by function. Most are expressed in inflammatory conditions and are termed inflammatory chemokines, whereas others are produced constitutively and take part in leukocyte trafficking; these are the homeostatic chemokines (Figure 1). Dual chemokines exert both functions.

A characteristic of the chemokine ligand-receptor system is its redundancy (Mellado *et al.*, 2001). A given chemokine can bind different receptors of the same family, and vice versa. This redundancy has been explained as a result of genomic evolution; clusters of chemokines have arisen from duplication of shorter units, maintaining minimum structural characteristics that allow for common receptors (Zlotnik *et al.*, 2006). Indeed, chemokines in the same gene cluster share a set of receptors (Figure 1). Other chemokines do not form gene clusters and tend to have a unique receptor, indicating strong evolutionary pressure against duplication and subsequent mutation (Figure 1) (Zlotnik *et al.*, 2006). This redundancy could be responsible for the apparent lack of functional specificity among chemokines that share a common receptor. Precise spatial and temporal control of gene expression nonetheless confers specificity on this ligand-receptor system (Mellado *et al.*, 2001).

An additional level of complexity in chemokine-receptor association is the ability of receptors and ligands to homo- or heterodimerize. It is suggested that homo- and heterodimers have distinct functional properties (Mellado *et al.*, 2001; Zaitseva *et al.*, 1997). In this way, a given receptor can integrate the signaling of different chemokines to produce distinct effects (Zhang *et al.*, 1999), and different receptors coexpressed in the same cell can integrate distinct chemokine signals for a shared function (Mellado *et al.*, 2001). The activation of chemokine receptors can also transactivate other signaling modules, as reported for the JAK/STAT pathway (Mellado *et al.*, 2001) and ErbB receptors (Lazennec & Richmond, 2010; Tardáguila *et al.*, 2013; White *et al.*, 2009).

3   Chemokines in Cancer Progression

As the chief mediators of leukocyte recruitment, chemokines are paramount in shaping the tumor microenvironment and tumor progression (Allavena *et al.*, 2011; Balkwill, 2012) (Figure 2). Nonetheless, chemokines also participate in the balance between angiogenic and anti-angiogenic signals in the tumor milieu (Lazennec & Richmond, 2010) and act directly on tumor cells to promote survival and proliferation or senescence (Acharyya *et al.*, 2012; Acosta *et al.*, 2008; Allavena *et al.*, 2011; Balkwill, 2012). *De novo* or increased expression of chemokine receptors allows tumor cells to migrate and colonize distant tissues, a process involved in the metastasis of various tumor types (Balkwill, 2012; Mañes *et al.*, 2001; Mira *et al.*, 2001). It is therefore not surprising that causative genetic lesions of human cancers, such as activating mutations in the oncogenes *Ras, Ret* and *Myc*, induce upregulation of certain sets of chemokines (Balkwill, 2012).

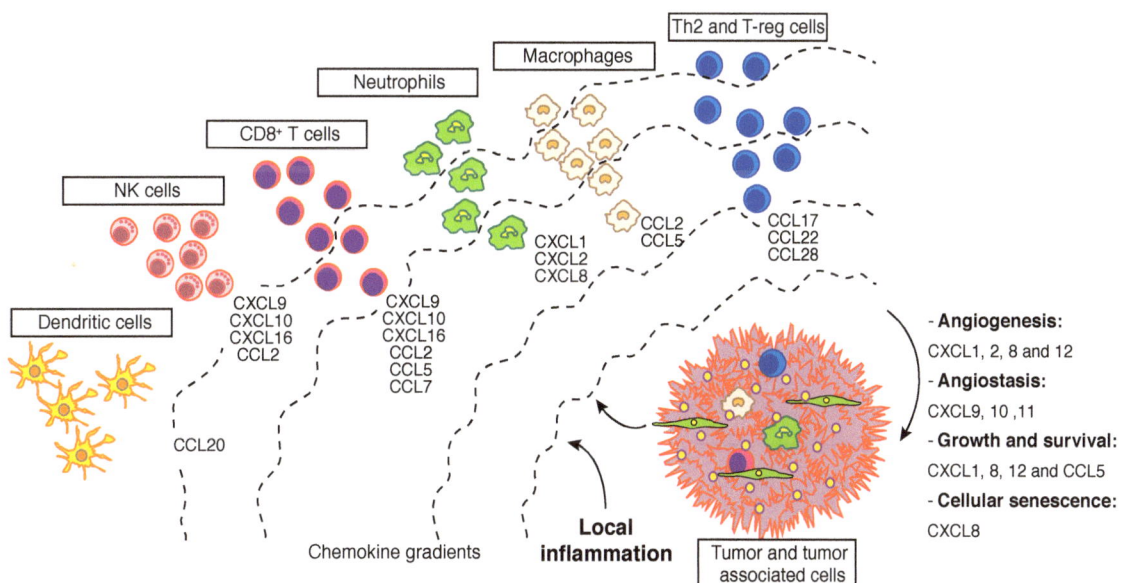

Figure 2: **Chemokines and chemokine receptors in cancer.** Chemokine gradients produced by neoplastic and tumor-associated cells are depicted as dashed lines. Specific chemokines that attract different leukocyte subpopulations are indicated. In addition to directing leukocyte infiltration, chemokines can have pro- or anti-angiogenic effects, stimulate proliferation and survival, or induce cell senescence (left).

3.1   Shaping the Tumor Microenvironment

The leukocyte compartment constitutes a key element of the tumor microenvironment. The complex assembly of cells and molecules that make up this compartment contributes to develop and maintain most hallmarks of cancer. Chemokines are well characterized as cues for leukocyte recruitment to the vicinity of the tumor. Examples of chemokine-mediated leukocyte attraction to tumors include the CXCL8-, CXCL1- and CXCL2-mediated chemoattraction of $CXCR2^+$ neutrophils (Hirose et al., 1995), CCL2- and CCL5-induced recruitment of macrophages that express CCR2, CCR1 and CCR5 (González-Martín et al., 2012), CCL20/CCR6-mediated dendritic cell infiltration (Vicari et al., 2004), or CXCL9, CXCL10 and CXCL16-induced recruitment of $CXCR3^+/CXCR5^+$ NK and $CD8^+$ T cells (Nokihara et al., 2000; Sallusto et al., 1998).

CCR7-expressing naive T cells and mature dendritic cells migrate to lymph nodes adjacent to tumors, guided by gradients of the homeostatic chemokines CCL19 and CCL21 (Forster et al., 2008). Leukocyte infiltration of tumors is nonetheless a double-edged sword. Many tumor cells, as well as cells of the tumor stroma such as cancer-associated fibroblasts (CAF) or mesenchymal stem cells (MSC), produce chemokines that attract and later subvert immune cells (Allavena et al., 2011; Balkwill, 2012), as shown with CXCL1 and CXCL2 for neutrophils (Acharyya et al., 2012; Fridlender et al., 2009) or CCL2 and CCL5 for macrophages (Bailey et al., 2007; Balkwill & Mantovani, 2012). In addition, certain chemokines attract immunosuppressive cells that promote tumor growth; these include Th2 cells that migrate towards CCL17 and CCL22, as well as regulatory T cells, which respond to CCL22 and CCL28 (Allavena et al., 2011; Budhu and Wang, 2012). Whereas chemokines should act as a protective system against cancer, in aid of immune cells to seek and destroy transformed cells, progressing tumors hijack the chemokine system to manipulate the tumor microenvironment and support their own advance. New chemokine receptor-based therapeutic approaches target leukocyte recruitment to curb tumor growth. For instance, CCL2 blockade by neutralizing antibodies inhibits monocyte recruitment and prolongs survival of mice with prostate tumors (Loberg et al., 2007); a similar strategy is currently undergoing clinical evaluation in ovarian and prostate cancer patients (Allavena et al., 2011). Another chemokine-centered approach under study is the blockade of immunosuppressive cell infiltration into tumors; CCR4 inhibition using antagonistic antibodies reduces recruitment of regulatory T cells, which boosts the anti-tumor immune response and inhibits tumor growth (Ito et al., 2009).

3.2   Chemokine Function in Tumor Angiogenesis

As we comment above, chemokines can act as pro-angiogenic or angiostatic molecules. The CXC ELR^+ chemokines CXCL1, 2, 8 and 12 promote angiogenesis by inducing migration, proliferation and survival signals to endothelial cells that express CXCR2 or CXCR4 (Mehrad et al., 2007; Wang et al., 2007). In contrast, the CXC ELR^- chemokines CXCL9, 10 and 11 act through CXCR3 to inhibit the pro-angiogenic effects of basic fibroblast growth factor (bFGF) and vascular-endothelial growth factor (VEGF), and to antagonize CXC ELR^+ chemokines (Rosenkilde & Schwartz, 2004; Salcedo et al., 2000). The atypical chemokine receptor Duffy binds ELR^+ chemokines and counterbalances their action (Rosenkilde & Schwartz, 2004). The chemokines can thus be considered critical mediators of angiogenesis; indeed, the combined increase in pro-angiogenic chemokine production and repression of the Duffy receptor are thought to be a key step in the "angiogenic switch" in tumors (Huang et al., 2002).

3.3   Chemokine Activities in Cell Cycle Progression and Senescence

Reports of their ability to induce *in vitro* proliferation and/or survival of a variety of tumor cell types led to the assumption that chemokines can act as paracrine or autocrine proliferation factors (Balkwill, 2012). Chemokine receptor engagement activates PI3K (phosphoinositide 3-kinase), an important pathway in apoptosis resistance, and ERK/MAPK (extracellular signal-regulated kinases/mitogen-activated protein kinases), a route involved in cell proliferation (Mellado *et al.*, 2001). Chemokine influence on tumor cell proliferation has been demonstrated for the CXCL12/CXCR4 pair (Balkwill, 2012; Barbero *et al.*, 2003; Hartmann *et al.*, 2005; Juarez *et al.*, 2003; Zhou *et al.*, 2002); the CXCR4 antagonist AMD3100 inhibits growth of primary tumors in models of melanoma, osteosarcoma, breast and prostate cancer, suggesting therapeutic utility (Balkwill & Mantovani, 2012). Other chemokine/receptor pairs include CXCL1/CXCL8 with CXCR2 in colon carcinoma (Brew *et al.*, 2000), CCL5/CCR5 in prostate cancer (Vaday *et al.*, 2006), CCL6/CCR6 in colorectal cancer (Balkwill, 2012) and CCL21/CCR7 in squamous cell carcinoma (Wang *et al.*, 2008).

Chemokines and their receptors can nonetheless also restrain tumor growth. For instance, the CCL5/CCR5 pair activates p53 signaling in breast cancer cell lines, leading to upregulation of the cell cycle inhibitor p21 and reduced *in vivo* proliferation (Mañes *et al.*, 2003). In breast cancer patients bearing the *ccr5D32* CCR5 polymorphism, which renders a non-functional receptor, disease-free survival time is shorter than for those who express functional CCR5 and have tumors with unmutated p53 (Mañes *et al.*, 2003). Surprisingly, the mutation rate of the tumor suppressor p53 is lower in tumors from *ccr5D32* patients compared with those bearing wild-type CCR5 alleles (Aoki *et al.*, 2009; Mañes *et al.*, 2003); this suggests that selective pressure for p53 mutation is lower in tumors from *ccr5Δ32* individuals. Since ~50% of tumors have developed mechanisms other than mutation to suppress p53 function, it is possible that p53 silencing in ccr5Δ32 tumors occurs in conditions in which this tumor suppressor gene is activated in CCR5 wild-type individuals.

CXCR2 signaling increases the rate of cell senescence induced by oncogenic stress, also via a p53-dependent mechanism (Acosta *et al.*, 2008). CXCR2 ligands such as CXCL8 paradoxically promote cell survival and proliferation as well as cell senescence. Mutation of p53 or its functional inactivation in tumor cells might lead to the loss of this CXCR2-mediated senescence checkpoint; in such circumstances, CXCR2 ligands would have predominantly pro-survival and pro-mitogenic activities (Allavena *et al.*, 2011).

3.4   Chemokines as Inducers of Organ-specific Tumor Metastasis

Receptor-expressing tumor cells can use chemokine gradients to migrate and colonize distant tissues. One of the most important pathways in metastasis involves homeostatic chemokine gradients and their receptors (Zlotnik *et al.*, 2011). These gradients act as "cell highways", providing routes for cell homing to specific anatomical locations (Figure 3). The first such observation was the specific metastasis of CXCR4[+] tumor cells from melanoma, glioblastoma, breast, ovarian, prostate and pancreatic cancers in lung, bone and liver, as these organs express high levels of CXCL12, the CXCR4 ligand (Jankowski *et al.*, 2003; Kang *et al.*, 2003; Müller *et al.*, 2001; Murakami *et al.*, 2002; Zeelenberg *et al.*, 2001). Other CXC receptors including CXCR1, CXCR2, CXCR3 and CXCR5 have been implicated in the metastasis of malignant melanoma, colorectal, gastric, and renal carcinomas to the liver (Tsaur *et al.*, 2011; Varney *et al.*, 2011; Wang *et al.*, 2013). In the case of CC chemokines, various tumor cell types express CCR7 and use CCL19 and CCL21 gradients to migrate to lymph nodes (Allavena *et al.*, 2011; Oliveira-Neto *et*

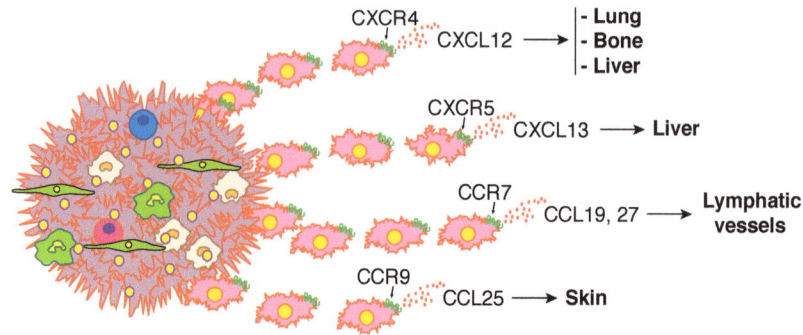

Figure 3. Tumors hijack the chemokine system to trigger organ-specific metastasis. Several chemokine receptors expressed by tumor cells allow these cells to migrate and to colonize specific anatomical sites.

al., 2013; Raman *et al.*, 2007; Takanami, 2003; Wiley *et al.*, 2001). CCR7 use in lymph node metastasis is consistent with elevated expression of its ligands in secondary lymphoid organs. Shields et al. nonetheless showed that tumor cells themselves can generate chemokine gradients that stimulate autocrine CCR7 signaling, which greatly enhances their migration to lymph nodes (Shields *et al.*, 2007). Autocrine production of chemokines might give a permissive signal for acquisition of the motility program needed for metastasis. Autocrine CCL5 production after growth factor stimulation provides a necessary signal for acquisition of a polarized morphology by breast cancer cells (Mira *et al.*, 2001).

CCR receptors other than CCR5 are also implicated in the metastatic process. Melanoma cells upregulate CCR9 to metastasize to small intestine via CCL25 gradients (Amersi *et al.*, 2008), whereas CCR10 and CCR4 promote skin metastasis of lymphoma (Allavena *et al.*, 2011). These examples illustrate the importance of chemokine gradients for organ-specific tumor dissemination. Whether the chemokine system has clinical utility in the prevention of tumor metastasis remain to be determined, although preclinical studies have shown positive results. AMD3100 inhibits the CXCR4-mediated metastatic process in several murine models of melanoma, osteosarcoma, breast and prostate cancer (Balkwill and Mantovani, 2012). Interestingly, AMD3100 also induces $CD34^+$ stem cell mobilization in bone marrow; it is currently used to treat multiple myeloma and acute myeloid leukemia, as it marshals malignant cells and increases their sensitivity to chemotherapy (Balkwill & Mantovani, 2012).

4   The CX3CL1/CX3CR1 Axis in Cancer Biology

4.1   CX3CL1, An Atypical Chemokine

CX3CL1, also known as fractalkine, is the sole member of the CX3C d-chemokine family (Bazan *et al.*, 1997; Pan *et al.*, 1997). It is a 95 kDa type I transmembrane protein that can be processed by ADAM proteases to give rise to an 80 kDa soluble form (Hermand *et al.*, 2008). The protein has four domains (Figure 4). The first 76 N-terminal amino acids form the chemokine domain, which faces the extracellular space and contains the C-XXX-C motif. This domain alone is responsible for engaging CX3CR1, the sole CX3CL1 receptor (see below). The chemokine moiety is followed by a "mucin-like stalk" (Figure 4), a long protein stem (26 nm) enriched in mucin-like repeats. The only known function of this stalk is to project the chemokine domain far beyond the plasma membrane; the mucin stalk does not participate in binding to or signaling through CX3CR1 (Fong *et al.*, 1998). At the base of the stalk lies the target sequence for the ADAM proteases. A short, 18-amino-acid transmembrane domain connects the extracellular domains to a 40-amino-acid cytoplasmic tail (Hermand *et al.*, 2008) (Figure 4). This intracellular tail has binding sites for the adaptor protein AP-2, which is implicated in the constitutive endocytosis of the chemokine (Andrzejewski *et al.*, 2010; Huang *et al.*, 2009).

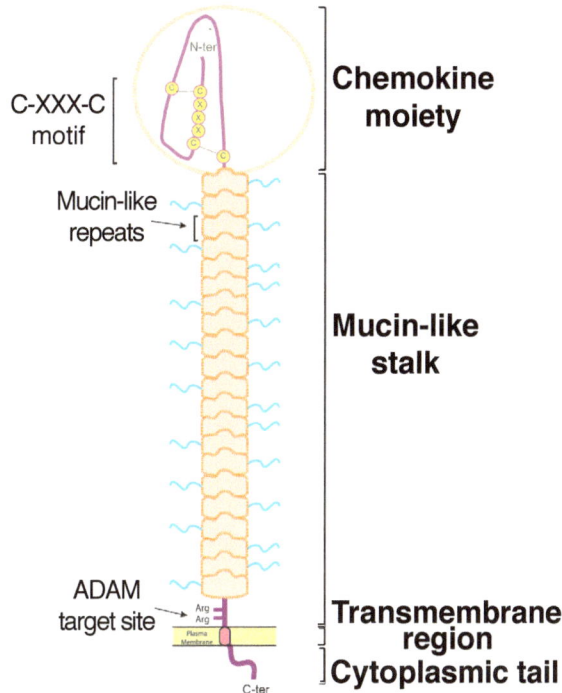

Figure 4. CX3CL1 structure. Scheme showing the four functional CX3CL1 domains and the cleavage site for ADAM proteases.

CX3CL1 is expressed in several cell types including endothelial (Bazan *et al.*, 1997), epithelial (Lucas *et al.*, 2001; Muehlhoefer *et al.*, 2000) and dendritic cells (Papadopoulos *et al.*, 1999), neurons (Pan *et al.*, 1997), osteoblasts (Koizumi *et al.*, 2009) and keratinocytes (Sugaya *et al.*, 2003). CX3CL1 transcription in these cells is controlled by pro-inflammatory cytokines such as TNFa, IL-1b and IFNg *via* the NF-kB pathway (Imaizumi *et al.*, 2002; Marchesi *et al.*, 2010). Other stimuli that increase CX3CL1 expression are gonadotropins (Zhao *et al.*, 2008) and the combination of high glucose with the cytokine resistin (Manduteanu *et al.*, 2009). CX3CL1 expression is repressed by inhibitors of the NF-kB pathway, agonists of the peroxisome proliferator-activated receptor gamma (PPARg) (Imaizumi *et al.*, 2002) and the glucocorticoid receptor (Bhavsar *et al.*, 2008). CX3CL1 expression is also regulated posttranscriptionally by TNFa, which stabilizes mRNA through the p38 MAPK pathway (Matsumiya *et al.*, 2010); notably, IFNg does not trigger CX3CL1 mRNA stabilization.

4.2   CX3CR1, the CX3CL1 Receptor

The only known physiological receptor for CX3CL1 is CX3CR1 (Imai *et al.*, 1997), a classical seven-transmembrane GPCR (Figure 5). As for other chemokine receptors, CX3CR1 has a DRYLAIV motif in the second intracellular loop, which is essential for receptor signaling; it likewise has abundant serine residues at the C terminus, which are targeted by GPCR kinases (GRK) for receptor endocytosis (Haskell *et al.*, 1999; Schwarz *et al.*, 2010).

CX3CR1 has several sequence polymorphisms (Figure 5), and some are thought to have important functional consequences. An isoleucine residue rather than valine at position 249 (V249I) has been linked to low receptor availability at the cell surface, whereas methionine instead of threonine at position 280 (T280M) reduces receptor affinity for CX3CL1 (Faure *et al.*, 2000). In murine CX3CR1, which shares 83% identity with the human gene (Combadiere *et al.*, 1998), a proline in position 326 is hypothesized to prevent the murine receptor from activating the PI3K pathway directly (Davis and Harrison, 2006). In an apparent contradiction, the CX3CL1/CX3CR1 axis promotes survival in various murine cell types (Landsman *et al.*, 2009). One explanation lies in its ability to transactivate other receptors, such as those of the epidermal growth factor (EGF) family, that ultimately trigger PI3K activation (White *et al.*, 2009). As discussed below, CX3CR1 transactivation of EGF receptors could have important implications for cancer biology.

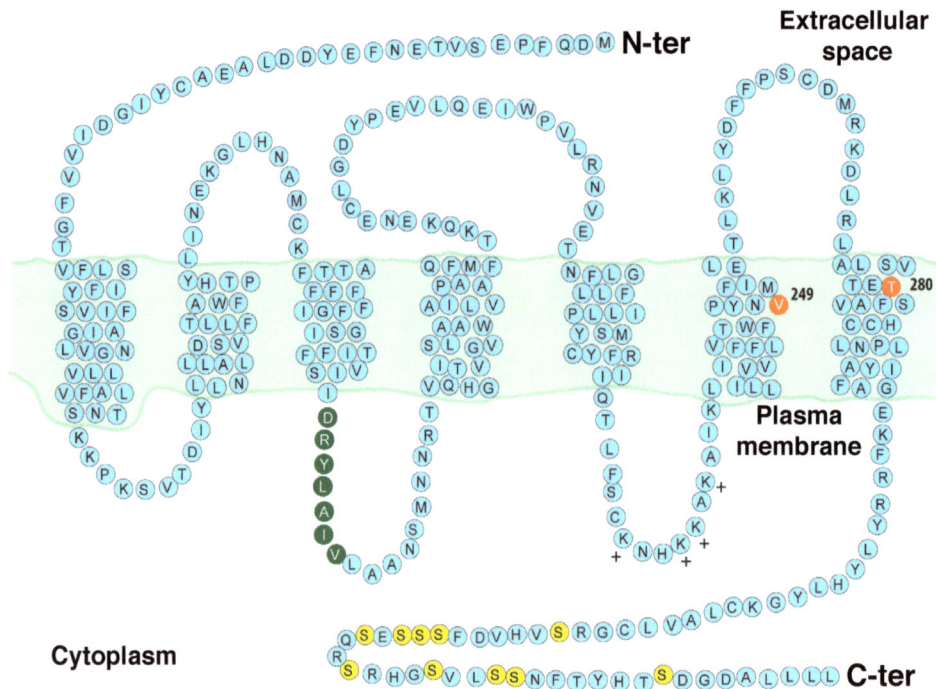

Figure 5: CX3CR1 structure. Primary structure of CX3CR1 (adapted from Schwarz *et al.* (Schwarz *et al.*, 2010)). The DRYLAIV motif (green) interacts with G proteins; the C-terminal serine residues (yellow) are susceptible to GRK phosphorylation. The polymorphic residues at position 249 and 280 (red) give rise to hypofunctional receptor variants.

In vivo CX3CR1 expression has been studied extensively using a knock-in mouse model that mirrors receptor expression with the green fluorescent protein (GFP) reporter (Jung *et al.*, 2000). In this model, CX3CR1 is expressed by the GR1⁻ monocyte subpopulation (Geissmann *et al.*, 2003), by resident dendritic cells of the olfactory (Ruitenberg *et al.*, 2008) and intestinal (Niess *et al.*, 2005) epithelia, by bone marrow precursors of smooth muscle cells (Kumar *et al.*, 2010) and by osteoclasts (Koizumi *et al.*, 2009). In humans, CX3CR1 is also expressed by different subsets of CTL (Nishimura *et al.*, 2002) and CD4⁺ T lymphocytes, including Th2 cells (Foussat *et al.*, 2000; Mionnet *et al.*, 2010; Nishimura *et al.*, 2002; Sawai *et al.*, 2005), by B lymphocytes (Corcione *et al.*, 2009), CD16⁺ monocytes (Ancuta *et al.*, 2003) and NK cells (Robinson *et al.*, 2003). In the human and murine central nervous systems, CX3CR1 is expressed specifically in microglial cells (Jung *et al.*, 2000; Ludwig & Mentlein, 2008).

As for CX3CL1, CX3CR1 expression at the cell surface is regulated by various factors. At the transcriptional level, the cytokine RANKL represses CX3CR1 expression in osteoclasts (Saitoh *et al.*, 2007); at the posttranslational level, membrane CX3CR1 levels are increased by IL-2, CCL2 and hypoxia, whereas IL-15 reduces receptor expression (Barlic *et al.*, 2004; Green *et al.*, 2006; Hung *et al.*, 2007).

4.3   Posttranslational Regulation of the CX3CL1/CX3CR1 Axis

A peculiarity of CX3CL1 is its synthesis as a transmembrane precursor, which constitutes an additional regulatory level for its biological activity. Although *in vitro* results suggested that soluble and membrane-anchored CX3CL1 forms are equally effective in attracting CX3CR1⁺ cells, recent evidence from transgenic mice that express the wild-type precursor or an obligatory soluble CX3CL1 mutant showed that membrane-tethered and shed CX3CL1 forms are not totally interchangeable *in vivo*. Monocyte survival specifically requires membrane-bound CX3CL1, whereas the obligatory soluble CX3CL1 mutant can induce transepithelial dendrite formation by intestinal macrophages (Kim *et al.*, 2011). Regulation of CX3CL1 availability at the plasma membrane might thus be central to the biological function of this axis.

An important regulatory step for CX3CL1 availability is its shedding by ADAM proteases. ADAM10 cleaves the chemokine constitutively, whereas ADAM17 does so in an inflammation-induced manner (Hundhausen *et al.*, 2007; Schulte *et al.*, 2007). Pro-shedding stimuli include TNFa, thromboxane A2 (Tole *et al.*, 2010) and CXCL12 (Cook *et al.*, 2010); in contrast, vitamin D receptor ligands inhibit CX3CL1 membrane shedding (Banerjee *et al.*, 2008). Cathepsin S is also reported to be a major regulator of neuron-microglia communication, as it releases membrane-bound CX3CL1 in dorsal horn neurons (Clark *et al.*, 2009); indeed, cathepsin S-mediated liberation of CX3CL1 is thought to contribute to the amplification and maintenance of chronic pain.

Membrane-tethered CX3CL1 can be regulated by other mechanisms in addition to proteolytic cleavage; these include constitutive endocytosis and recycling of chemokine-filled vesicles (Huang *et al.*, 2009) and chemokine clustering mediated by lateral interactions (Hermand *et al.*, 2008). Finally, the amount of soluble chemokine can also be modulated; receptor engagement and later endocytosis allow CX3CR1 to scavenge soluble ligand from the extracellular medium (Cardona *et al.*, 2008).

4.4   Functions of the CX3CL1/CX3CR1 Axis

CX3CL1 was originally discovered in endothelial cells as a gene upregulated by pro-inflammatory stimuli (Bazan *et al.*, 1997); it can therefore be predicted to act in leukocyte infiltration into inflamed tissues. Leukocyte transendothelial migration (TEM) is initiated by weak affinity interactions between selectins, which cause leukocytes to roll over the endothelial layer. Chemokines expressed by the endothelium activate integrins expressed on leukocytes, triggering their firm adhesion; the cells then transmigrate through the endothelial layer into the tissue (Mellado *et al.*, 2001). This picture can change when membrane-bound CX3CL1 is present, since binding to its receptor can act as an adhesive mechanism, independently of CX3CR1 signaling and integrin activation (Haskell *et al.*, 1999; Mionnet *et al.*, 2010). CX3CL1/CX3CR1 binding has a dissociation constant in the range of 100 pM, which is strong enough to allow cell-to-cell adhesion, even in blood flow conditions (Harrison *et al.*, 2001; Haskell *et al.*, 2000). Indeed, inhibition of CX3CL1 cleavage increases leukocyte retention on the surface of endothelial layers, inhibiting TEM. This observation has prompted Schwarz et al. (Schwarz *et al.*, 2010) to propose a three-step model for CX3CL1-mediated leukocyte transmigration (Figure 6A).

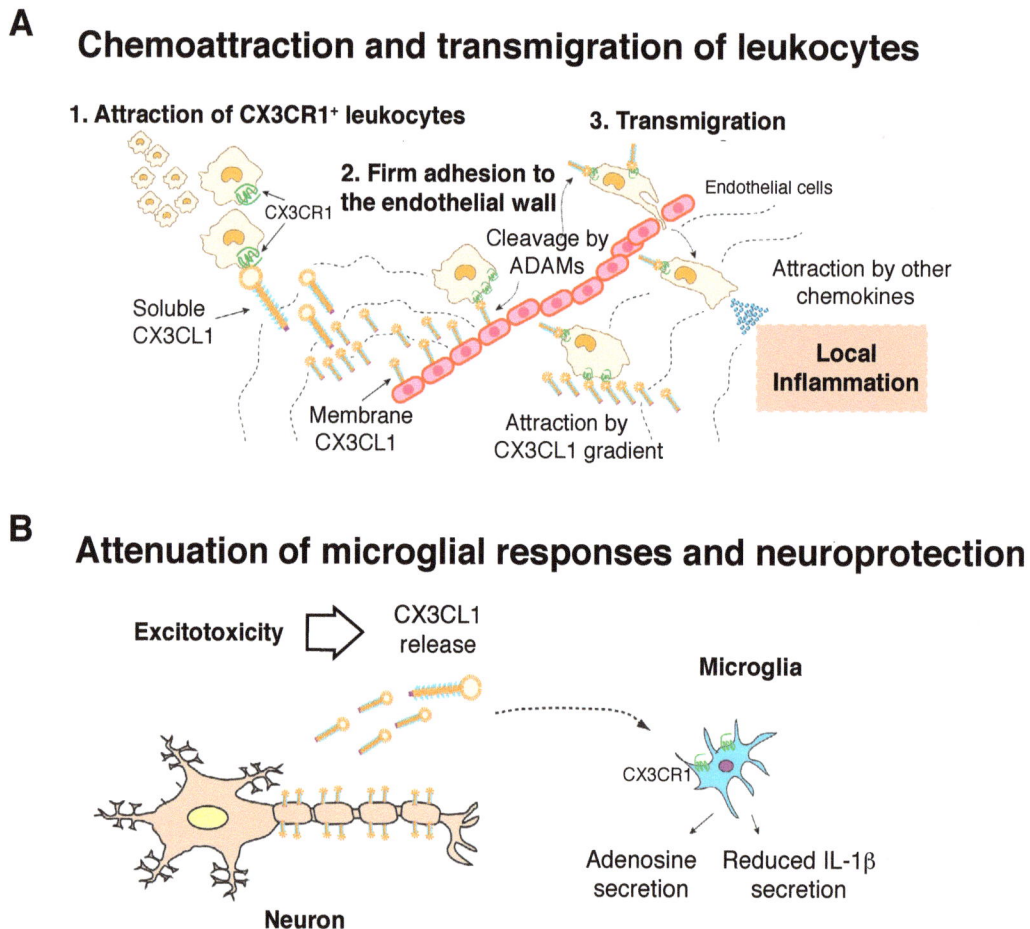

A   Chemoattraction and transmigration of leukocytes

B   Attenuation of microglial responses and neuroprotection

Figure 6: The CX3CL1/CX3CR1 axis is a paracrine communication system in inflammation. A) CX3CL1-induced leukocyte attraction and transmigration. Soluble CX3CL1 attracts CX3CR1[+] leukocytes, whereas membrane-tethered CX3CL1 mediates their adhesion to endothelial cells. Leukocyte transmigration requires CX3CL1 shedding; leukocytes can then follow CX3CL1 or secondary chemokine gradients. B) In the central nervous system, CX3CL1 released from neurons attenuates the inflammatory reaction of CX3CR1[+]-expressing microglial cells and stimulates secretion of neuroprotective factors.

In this model, soluble CX3CL1 first attracts CX3CR1-expresing leukocytes to the inflammation site; binding of membrane-tethered CX3CL1 on the endothelial surface to leukocyte-expressed CX3CR1 would lead to firm adhesion to the endothelial layer. CX3CL1/CX3CR1 interaction can also increase affinity of leukocyte integrins, enabling much firmer adhesion to the activated endothelium. Finally, ADAM protease cleavage of transmembrane CX3CL1 releases leukocytes, allowing transmigration through the endothelium (Hundhausen et al., 2007); transmigrated cells can then follow secondary chemokine gradients in the inflamed tissue (Nishimura et al., 2002).

The firm cell-cell adhesion induced by engagement of membrane-bound CX3CL1 and CX3CR1 is not limited to leukocyte-endothelial interactions. In embryo implantation, CX3CL1 promotes migration and adhesion of trophoblastic cells to the vascular cells of the endometrium (Dimitriadis et al., 2010; Hannan & Salamonsen, 2008). CX3CL1 binding to its receptor not only induces cell-cell adhesion but also triggers receptor signaling, as shown by the opening of calcium channels (Imai et al., 1997) and activation of the PI3K survival pathway in leukocytes (Landsman et al., 2009). In CX3CR1$^+$ bone marrow precursors, CX3CL1 can induce both PI3K/AKT and MAPK/ERK pathways, promoting differentiation to smooth muscle cells (Chandrasekar et al., 2003; White et al., 2009). In the context of rheumatoid arthritis, activation of these survival and proliferation pathways in endothelial cells has led to proposals of a pro-angiogenic function for CX3CL1 (Lee et al., 2006; Volin et al., 2001).

The role of the CX3CL1/CX3CR1 pair in mediating leukocyte infiltration has clinical consequences. CX3CL1-mediated leukocyte recruitment takes part in the immune response to Legionella pneumophila and in protection from septic shock (Ishida et al., 2008; Kikuchi et al., 2005; Pachot et al., 2008). CX3CL1-mediated leukocyte recruitment can nonetheless aggravate chronic and acute immune disorders such as lupus (Nakatani et al., 2010) and pancreatitis (Inoue et al., 2005). CX3CL1/CX3CR1 activity is also deleterious in atherosclerosis, in which this chemokine/receptor pair boosts monocyte/macrophage interaction with endothelial and smooth muscle cells at the vessel wall (Barlic et al., 2007; Lesnik et al., 2003). The hypofunctional polymorphic CX3CR1 V249I and T280M are associated with a lower risk of coronary disease (Moatti et al., 2001), which reinforces a role for CX3CL1 in atherogenesis.

Simultaneously with its identification in endothelial cells, CX3CL1 was isolated as an inflammation-induced gene from neurons, where it was called neurotactin (Pan et al., 1997); CX3CL1 is also expressed at high levels in human immunodeficiency virus-infected patients in which the virus invades the central nervous system (Tong et al., 2000). Various studies have described the CX3CL1/CX3CR1 axis as an important paracrine communication system for neuroprotection in inflammatory situations (Harrison et al., 1998; Zujovic et al., 2000; Zujovic et al., 2001). As mentioned above, CX3CL1 and CX3CR1 show complementary expression in the central nervous system; the ligand is expressed in neurons, whereas the receptor is expressed in the microglia, a type of resident immune cells that act as macrophages (Harrison et al., 1998). Microglia respond rapidly to homeostatic disturbance by upregulating inflammatory molecules such as TNFα, IL-1b, IL-6 and inducible nitric oxide oxidase (iNOS), all of which cause neurotoxicity (Colton and Gilbert, 1987). The CX3CL1/CX3CR1 axis acts as a neuronal regulatory system that controls the overproduction of inflammatory mediators, inducing neuroprotection (Garcia et al., 2000; Lyons et al., 2009; Mizuno et al., 2003; Ransohoff et al., 2007; Re & Przedborski, 2006; Zujovic et al., 2000; Zujovic et al., 2001). CX3CL1 attenuates microglial activation, maintaining these cells in a resting phenotype (Figure 6). Factors that induce neuron injury cause shedding of membrane-bound CX3CL1 in neurons, attenuating microglial activation. Systemic LPS administration in CX3CR1-deficient mice increases the extent of neuronal lesions in the brain, concomitant with an increase in microglial cell production of IL-1b (Cardona *et al.*, 2006). CX3CL1-mediated neuroprotection is also active in conditions of excitotoxic stress, in which neurons secrete CX3CL1, triggering release of neuroprotective factors by the microglia (Lauro *et al.*, 2008). The mechanism by which the CX3CL1/CX3CR1 axis controls microglial activation is nonetheless complex, as it has the reverse effect in the dorsal horn of the spinal cord, where CX3CL1 stimulates microglial synthesis of pro-inflammatory mediators (Gao & Ji, 2010).

The CX3CL1/CX3CR1 system also appears to be involved in human neurodegeneration. The CX3CR1 polymorphisms V249I and T280M are associated with age-related macular degeneration (Chan *et al.*, 2005; Tuo *et al.*, 2004). CX3CL1 also acts as a neuroprotector in Parkinson's disease and amyotrophic lateral sclerosis (ALS) (Cardona *et al.*, 2006). In the case of Alzheimer's disease, the role of CX3CL1 is debated. An initial report indicated that CX3CL1 increases neuron loss (Fuhrmann *et al.*, 2010), whereas other studies suggest that CX3CL1/CX3CR1 function depends on the model. Using two mouse models of Alzheimer's, Lee et al. showed that loss of CX3CR1 increases the phagocytic capacity of the microglia, which reduces beta-amyloid deposition (Lee *et al.*, 2010); nonetheless, the neuroinflammatory milieu in these models is atypical, with notable upregulation of IL-1b. In contrast, loss of CX3CR1 in a murine model of Tau overexpression increases Tau phosphorylation in neurons, leading to enhanced microglial activity (Bhaskar *et al.*, 2010). In summary, CX3CL1 regulates microglial activation in opposite ways in two processes, amyloid deposition and Tau phosphorylation, that are intimately linked to Alzheimer's disease progression.

5   The CX3CL1/CX3CR1 Axis in Cancer Progression

5.1   Anti-tumor Effects of CX3CL1 Mediated by the Immune System

The ability of CX3CL1 to attract distinct leukocyte subsets, including CTL and NK cells, suggests that it inhibits tumor growth by boosting anti-tumor immune responses (Figure 7). Initial studies showed that forced CX3CL1 overexpression leads to reduced tumor growth or even to tumor eradication in murine models of lymphoblastoma (Lavergne *et al.*, 2003), lung (Guo *et al.*, 2003a; Guo *et al.*, 2003b), hepatocellular (Tang *et al.*, 2007) and colon carcinomas (Vitale *et al.*, 2007), and neuroblastoma (Zeng *et al.*, 2007). Loss-of-function approaches also indicate an anti-tumor role for the CX3CL1/CX3CR1 axis. CX3CR1-deficient mice had a larger number of lung metastases than wild type controls after tail-vein injection of melanoma cells; this effect is again a result of reduced anti-tumor immunity in the receptor-null mice (Yu *et al.*, 2007). Other studies nonetheless found no effect of CX3CR1 deficiency on the growth of tumors induced by injection of lymphoblastoma cells (Lavergne *et al.*, 2003).

The CX3CL1 anti-tumor effect in these models depends chiefly on CD8[+] lymphocytes and NK cells and, to a lesser extent, on dendritic cells and CD4[+] lymphocytes. It appears that CX3CL1 subcellular location might also be relevant to this anti-tumor activity. Experiments in a syngeneic mouse model of colon cancer showed that the native CX3CL1 form, which is produced as a membrane-anchored precursor, has a more potent effect on stem tumor growth than membrane-restricted or obligatory soluble CX3CL1 mutants (Vitale *et al.*, 2007); the three forms have distinct effects on lung metastases. Results from these preclinical models and from epidemiological studies that associate high CX3CL1 expression with improved prognosis in gastric (Hyakudomi *et al.*, 2008) and breast cancers (Park *et al.*, 2012) have motivated the development of strategies to engineer tumors that overexpress CX3CL1. Gene therapy approaches used to deliver CX3CL1 into tumors transplanted in mice include adenoviral vectors (Xin *et*

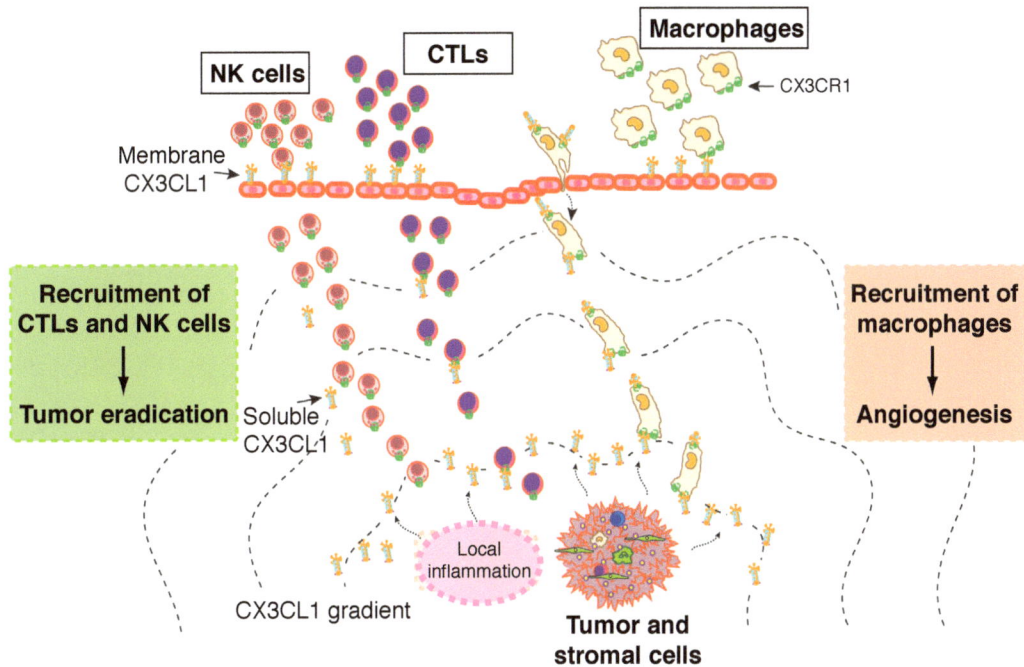

Figure 7: The CX3CL1/CX3CR1 axis influences tumor-associated inflammation. Neoplastic and stromal cells secrete CX3CL1, which attract CX3CR1-expressing leukocytes. CX3CR1[+] leukocytes of the innate immune system, such as monocytes/macrophages, enhance angiogenesis (Reed *et al*., 2012). In contrast, CX3CR1-expressing CTL and NK cells lead to tumor inhibition or eradication. In the latter case, CX3CL1 would act as an external tumor suppressor, given its transcriptional link with the tumor suppressor gene p53 (Shiraishi *et al*., 2000).

al., 2005) and mesenchymal stem cells (Xin *et al*., 2007); in both cases, strong CTL- and NK cell-dependent responses were reported.

Other tumor models have nonetheless failed to demonstrate anti-tumorigenic activity of CX3CL1/CX3CR1. In an inducible fibroblast growth factor receptor (iFGFR)1 transgenic mouse model of mammary carcinogenesis, onset of pre-neoplastic lesions coincided with NF-kB-dependent upregulation of CX3CL1; increased CX3CL1 levels in turn induced macrophage recruitment, which correlated with enhanced vessel formation and tumor progression (Reed *et al*., 2012). As suggested for rheumatoid arthritis, CX3CL1/CX3CR1 might also regulate angiogenesis in tumors, in this case indirectly. In another model of spontaneous mammary tumors caused by overexpression of the proto-oncogene *neu* (MMTV-neu) injection of adenoviral particles that encode the native CX3CL1 form did not reduce the tumor growth rate or alter the inflammatory infiltrate compared to controls (Tardáguila *et al*., 2013). Spontaneous mammary tumors in MMTV-neu mice develop central and peripheral tolerance, which might reduce their immunogenicity compared to tumor graft models. Further research is needed to understand the contrasting outcomes of elevated intratumor CX3CL1 levels.

5.2   CX3CL1 as a Cell-intrinsic Tumor Promoter

In addition to regulating tumor-associated inflammation, CX3CL1 can activate pro-tumorigenic pathways by acting on CX3CR1-expressing cancer cell lines from prostate (Shulby *et al.*, 2004), pancreas (Marchesi *et al.*, 2008), breast (Jamieson-Gladney *et al.*, 2011; Tardáguila *et al.*, 2013) ovary (Gaudin *et al.*, 2011) and neuroblastoma (Nevo *et al.*, 2009). CX3CR1 expression is also elevated in clinical samples from glioblastoma (Erreni *et al.*, 2010; Locatelli *et al.*, 2010), prostate (Jamieson *et al.*, 2008) and pancreatic cancers (Marchesi *et al.*, 2008). It is postulated that CX3CL1/CX3CR1 mediate pro-survival and pro-mitogenic signals in these cells. In human prostate cancer cells, for instance, soluble CX3CL1 induces phosphorylation of AKT and its downstream substrate GSK3b, which promotes cell survival (Shulby *et al.*, 2004). Enhanced apoptosis resistance and activation of the pro-mitogenic MAPK/ERK pathway is reported in stable CX3CR1 transfectants of pancreatic (Marchesi *et al.*, 2008), ovary (Gaudin *et al.*, 2011) and breast cancer cells (Jamieson-Gladney *et al.*, 2011). The MAPK/ERK pathway is also implicated in CX3CR1-induced expression of hypoxia-inducible factor (HIF)-1α, which reprograms glucose metabolism in pancreatic adenocarcinoma cells (Ren *et al.*, 2013).

In other cancer models, activation of pro-tumorigenic signals by this chemokine axis depends on transactivation of structurally distinct receptors (Figure 8). Although CX3CR1, like other GPCR, signals through activation of pertussis toxin (PTx)-sensitive heterotrimeric G proteins, CX3CL1-induced MAPK/ERK activation in the T47-D human cancer cell line and in primary cultures of mammary cells from transgenic MMTV-neu mice is unaffected by PTx treatment (Tardáguila *et al.*, 2013). This PTx insensitivity is caused by CX3CL1-induced transactivation of EGFR (also called HER1 or ErbB1) through the proteolytic shedding of membrane-tethered EGF precursors (Figure 8). In this manner, a GPCR (in this case CX3CR1) can induce potent MAPK/ERK pathway activation by transactivating a tyrosine kinase receptor (RTK, in this case the EGFR). This triple membrane-passing signaling mechanism is found for other GPCR and RTK (Liebmann, 2011), although its relevance in the carcinogenic process has not been fully defined (Prenzel *et al.*, 1999). Cross-communication between CX3CL1 and the EGF pathway is nonetheless important in mammary carcinogenesis; indeed, mammary tumor onset is delayed in CX3CL1-deficient transgenic MMTV-neu mice, which also have fewer tumors per mouse than wild-type littermates (Tardáguila *et al.*, 2013). The delay in tumor onset and reduced tumor multiplicity are also observed in heterozygous CX3CL1$^{+/-}$-MMTV-neu mice, which express CX3CL1 hemizygously in the mammary gland. CX3CL1 deficiency does not affect mammary carcinogenesis in MMTV-PyMT mice, which express the polyoma middle T (PyMT) oncogene that induces mammary carcinogenesis through an EGFR-independent pathway (Tardáguila *et al.*, 2013). These findings implicate CX3CL1 as a breast cancer promoter that acts in concert with the EGFR signaling pathway.

CX3CR1/EGFR crosstalk might influence human breast cancer, in which ~30% of tumors show HER2/*neu* oncogene amplification, and ~50% overexpress EGFR and EGFRvIII receptors (Arribas *et al.*, 2011; Rae *et al.*, 2004). CX3CL1/CX3CR1 might accelerate the development of incipient neoplastic lesions by causing qualitative and quantitative changes in the strength, frequency or adaptation of the MAPK/ERK pathway through EGFR transactivation. Some reports indicate that these MAPK/ERK signaling parameters are central relays in cell fate decisions (Avraham and Yarden, 2011; von Kriegsheim *et al.*, 2009).

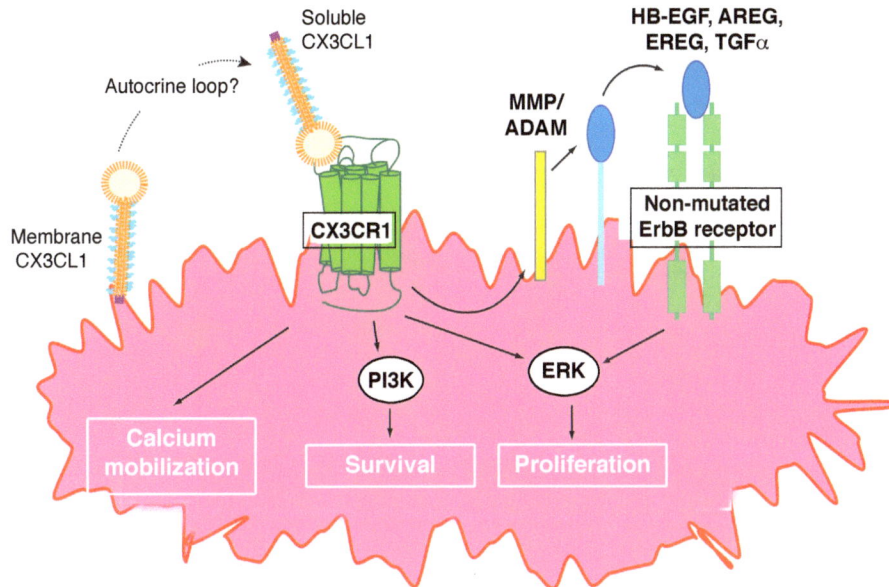

Figure 8: CX3CL1/CX3CR1 promotes mammary carcinogenesis through transactivation of the EGFR pathway. CX3CL1 can signal in a paracrine or autocrine manner to induce transactivation of EGFR through a triple membrane-passing signaling mechanism. This transactivation step is proposed to lead to quantitative and qualitative changes in MAPK/ERK activation, which accelerates growth of incipient neoplastic lesions (Tardáguila *et al.*, 2013). MMP, matrix metalloprotease; ADAM, a disintegrin and metalloproteinase; HB-EGF, heparin-binding EGF-like growth factor; AREG, amphiregulin; EREG, epiregulin; TGFa, transforming growth factor-alpha.

5.3   CX3CL1/CX3CR1 in Metastasis

Tumor cells are thought to use CX3CL1 expression in lung, bone or brain to form metastases in these organs (Figure 9). Engagement of CX3CR1-expressing prostate cancer cells with the membrane-tethered CX3CL1 on endothelial cells is a signal that retains neoplastic cells in bone marrow, thus explaining prostate tumor cell tropism for bone (Jamieson *et al.*, 2008; Shulby *et al.*, 2004). In this model, CX3CL1 would provide two signals, a "stop signal" delivered by the transmembrane CX3CL1 expressed in the endothelium, which arrests circulating prostate cancer cells, and a second "go signal" provided by soluble CX3CL1 released from osteoblasts, which induces tumor cell transmigration into the bone matrix. Androgens are key regulators of bone metastasis; they stimulate CX3CL1 shedding in androgen receptor-positive osteoblasts, but do not affect membrane-anchored CX3CL1 in endothelial cells, which are negative for androgen receptor expression.

The CX3CL1/CX3CR1 axis is also implicated in the bone tropism of breast cancers. Intracardiac injection of breast cancer cell lines stably transfected with CX3CR1 gave rise to a larger number of skeletal metastases than mock-transfected controls (Jamieson-Gladney *et al.*, 2011). Breast cancer cell homing to bone is significantly reduced in CX3CL1-deficient mice, indicating that CX3CL1 produced by the bone matrix is a causative agent for the bone tropism of CX3CR1-expressing cancer cells.

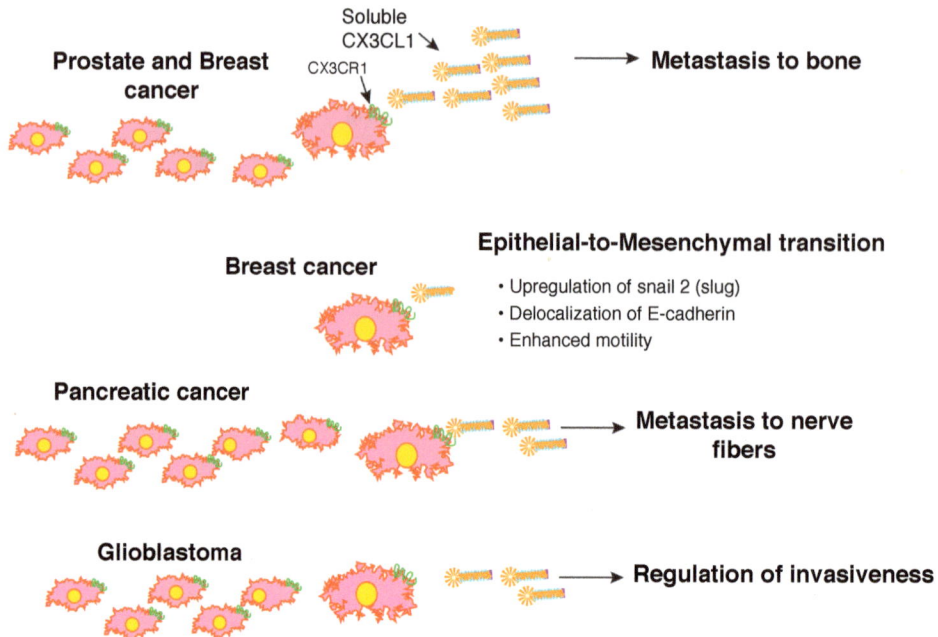

Figure 9: CX3CL1/CX3CR1 regulate the metastatic behavior of cancer cells. CX3CR1 expression can be instrumental in the colonization of distant tissues, as shown for the bone tropism of prostate and breast cancer cells and peri-neural invasion by pancreatic adenocarcinoma cells. CX3CL1/CX3CR1 activation might also activate a built-in invasive capacity and aggressiveness in cancer cells by triggering EMT, as demonstrated for breast cancer cells.

As is the case for bone metastasis, there is also evidence for CX3CL1/CX3CR1 activity in the neural tropism of some cancer cell lines. An *in vitro* and *in vivo* proof-of-concept study showed that CX3CL1 attracts CX3CR1-expressing pancreatic tumor cell lines, which migrate to and disseminate along peripheral nerves (Marchesi *et al*., 2010). Although CX3CL1 is an attractant for pancreatic cancer cells, it appears to negatively regulate glioblastoma cell invasiveness by increasing cell-cell adhesion (Sciume *et al*., 2010). High levels of CX3CL1 and its receptor are nonetheless associated with aggressive stages in glioblastoma (Erreni *et al*., 2010).

One fact that reconciles the apparent contradiction in these two results is the participation of the CX3CL1/CX3CR1 axis in different stages of the metastatic process. In breast cancer cells, CX3CL1 is involved in provoking the epithelial-to-mesenchymal transition (EMT) (Tardáguila *et al*., 2013), a developmental program by which epithelial cells transdifferentiate to mesenchymal cells; EMT is considered a central step in breast cancer dissemination (Drasin *et al*., 2011; Mani *et al*., 2008). CX3CL1 stimulation of breast cancer cells elicited changes in gene expression reminiscent of EMT, as well as delocalization of the intercellular adhesion molecule E-cadherin, both of which enhance cancer cell motility (Tardáguila *et al*., 2013). The CX3CL1/CX3CR1 axis thus induces a cell plasticity program that endows neoplastic cells with greater motility and a metastatic-prone phenotype.

6   Conclusion

The dual nature of CX3CL1 at different stages of cancer progression is an example of the interplay between neoplastic cells and the tumor stroma. As discussed above, CX3CL1 is an integral element of the immune system that is instrumental in effector cell recruitment to the tumor parenchyma. In many cases, however, CX3CL1 is abducted by incipient neoplasias to promote their own growth to established tumors by stimulating survival, proliferation, angiogenesis and finally, colonization of distant tissues. The use of this chemokine system to boost anti-tumor immune responses must therefore consider the risk of adverse effects. Exhaustive information on the tumor microenvironment is central to clinical decision-making, and requires studies of the quality and type of tumor-infiltrating cells, particularly immune cells, and of the complex assembly of cytokines and chemokines in each tumor microenvironment.

Another conclusion of this review is that research to characterize the role of a molecule in cancer, in this case of a chemokine/receptor pair, should take advantage of the wide variety of murine models now available. We must focus especially on models of spontaneous tumorigenesis that closely recapitulate the clinical features in patients, in which tumor onset and the tumor niche mirror the conditions of human cancer. CX3CL1 is an illustrative case; the use of spontaneous carcinogenic models has enabled identification of key aspects of the biology of this chemokine in tumor promotion.

About 25 centuries ago, the Chinese master strategist Sun Tzu wrote "If you know the enemy and know yourself, you need not fear the results of a hundred battles". Cancer poses a threat because it is both an adversary and part of our own nature, and can bend the body's mechanisms, including the immune system, to its own benefit. Our quest is to understand and disarm this formidable enemy within.

Acknowledgments

We are grateful to our lab-mates and collaborators for valuable discussions and help, and to C. Mark for editorial assistance. Our work is supported by the Spanish Ministry of Science and Innovation (SAF2011-24453) and the Comunidad de Madrid (IMMUNOTHERCAN; S2010/BMD-2326).

References

Acharyya, S., Oskarsson, T., Vanharanta, S., Malladi, S., Kim, J., Morris, P.G., Manova-Todorova, K., Leversha, M., Hogg, N., Seshan, V.E., et al. (2012). A CXCL1 paracrine network links cancer chemoresistance and metastasis. Cell 150(1), 165-178.

Acosta, J.C., O'Loghlen, A., Banito, A., Guijarro, M.V., Augert, A., Raguz, S., Fumagalli, M., Da Costa, M., Brown, C., Popov, N., et al. (2008). Chemokine signaling via the CXCR2 receptor reinforces senescence. Cell 133(6), 1006-1018.

Allavena, P., Garlanda, C., Borrello, M.G., Sica, A., and Mantovani, A. (2008). Pathways connecting inflammation and cancer. Curr Opin Genet Dev 18(1), 3-10.

Allavena, P., Germano, G., Marchesi, F., and Mantovani, A. (2011). Chemokines in cancer related inflammation. Exp Cell Res 317(5), 664-673.

Amersi, F.F., Terando, A.M., Goto, Y., Scolyer, R.A., Thompson, J.F., Tran, A.N., Faries, M.B., Morton, D.L., and Hoon, D.S. (2008). Activation of CCR9/CCL25 in cutaneous melanoma mediates preferential metastasis to the small intestine. Clin Cancer Res 14(3), 638-645.

Ancuta, P., Rao, R., Moses, A., Mehle, A., Shaw, S.K., Luscinskas, F.W., and Gabuzda, D. (2003). Fractalkine preferentially mediates arrest and migration of CD16+ monocytes. J Exp Med 197(12), 1701-1707.

Andrzejewski, M.G., Koelsch, A., Kogel, T., Dreymueller, D., Schwarz, N., and Ludwig, A. (2010). Distinct role of the intracellular C-terminus for subcellular expression, shedding and function of the murine transmembrane chemokine CX3CL1. Biochem Biophys Res Commun 395(2), 178-184.

Angiolillo, A.L., Sgadari, C., Taub, D.D., Liao, F., Farber, J.M., Maheshwari, S., Kleinman, H.K., Reaman, G.H., and Tosato, G. (1995). Human interferon-inducible protein 10 is a potent inhibitor of angiogenesis in vivo. J Exp Med 182(1), 155-162.

Aoki, M.N., da Silva do Amaral Herrera, A.C., Amarante, M.K., do Val Carneiro, J.L., Fungaro, M.H., and Watanabe, M.A. (2009). CCR5 and p53 codon 72 gene polymorphisms: implications in breast cancer development. Int J Mol Med 23(3), 429-435.

Arenberg, D.A., Polverini, P.J., Kunkel, S.L., Shanafelt, A., Hesselgesser, J., Horuk, R., and Strieter, R.M. (1997). The role of CXC chemokines in the regulation of angiogenesis in non-small cell lung cancer. J Leukoc Biol 62(5), 554-562.

Arribas, J., Baselga, J., Pedersen, K., and Parra-Palau, J.L. (2011). p95HER2 and breast cancer. Cancer Res 71(5), 1515-1519.

Avraham, R., and Yarden, Y. (2011). Feedback regulation of EGFR signalling: decision making by early and delayed loops. Nat Rev Mol Cell Biol 12(2), 104-117.

Baggiolini, M., Dewald, B., and Moser, B. (1994). Interleukin-8 and related chemotactic cytokines--CXC and CC chemokines. Adv Immunol 5597-179.

Baggiolini, M., Dewald, B., and Moser, B. (1997). Human chemokines: an update. Annu Rev Immunol 15675-705.

Bailey, C., Negus, R., Morris, A., Ziprin, P., Goldin, R., Allavena, P., Peck, D., and Darzi, A. (2007). Chemokine expression is associated with the accumulation of tumour associated macrophages (TAMs) and progression in human colorectal cancer. Clin Exp Metastasis 24(2), 121-130.

Balkwill, F., and Mantovani, A. (2001). Inflammation and cancer: back to Virchow? Lancet 357(9255), 539-545.

Balkwill, F.R. (2012). The chemokine system and cancer. J Pathol 226(2), 148-157.

Balkwill, F.R., and Mantovani, A. (2012). Cancer-related inflammation: common themes and therapeutic opportunities. Semin Cancer Biol 22(1), 33-40.

Ballas, Z.K., and Rasmussen, W. (1990). NK1.1+ thymocytes. Adult murine CD4-, CD8- thymocytes contain an NK1.1+, CD3+, CD5hi, CD44hi, TCR-V beta 8+ subset. J Immunol 145(4), 1039-1045.

Banerjee, A., Damera, G., Bhandare, R., Gu, S., Lopez-Boado, Y., Panettieri, R., Jr., and Tliba, O. (2008). Vitamin D and glucocorticoids differentially modulate chemokine expression in human airway smooth muscle cells. Br J Pharmacol 155(1), 84-92.

Barbero, S., Bonavia, R., Bajetto, A., Porcile, C., Pirani, P., Ravetti, J.L., Zona, G.L., Spaziante, R., Florio, T., and Schettini, G. (2003). Stromal cell-derived factor 1alpha stimulates human glioblastoma cell growth through the activation of both extracellular signal-regulated kinases 1/2 and Akt. Cancer Res 63(8), 1969-1974.

Barlic, J., McDermott, D.H., Merrell, M.N., Gonzales, J., Via, L.E., and Murphy, P.M. (2004). Interleukin (IL)-15 and IL-2 reciprocally regulate expression of the chemokine receptor CX3CR1 through selective NFAT1- and NFAT2-dependent mechanisms. J Biol Chem 279(47), 48520-48534.

Barlic, J., Zhang, Y., and Murphy, P.M. (2007). Atherogenic lipids induce adhesion of human coronary artery smooth muscle cells to macrophages by up-regulating chemokine CX3CL1 on smooth muscle cells in a TNFalpha-NFkappaB-dependent manner. J Biol Chem 282(26), 19167-19176.

Bazan, J.F., Bacon, K.B., Hardiman, G., Wang, W., Soo, K., Rossi, D., Greaves, D.R., Zlotnik, A., and Schall, T.J. (1997). A new class of membrane-bound chemokine with a CX3C motif. Nature 385(6617), 640-644.

Bhaskar, K., Konerth, M., Kokiko-Cochran, O.N., Cardona, A., Ransohoff, R.M., and Lamb, B.T. (2010). Regulation of tau pathology by the microglial fractalkine receptor. Neuron 68(1), 19-31.

Bhavsar, P.K., Sukkar, M.B., Khorasani, N., Lee, K.Y., and Chung, K.F. (2008). Glucocorticoid suppression of CX3CL1 (fractalkine) by reduced gene promoter recruitment of NF-kappaB. FASEB J 22(6), 1807-1816.

Bissell, M.J., and Hines, W.C. (2011). Why don't we get more cancer? A proposed role of the microenvironment in restraining cancer progression. Nat Med 17(3), 320-329.

Bonecchi, R., Locati, M., and Mantovani, A. (2011). Chemokines and cancer: a fatal attraction. Cancer Cell 19(4), 434-435.

Brew, R., Erikson, J.S., West, D.C., Kinsella, A.R., Slavin, J., and Christmas, S.E. (2000). Interleukin-8 as an autocrine growth factor for human colon carcinoma cells in vitro. Cytokine 12(1), 78-85.

Budhu, A., and Wang, X.W. (2012). Transforming the microenvironment: a trick of the metastatic cancer cell. Cancer Cell 22(3), 279-280.

Cardona, A.E., Pioro, E.P., Sasse, M.E., Kostenko, V., Cardona, S.M., Dijkstra, I.M., Huang, D., Kidd, G., Dombrowski, S., Dutta, R., et al. (2006). Control of microglial neurotoxicity by the fractalkine receptor. Nat Neurosci 9(7), 917-924.

Cardona, A.E., Sasse, M.E., Liu, L., Cardona, S.M., Mizutani, M., Savarin, C., Hu, T., and Ransohoff, R.M. (2008). Scavenging roles of chemokine receptors: chemokine receptor deficiency is associated with increased levels of ligand in circulation and tissues. Blood 112(2), 256-263.

Chan, C.C., Tuo, J., Bojanowski, C.M., Csaky, K.G., and Green, W.R. (2005). Detection of CX3CR1 single nucleotide polymorphism and expression on archived eyes with age-related macular degeneration. Histol Histopathol 20(3), 857-863.

Chandrasekar, B., Mummidi, S., Perla, R.P., Bysani, S., Dulin, N.O., Liu, F., and Melby, P.C. (2003). Fractalkine (CX3CL1) stimulated by nuclear factor kappaB (NF-kappaB)-dependent inflammatory signals induces aortic smooth muscle cell proliferation through an autocrine pathway. Biochem J 373(Pt 2), 547-558.

Clark, A.K., Yip, P.K., and Malcangio, M. (2009). The liberation of fractalkine in the dorsal horn requires microglial cathepsin S. J Neurosci 29(21), 6945-6954.

Clark-Lewis, I., Schumacher, C., Baggiolini, M., and Moser, B. (1991). Structure-activity relationships of interleukin-8 determined using chemically synthesized analogs. Critical role of NH2-terminal residues and evidence for uncoupling of neutrophil chemotaxis, exocytosis, and receptor binding activities. J Biol Chem 266(34), 23128-23134.

Colton, C.A., and Gilbert, D.L. (1987). Production of superoxide anions by a CNS macrophage, the microglia. FEBS Lett 223(2), 284-288.

Combadiere, C., Gao, J., Tiffany, H.L., and Murphy, P.M. (1998). Gene cloning, RNA distribution, and functional expression of mCX3CR1, a mouse chemotactic receptor for the CX3C chemokine fractalkine. Biochem Biophys Res Commun 253(3), 728-732.

Contento, R.L., Molon, B., Boularan, C., Pozzan, T., Mañes, S., Marullo, S., and Viola, A. (2008). CXCR4-CCR5: a couple modulating T cell functions. Proc Natl Acad Sci USA 105(29), 10101-10106.

Cook, A., Hippensteel, R., Shimizu, S., Nicolai, J., Fatatis, A., and Meucci, O. (2010). Interactions between chemokines: regulation of fractalkine/CX3CL1 homeostasis by SDF/CXCL12 in cortical neurons. J Biol Chem 285(14), 10563-10571.

Corcione, A., Ferretti, E., Bertolotto, M., Fais, F., Raffaghello, L., Gregorio, A., Tenca, C., Ottonello, L., Gambini, C., Furtado, G., et al. (2009). CX3CR1 is expressed by human B lymphocytes and mediates [corrected] CX3CL1 driven chemotaxis of tonsil centrocytes. PLoS One 4(12), e8485.

Davis, C.N., and Harrison, J.K. (2006). Proline 326 in the C terminus of murine CX3CR1 prevents G-protein and phosphatidylinositol 3-kinase-dependent stimulation of Akt and extracellular signal-regulated kinase in Chinese hamster ovary cells. J Pharmacol Exp Ther 316(1), 356-363.

de Brevern, A.G., Wong, H., Tournamille, C., Colin, Y., Le Van Kim, C., and Etchebest, C. (2005). A structural model of a seven-transmembrane helix receptor: the Duffy antigen/receptor for chemokine (DARC). Biochim Biophys Acta 1724(3), 288-306.

DeNardo, D.G., and Coussens, L.M. (2007). Inflammation and breast cancer. Balancing immune response: crosstalk between adaptive and innate immune cells during breast cancer progression. Breast Cancer Res 9(4), 212.

Dimitriadis, E., Nie, G., Hannan, N.J., Paiva, P., and Salamonsen, L.A. (2010). Local regulation of implantation at the human fetal-maternal interface. Int J Dev Biol 54(2-3), 313-322.

Drasin, D.J., Robin, T.P., and Ford, H.L. (2011). Breast cancer epithelial-to-mesenchymal transition: examining the functional consequences of plasticity. Breast Cancer Res 13(6), 226.

Erreni, M., Solinas, G., Brescia, P., Osti, D., Zunino, F., Colombo, P., Destro, A., Roncalli, M., Mantovani, A., Draghi, R., et al. (2010). Human glioblastoma tumours and neural cancer stem cells express the chemokine CX3CL1 and its receptor CX3CR1. Eur J Cancer 46(18), 3383-3392.

Faure, S., Meyer, L., Costagliola, D., Vaneensberghe, C., Genin, E., Autran, B., Delfraissy, J.F., McDermott, D.H., Murphy, P.M., Debre, P., et al. (2000). Rapid progression to AIDS in HIV+ individuals with a structural variant of the chemokine receptor CX3CR1. Science 287(5461), 2274-2277.

Fong, A.M., Robinson, L.A., Steeber, D.A., Tedder, T.F., Yoshie, O., Imai, T., and Patel, D.D. (1998). Fractalkine and CX3CR1 mediate a novel mechanism of leukocyte capture, firm adhesion, and activation under physiologic flow. J Exp Med 188(8), 1413-1419.

Forster, R., Davalos-Misslitz, A.C., and Rot, A. (2008). CCR7 and its ligands: balancing immunity and tolerance. Nat Rev Immunol 8(5), 362-371.

Foussat, A., Coulomb-L'Hermine, A., Gosling, J., Krzysiek, R., Durand-Gasselin, I., Schall, T., Balian, A., Richard, Y., Galanaud, P., and Emilie, D. (2000). Fractalkine receptor expression by T lymphocyte subpopulations and in vivo production of fractalkine in human. Eur J Immunol 30(1), 87-97.

Fridlender, Z.G., Sun, J., Kim, S., Kapoor, V., Cheng, G., Ling, L., Worthen, G.S., and Albelda, S.M. (2009). Polarization of tumor-associated neutrophil phenotype by TGF-beta: "N1" versus "N2" TAN. Cancer Cell 16(3), 183-194.

Fuhrmann, M., Bittner, T., Jung, C.K., Burgold, S., Page, R.M., Mitteregger, G., Haass, C., LaFerla, F.M., Kretzschmar, H., and Herms, J. (2010). Microglial Cx3cr1 knockout prevents neuron loss in a mouse model of Alzheimer's disease. Nat Neurosci 13(4), 411-413.

Gao, Y.J., and Ji, R.R. (2010). Chemokines, neuronal-glial interactions, and central processing of neuropathic pain. Pharmacol Ther 126(1), 56-68.

Garcia, G.E., Xia, Y., Chen, S., Wang, Y., Ye, R.D., Harrison, J.K., Bacon, K.B., Zerwes, H.G., and Feng, L. (2000). NF-kappaB-dependent fractalkine induction in rat aortic endothelial cells stimulated by IL-1beta, TNF-alpha, and LPS. J Leukoc Biol 67(4), 577-584.

Gaudin, F., Nasreddine, S., Donnadieu, A.C., Emilie, D., Combadiere, C., Prevot, S., Machelon, V., and Balabanian, K. (2011). Identification of the chemokine CX3CL1 as a new regulator of malignant cell proliferation in epithelial ovarian cancer. PLoS One 6(7), e21546.

Geissmann, F., Jung, S., and Littman, D.R. (2003). Blood monocytes consist of two principal subsets with distinct migratory properties. Immunity 19(1), 71-82.

González-Martín, A., Gómez, L., Lustgarten, J., Mira, E., and Mañes, S. (2011). Maximal T cell-mediated antitumor responses rely upon CCR5 expression in both CD4(+) and CD8(+) T cells. Cancer Res 71(16), 5455-5466.

González-Martín, A., Mira, E., and Mañes, S. (2012). CCR5 as a potential target in cancer therapy: inhibition or stimulation? Anticancer Agents Med Chem 12(9), 1045-1057.

Green, S.R., Han, K.H., Chen, Y., Almazan, F., Charo, I.F., Miller, Y.I., and Quehenberger, O. (2006). The CC chemokine MCP-1 stimulates surface expression of CX3CR1 and enhances the adhesion of monocytes to fractalkine/CX3CL1 via p38 MAPK. J Immunol 176(12), 7412-7420.

Gu, L., Tseng, S., Horner, R.M., Tam, C., Loda, M., and Rollins, B.J. (2000). Control of TH2 polarization by the chemokine monocyte chemoattractant protein-1. Nature 404(6776), 407-411.

Guo, J., Chen, T., Wang, B., Zhang, M., An, H., Guo, Z., Yu, Y., Qin, Z., and Cao, X. (2003a). Chemoattraction, adhesion and activation of natural killer cells are involved in the antitumor immune response induced by fractalkine/CX3CL1. Immunol Lett 89(1), 1-7.

Guo, J., Zhang, M., Wang, B., Yuan, Z., Guo, Z., Chen, T., Yu, Y., Qin, Z., and Cao, X. (2003b). Fractalkine transgene induces T-cell-dependent antitumor immunity through chemoattraction and activation of dendritic cells. Int J Cancer 103(2), 212-220.

Gupta, S.K., Lysko, P.G., Pillarisetti, K., Ohlstein, E., and Stadel, J.M. (1998). Chemokine receptors in human endothelial cells. Functional expression of CXCR4 and its transcriptional regulation by inflammatory cytokines. J Biol Chem 273(7), 4282-4287.

Hanahan, D., and Weinberg, R.A. (2000). The hallmarks of cancer. Cell 100(1), 57-70.

Hanahan, D., and Weinberg, R.A. (2011). Hallmarks of cancer: the next generation. Cell 144(5), 646-674.

Handel, T.M., Johnson, Z., Crown, S.E., Lau, E.K., and Proudfoot, A.E. (2005). Regulation of protein function by glycosaminoglycans--as exemplified by chemokines. Annu Rev Biochem 74385-410.

Hannan, N.J., and Salamonsen, L.A. (2008). CX3CL1 and CCL14 regulate extracellular matrix and adhesion molecules in the trophoblast: potential roles in human embryo implantation. Biol Reprod 79(1), 58-65.

Hansell, C.A., Simpson, C.V., and Nibbs, R.J. (2006). Chemokine sequestration by atypical chemokine receptors. Biochem Soc Trans 34(Pt 6), 1009-1013.

Harrison, J.K., Fong, A.M., Swain, P.A., Chen, S., Yu, Y.R., Salafranca, M.N., Greenleaf, W.B., Imai, T., and Patel, D.D. (2001). Mutational analysis of the fractalkine chemokine domain. Basic amino acid residues differentially contribute to CX3CR1 binding, signaling, and cell adhesion. J Biol Chem 276(24), 21632-21641.

Harrison, J.K., Jiang, Y., Chen, S., Xia, Y., Maciejewski, D., McNamara, R.K., Streit, W.J., Salafranca, M.N., Adhikari, S., Thompson, D.A., et al. (1998). Role for neuronally derived fractalkine in mediating interactions between neurons and CX3CR1-expressing microglia. Proc Natl Acad Sci USA 95(18), 10896-10901.

Hartmann, T.N., Burger, J.A., Glodek, A., Fujii, N., and Burger, M. (2005). CXCR4 chemokine receptor and integrin signaling co-operate in mediating adhesion and chemoresistance in small cell lung cancer (SCLC) cells. Oncogene 24(27), 4462-4471.

Haskell, C.A., Cleary, M.D., and Charo, I.F. (1999). Molecular uncoupling of fractalkine-mediated cell adhesion and signal transduction. Rapid flow arrest of CX3CR1-expressing cells is independent of G-protein activation. J Biol Chem 274(15), 10053-10058.

Haskell, C.A., Cleary, M.D., and Charo, I.F. (2000). Unique role of the chemokine domain of fractalkine in cell capture. Kinetics of receptor dissociation correlate with cell adhesion. J Biol Chem 275(44), 34183-34189.

Hermand, P., Pincet, F., Carvalho, S., Ansanay, H., Trinquet, E., Daoudi, M., Combadiere, C., and Deterre, P. (2008). Functional adhesiveness of the CX3CL1 chemokine requires its aggregation. Role of the transmembrane domain. J Biol Chem 283(44), 30225-30234.

Hirose, K., Hakozaki, M., Nyunoya, Y., Kobayashi, Y., Matsushita, K., Takenouchi, T., Mikata, A., Mukaida, N., and Matsushima, K. (1995). Chemokine gene transfection into tumour cells reduced tumorigenicity in nude mice in association with neutrophilic infiltration. Br J Cancer 72(3), 708-714.

Huang, S., Mills, L., Mian, B., Tellez, C., McCarty, M., Yang, X.D., Gudas, J.M., and Bar-Eli, M. (2002). *Fully humanized neutralizing antibodies to interleukin-8 (ABX-IL8) inhibit angiogenesis, tumor growth, and metastasis of human melanoma. Am J Pathol 161(1), 125-134.*

Huang, Y.W., Su, P., Liu, G.Y., Crow, M.R., Chaukos, D., Yan, H., and Robinson, L.A. (2009). *Constitutive endocytosis of the chemokine CX3CL1 prevents its degradation by cell surface metalloproteases. J Biol Chem 284(43), 29644-29653.*

Hundhausen, C., Schulte, A., Schulz, B., Andrzejewski, M.G., Schwarz, N., von Hundelshausen, P., Winter, U., Paliga, K., Reiss, K., Saftig, P., et al. (2007). *Regulated shedding of transmembrane chemokines by the disintegrin and metalloproteinase 10 facilitates detachment of adherent leukocytes. J Immunol 178(12), 8064-8072.*

Hung, S.C., Pochampally, R.R., Hsu, S.C., Sanchez, C., Chen, S.C., Spees, J., and Prockop, D.J. (2007). *Short-term exposure of multipotent stromal cells to low oxygen increases their expression of CX3CR1 and CXCR4 and their engraftment in vivo. PLoS One 2(5), e416.*

Hyakudomi, M., Matsubara, T., Hyakudomi, R., Yamamoto, T., Kinugasa, S., Yamanoi, A., Maruyama, R., and Tanaka, T. (2008). *Increased expression of fractalkine is correlated with a better prognosis and an increased number of both CD8+ T cells and natural killer cells in gastric adenocarcinoma. Ann Surg Oncol 15(6), 1775-1782.*

Imai, T., Hieshima, K., Haskell, C., Baba, M., Nagira, M., Nishimura, M., Kakizaki, M., Takagi, S., Nomiyama, H., Schall, T.J., et al. (1997). *Identification and molecular characterization of fractalkine receptor CX3CR1, which mediates both leukocyte migration and adhesion. Cell 91(4), 521-530.*

Imaizumi, T., Matsumiya, T., Tamo, W., Shibata, T., Fujimoto, K., Kumagai, M., Yoshida, H., Cui, X.F., Tanji, K., Hatakeyama, M., et al. (2002). *15-Deoxy-D12,14-prostaglandin J2 inhibits CX3CL1/fractalkine expression in human endothelial cells. Immunol Cell Biol 80(6), 531-536.*

Inoue, A., Hasegawa, H., Kohno, M., Ito, M.R., Terada, M., Imai, T., Yoshie, O., Nose, M., and Fujita, S. (2005). *Antagonist of fractalkine (CX3CL1) delays the initiation and ameliorates the progression of lupus nephritis in MRL/lpr mice. Arthritis Rheum 52(5), 1522-1533.*

Ishida, Y., Hayashi, T., Goto, T., Kimura, A., Akimoto, S., Mukaida, N., and Kondo, T. (2008). *Essential involvement of CX3CR1-mediated signals in the bactericidal host defense during septic peritonitis. J Immunol 181(6), 4208-4218.*

Ito, A., Ishida, T., Yano, H., Inagaki, A., Suzuki, S., Sato, F., Takino, H., Mori, F., Ri, M., Kusumoto, S., et al. (2009). *Defucosylated anti-CCR4 monoclonal antibody exercises potent ADCC-mediated antitumor effect in the novel tumor-bearing humanized NOD/Shi-scid, IL-2Rgamma(null) mouse model. Cancer Immunol Immun 58(8), 1195-1206.*

Jamieson, W.L., Shimizu, S., D'Ambrosio, J.A., Meucci, O., and Fatatis, A. (2008). *CX3CR1 is expressed by prostate epithelial cells and androgens regulate the levels of CX3CL1/fractalkine in the bone marrow: potential role in prostate cancer bone tropism. Cancer Res 68(6), 1715-1722.*

Jamieson-Gladney, W.L., Zhang, Y., Fong, A.M., Meucci, O., and Fatatis, A. (2011). *The chemokine receptor CX(3)CR1 is directly involved in the arrest of breast cancer cells to the skeleton. Breast Cancer Res 13(5), R91.*

Jankowski, K., Kucia, M., Wysoczynski, M., Reca, R., Zhao, D., Trzyna, E., Trent, J., Peiper, S., Zembala, M., Ratajczak, J., et al. (2003). *Both hepatocyte growth factor (HGF) and stromal-derived factor-1 regulate the metastatic behavior of human rhabdomyosarcoma cells, but only HGF enhances their resistance to radiochemotherapy. Cancer Res 63(22), 7926-7935.*

Juarez, J., Bradstock, K.F., Gottlieb, D.J., and Bendall, L.J. (2003). *Effects of inhibitors of the chemokine receptor CXCR4 on acute lymphoblastic leukemia cells in vitro. Leukemia 17(7), 1294-1300.*

Jung, S., Aliberti, J., Graemmel, P., Sunshine, M.J., Kreutzberg, G.W., Sher, A., and Littman, D.R. (2000). *Analysis of fractalkine receptor CX(3)CR1 function by targeted deletion and green fluorescent protein reporter gene insertion. Mol Cell Biol 20(11), 4106-4114.*

Kang, Y., Siegel, P.M., Shu, W., Drobnjak, M., Kakonen, S.M., Cordon-Cardo, C., Guise, T.A., and Massague, J. (2003). *A multigenic program mediating breast cancer metastasis to bone. Cancer Cell 3(6), 537-549.*

Kelner, G.S., Kennedy, J., Bacon, K.B., Kleyensteuber, S., Largaespada, D.A., Jenkins, N.A., Copeland, N.G., Bazan, J.F., Moore, K.W., Schall, T.J., et al. (1994). Lymphotactin: a cytokine that represents a new class of chemokine. Science 266(5189), 1395-1399.

Kikuchi, T., Andarini, S., Xin, H., Gomi, K., Tokue, Y., Saijo, Y., Honjo, T., Watanabe, A., and Nukiwa, T. (2005). Involvement of fractalkine/CX3CL1 expression by dendritic cells in the enhancement of host immunity against Legionella pneumophila. Infect Immun 73(9), 5350-5357.

Kim, K.W., Vallon-Eberhard, A., Zigmond, E., Farache, J., Shezen, E., Shakhar, G., Ludwig, A., Lira, S.A., and Jung, S. (2011). In vivo structure/function and expression analysis of the CX3C chemokine fractalkine. Blood 118(22), e156-167.

Koizumi, K., Saitoh, Y., Minami, T., Takeno, N., Tsuneyama, K., Miyahara, T., Nakayama, T., Sakurai, H., Takano, Y., Nishimura, M., et al. (2009). Role of CX3CL1/fractalkine in osteoclast differentiation and bone resorption. J Immunol 183(12), 7825-7831.

Kumar, A.H., Metharom, P., Schmeckpeper, J., Weiss, S., Martin, K., and Caplice, N.M. (2010). Bone marrow-derived CX3CR1 progenitors contribute to neointimal smooth muscle cells via fractalkine CX3CR1 interaction. FASEB J 24(1), 81-92.

Landsman, L., Bar-On, L., Zernecke, A., Kim, K.W., Krauthgamer, R., Shagdarsuren, E., Lira, S.A., Weissman, I.L., Weber, C., and Jung, S. (2009). CX3CR1 is required for monocyte homeostasis and atherogenesis by promoting cell survival. Blood 113(4), 963-972.

Lauro, C., Di Angelantonio, S., Cipriani, R., Sobrero, F., Antonilli, L., Brusadin, V., Ragozzino, D., and Limatola, C. (2008). Activity of adenosine receptors type 1 Is required for CX3CL1-mediated neuroprotection and neuromodulation in hippocampal neurons. J Immunol 180(11), 7590-7596.

Lavergne, E., Combadiere, B., Bonduelle, O., Iga, M., Gao, J.L., Maho, M., Boissonnas, A., Murphy, P.M., Debre, P., and Combadiere, C. (2003). Fractalkine mediates natural killer-dependent antitumor responses in vivo. Cancer Res 63(21), 7468-7474.

Lazennec, G., and Richmond, A. (2010). Chemokines and chemokine receptors: new insights into cancer-related inflammation. Trends Mol Med 16(3), 133-144.

Lee, S., Varvel, N.H., Konerth, M.E., Xu, G., Cardona, A.E., Ransohoff, R.M., and Lamb, B.T. (2010). CX3CR1 deficiency alters microglial activation and reduces beta-amyloid deposition in two Alzheimer's disease mouse models. Am J Pathol 177(5), 2549-2562.

Lee, S.J., Namkoong, S., Kim, Y.M., Kim, C.K., Lee, H., Ha, K.S., Chung, H.T., and Kwon, Y.G. (2006). Fractalkine stimulates angiogenesis by activating the Raf-1/MEK/ERK- and PI3K/Akt/eNOS-dependent signal pathways. Am J Physiol Heart Circ Physiol 291(6), H2836-2846.

Lesnik, P., Haskell, C.A., and Charo, I.F. (2003). Decreased atherosclerosis in CX3CR1-/- mice reveals a role for fractalkine in atherogenesis. J Clin Invest 111(3), 333-340.

Liebmann, C. (2011). EGF receptor activation by GPCRs: an universal pathway reveals different versions. Mol Cell Endocrinol 331(2), 222-231.

Loberg, R.D., Ying, C., Craig, M., Yan, L., Snyder, L.A., and Pienta, K.J. (2007). CCL2 as an important mediator of prostate cancer growth in vivo through the regulation of macrophage infiltration. Neoplasia 9(7), 556-562.

Locatelli, M., Boiocchi, L., Ferrero, S., Martinelli Boneschi, F., Zavanone, M., Pesce, S., Allavena, P., Maria Gaini, S., Bello, L., and Mantovani, A. (2010). Human glioma tumors express high levels of the chemokine receptor CX3CR1. Eur Cytokine Netw 21(1), 27-33.

Lucas, A.D., Chadwick, N., Warren, B.F., Jewell, D.P., Gordon, S., Powrie, F., and Greaves, D.R. (2001). The transmembrane form of the CX3CL1 chemokine fractalkine is expressed predominantly by epithelial cells in vivo. Am J Pathol 158(3), 855-866.

Ludwig, A., and Mentlein, R. (2008). Glial cross-talk by transmembrane chemokines CX3CL1 and CXCL16. J Neuroimmunol 198(1-2), 92-97.

Lyons, A., Lynch, A.M., Downer, E.J., Hanley, R., O'Sullivan, J.B., Smith, A., and Lynch, M.A. (2009). Fractalkine-induced activation of the phosphatidylinositol-3 kinase pathway attenuates microglial activation in vivo and in vitro. J Neurochem 110(5), 1547-1556.

Manduteanu, I., Pirvulescu, M., Gan, A.M., Stan, D., Simion, V., Dragomir, E., Calin, M., Manea, A., and Simionescu, M. (2009). Similar effects of resistin and high glucose on P-selectin and fractalkine expression and monocyte adhesion in human endothelial cells. Biochem Biophys Res Commun 391(3), 1443-1448.

Mani, S.A., Guo, W., Liao, M.J., Eaton, E.N., Ayyanan, A., Zhou, A.Y., Brooks, M., Reinhard, F., Zhang, C.C., Shipitsin, M., et al. (2008). The epithelial-mesenchymal transition generates cells with properties of stem cells. Cell 133(4), 704-715.

Mañes, S., Lacalle, R.A., Gómez-Moutón, C., del Real, G., Mira, E., and Martínez, A.C. (2001). Membrane raft microdomains in chemokine receptor function. Semin Immunol 13(2), 147-157.

Mañes, S., Mira, E., Colomer, R., Montero, S., Real, L.M., Gómez-Moutón, C., Jiménez-Baranda, S., Garzón, A., Lacalle, R.A., Harshman, K., et al. (2003). CCR5 expression influences the progression of human breast cancer in a p53-dependent manner. J Exp Med 198(9), 1381-1389.

Marchesi, F., Locatelli, M., Solinas, G., Erreni, M., Allavena, P., and Mantovani, A. (2010). Role of CX3CR1/CX3CL1 axis in primary and secondary involvement of the nervous system by cancer. J Neuroimmunol 224(1-2), 39-44.

Marchesi, F., Piemonti, L., Fedele, G., Destro, A., Roncalli, M., Albarello, L., Doglioni, C., Anselmo, A., Doni, A., Bianchi, P., et al. (2008). The chemokine receptor CX3CR1 is involved in the neural tropism and malignant behavior of pancreatic ductal adenocarcinoma. Cancer Res 68(21), 9060-9069.

Matloubian, M., David, A., Engel, S., Ryan, J.E., and Cyster, J.G. (2000). A transmembrane CXC chemokine is a ligand for HIV-coreceptor Bonzo. Nat Immunol 1(4), 298-304.

Matsumiya, T., Ota, K., Imaizumi, T., Yoshida, H., Kimura, H., and Satoh, K. (2010). Characterization of synergistic induction of CX3CL1/fractalkine by TNF-alpha and IFN-gamma in vascular endothelial cells: an essential role for TNF-alpha in post-transcriptional regulation of CX3CL1. J Immunol 184(8), 4205-4214.

Mehrad, B., Keane, M.P., and Strieter, R.M. (2007). Chemokines as mediators of angiogenesis. Thromb Haemost 97(5), 755-762.

Mellado, M., Rodriguez-Frade, J.M., Mañes, S., and Martinez, A.C. (2001). Chemokine signaling and functional responses: the role of receptor dimerization and TK pathway activation. Annu Rev Immunol 19397-421.

Mionnet, C., Buatois, V., Kanda, A., Milcent, V., Fleury, S., Lair, D., Langelot, M., Lacoeuille, Y., Hessel, E., Coffman, R., et al. (2010). CX3CR1 is required for airway inflammation by promoting T helper cell survival and maintenance in inflamed lung. Nat Med 16(11), 1305-1312.

Mira, E., Lacalle, R.A., Gonzalez, M.A., Gómez-Moutón, C., Abad, J.L., Bernad, A., Martínez-A., C., and Manes, S. (2001). A role for chemokine receptor transactivation in growth factor signaling. EMBO Rep 2(2), 151-156.

Mizuno, T., Kawanokuchi, J., Numata, K., and Suzumura, A. (2003). Production and neuroprotective functions of fractalkine in the central nervous system. Brain Res 979(1-2), 65-70.

Moatti, D., Faure, S., Fumeron, F., Amara Mel, W., Seknadji, P., McDermott, D.H., Debre, P., Aumont, M.C., Murphy, P.M., de Prost, D., et al. (2001). Polymorphism in the fractalkine receptor CX3CR1 as a genetic risk factor for coronary artery disease. Blood 97(7), 1925-1928.

Molon, B., Gri, G., Bettella, M., Gomez-Mouton, C., Lanzavecchia, A., Martinez, A.C., Mañes, S., and Viola, A. (2005). T cell costimulation by chemokine receptors. Nat Immunol 6(5), 465-471.

Mosser, D.M., and Edwards, J.P. (2008). Exploring the full spectrum of macrophage activation. Nat Rev Immunol 8(12), 958-969.

Muehlhoefer, A., Saubermann, L.J., Gu, X., Luedtke-Heckenkamp, K., Xavier, R., Blumberg, R.S., Podolsky, D.K., Mac-Dermott, R.P., and Reinecker, H.C. (2000). Fractalkine is an epithelial and endothelial cell-derived chemoattractant for intraepithelial lymphocytes in the small intestinal mucosa. J Immunol 164(6), 3368-3376.

Müller, A., Homey, B., Soto, H., Ge, N., Catron, D., Buchanan, M.E., McClanahan, T., Murphy, E., Yuan, W., Wagner, S.N., et al. (2001). Involvement of chemokine receptors in breast cancer metastasis. Nature 410(6824), 50-56.

Murakami, T., Maki, W., Cardones, A.R., Fang, H., Tun Kyi, A., Nestle, F.O., and Hwang, S.T. (2002). Expression of CXC chemokine receptor-4 enhances the pulmonary metastatic potential of murine B16 melanoma cells. Cancer Res 62(24), 7328-7334.

Murphy, K., Travers, P., and Walport, M. (2008). Janeway's Immunobiology, Seventh edn (Garland Science).

Murphy, P.M. (1994). The molecular biology of leukocyte chemoattractant receptors. Annu Rev Immunol 12593-633.

Nakatani, K., Yoshimoto, S., Iwano, M., Asai, O., Samejima, K., Sakan, H., Terada, M., Hasegawa, H., Nose, M., and Saito, Y. (2010). Fractalkine expression and CD16+ monocyte accumulation in glomerular lesions: association with their severity and diversity in lupus models. Am J Physiol Renal Physiol 299(1), F207-216.

Nevo, I., Sagi-Assif, O., Meshel, T., Ben-Baruch, A., Johrer, K., Greil, R., Trejo, L.E., Kharenko, O., Feinmesser, M., Yron, I., et al. (2009). The involvement of the fractalkine receptor in the transmigration of neuroblastoma cells through bone-marrow endothelial cells. Cancer Lett 273(1), 127-139.

Niess, J.H., Brand, S., Gu, X., Landsman, L., Jung, S., McCormick, B.A., Vyas, J.M., Boes, M., Ploegh, H.L., Fox, J.G., et al. (2005). CX3CR1-mediated dendritic cell access to the intestinal lumen and bacterial clearance. Science 307(5707), 254-258.

Nishimura, M., Umehara, H., Nakayama, T., Yoneda, O., Hieshima, K., Kakizaki, M., Dohmae, N., Yoshie, O., and Imai, T. (2002). Dual functions of fractalkine/CX3C ligand 1 in trafficking of perforin+/granzyme B+ cytotoxic effector lymphocytes that are defined by CX3CR1 expression. J Immunol 168(12), 6173-6180.

Nokihara, H., Yanagawa, H., Nishioka, Y., Yano, S., Mukaida, N., Matsushima, K., and Sone, S. (2000). Natural killer cell-dependent suppression of systemic spread of human lung adenocarcinoma cells by monocyte chemoattractant protein-1 gene transfection in severe combined immunodeficient mice. Cancer Res 60(24), 7002-7007.

Oliveira-Neto, H.H., de Souza, P.P., da Silva, M.R., Mendonca, E.F., Silva, T.A., and Batista, A.C. (2013). The expression of chemokines CCL19, CCL21 and their receptor CCR7 in oral squamous cell carcinoma and its relevance to cervical lymph node metastasis. Tumour Biol 34(1), 65-70.

Pachot, A., Cazalis, M.A., Venet, F., Turrel, F., Faudot, C., Voirin, N., Diasparra, J., Bourgoin, N., Poitevin, F., Mougin, B., et al. (2008). Decreased expression of the fractalkine receptor CX3CR1 on circulating monocytes as new feature of sepsis-induced immunosuppression. J Immunol 180(9), 6421-6429.

Pan, Y., Lloyd, C., Zhou, H., Dolich, S., Deeds, J., Gonzalo, J.A., Vath, J., Gosselin, M., Ma, J., Dussault, B., et al. (1997). Neurotactin, a membrane-anchored chemokine upregulated in brain inflammation. Nature 387(6633), 611-617.

Papadopoulos, E.J., Sassetti, C., Saeki, H., Yamada, N., Kawamura, T., Fitzhugh, D.J., Saraf, M.A., Schall, T., Blauvelt, A., Rosen, S.D., et al. (1999). Fractalkine, a CX3C chemokine, is expressed by dendritic cells and is up-regulated upon dendritic cell maturation. Eur J Immunol 29(8), 2551-2559.

Pardoll, D. (2003). Does the immune system see tumors as foreign or self? Annu Rev Immunol 21807-839.

Park, M.H., Lee, J.S., and Yoon, J.H. (2012). High expression of CX3CL1 by tumor cells correlates with a good prognosis and increased tumor-infiltrating CD8+ T cells, natural killer cells, and dendritic cells in breast carcinoma. J Surg Oncol 106(4), 386-392.

Premack, B.A., and Schall, T.J. (1996). Chemokine receptors: gateways to inflammation and infection. Nat Med 2(11), 1174-1178.

Prenzel, N., Zwick, E., Daub, H., Leserer, M., Abraham, R., Wallasch, C., and Ullrich, A. (1999). EGF receptor transactivation by G-protein-coupled receptors requires metalloproteinase cleavage of proHB-EGF. Nature 402(6764), 884-888.

Rae, J.M., Scheys, J.O., Clark, K.M., Chadwick, R.B., Kiefer, M.C., and Lippman, M.E. (2004). EGFR and EGFRvIII expression in primary breast cancer and cell lines. Breast Cancer Res Treat 87(1), 87-95.

Raman, D., Baugher, P.J., Thu, Y.M., and Richmond, A. (2007). Role of chemokines in tumor growth. Cancer Lett 256(2), 137-165.

Ransohoff, R.M., Liu, L., and Cardona, A.E. (2007). Chemokines and chemokine receptors: multipurpose players in neuroinflammation. Int Rev Neurobiol 82, 187-204.

Re, D.B., and Przedborski, S. (2006). Fractalkine: moving from chemotaxis to neuroprotection. Nat Neurosci 9(7), 859-861.

Reed, J.R., Stone, M.D., Beadnell, T.C., Ryu, Y., Griffin, T.J., and Schwertfeger, K.L. (2012). Fibroblast growth factor receptor 1 activation in mammary tumor cells promotes macrophage recruitment in a CX3CL1-dependent manner. PLoS One 7(9), e45877.

Ren, H., Zhao, T., Sun, J., Wang, X., Liu, J., Gao, S., Yu, M., and Hao, J. (2013). The CX3CL1/CX3CR1 reprograms glucose metabolism through HIF-1 pathway in pancreatic adenocarcinoma, J Cell Biochem 114(11), 2603-2611.

Robinson, L.A., Nataraj, C., Thomas, D.W., Cosby, J.M., Griffiths, R., Bautch, V.L., Patel, D.D., and Coffman, T.M. (2003). The chemokine CX3CL1 regulates NK cell activity in vivo. Cell Immunol 225(2), 122-130.

Rosenkilde, M.M., and Schwartz, T.W. (2004). The chemokine system -- a major regulator of angiogenesis in health and disease. APMIS 112(7-8), 481-495.

Ruitenberg, M.J., Vukovic, J., Blomster, L., Hall, J.M., Jung, S., Filgueira, L., McMenamin, P.G., and Plant, G.W. (2008). CX3CL1/fractalkine regulates branching and migration of monocyte-derived cells in the mouse olfactory epithelium. J Neuroimmunol 205(1-2), 80-85.

Saitoh, Y., Koizumi, K., Sakurai, H., Minami, T., and Saiki, I. (2007). RANKL-induced down-regulation of CX3CR1 via PI3K/Akt signaling pathway suppresses Fractalkine/CX3CL1-induced cellular responses in RAW264.7 cells. Biochem Biophys Res Commun 364(3), 417-422.

Salcedo, R., Resau, J.H., Halverson, D., Hudson, E.A., Dambach, M., Powell, D., Wasserman, K., and Oppenheim, J.J. (2000). Differential expression and responsiveness of chemokine receptors (CXCR1-3) by human microvascular endothelial cells and umbilical vein endothelial cells. FASEB J 14(13), 2055-2064.

Sallusto, F., Lanzavecchia, A., and Mackay, C.R. (1998). Chemokines and chemokine receptors in T-cell priming and Th1/Th2-mediated responses. Immunol Today 19(12), 568-574.

Sawai, H., Park, Y.W., Roberson, J., Imai, T., Goronzy, J.J., and Weyand, C.M. (2005). T cell costimulation by fractalkine-expressing synoviocytes in rheumatoid arthritis. Arthritis Rheum 52(5), 1392-1401.

Schulte, A., Schulz, B., Andrzejewski, M.G., Hundhausen, C., Mletzko, S., Achilles, J., Reiss, K., Paliga, K., Weber, C., John, S.R., et al. (2007). Sequential processing of the transmembrane chemokines CX3CL1 and CXCL16 by alpha- and gamma-secretases. Biochem Biophys Res Commun 358(1), 233-240.

Schwarz, N., Pruessmeyer, J., Hess, F.M., Dreymueller, D., Pantaler, E., Koelsch, A., Windoffer, R., Voss, M., Sarabi, A., Weber, C., et al. (2010). Requirements for leukocyte transmigration via the transmembrane chemokine CX3CL1. Cell Mol Life Sci 67(24), 4233-4248.

Sciume, G., Soriani, A., Piccoli, M., Frati, L., Santoni, A., and Bernardini, G. (2010). CX3CR1/CX3CL1 axis negatively controls glioma cell invasion and is modulated by transforming growth factor-beta1. Neuro Oncol 12(7), 701-710.

Shields, J.D., Fleury, M.E., Yong, C., Tomei, A.A., Randolph, G.J., and Swartz, M.A. (2007). Autologous chemotaxis as a mechanism of tumor cell homing to lymphatics via interstitial flow and autocrine CCR7 signaling. Cancer Cell 11(6), 526-538.

Shiraishi, K., Fukuda, S., Mori, T., Matsuda, K., Yamaguchi, T., Tanikawa, C., Ogawa, M., Nakamura, Y., and Arakawa, H. (2000). Identification of fractalkine, a CX3C-type chemokine, as a direct target of p53. Cancer Res 60(14), 3722-3726.

Shulby, S.A., Dolloff, N.G., Stearns, M.E., Meucci, O., and Fatatis, A. (2004). CX3CR1-fractalkine expression regulates cellular mechanisms involved in adhesion, migration, and survival of human prostate cancer cells. Cancer Res 64(14), 4693-4698.

Smith, D.R., Polverini, P.J., Kunkel, S.L., Orringer, M.B., Whyte, R.I., Burdick, M.D., Wilke, C.A., and Strieter, R.M. (1994). Inhibition of interleukin 8 attenuates angiogenesis in bronchogenic carcinoma. J Exp Med 179(5), 1409-1415.

Strieter, R.M., Polverini, P.J., Kunkel, S.L., Arenberg, D.A., Burdick, M.D., Kasper, J., Dzuiba, J., Van Damme, J., Walz, A., Marriott, D., et al. (1995). The functional role of the ELR motif in CXC chemokine-mediated angiogenesis. J Biol Chem 270(45), 27348-27357.

Sugaya, M., Nakamura, K., Mitsui, H., Takekoshi, T., Saeki, H., and Tamaki, K. (2003). Human keratinocytes express fractalkine/CX3CL1. J Dermatol Sci 31(3), 179-187.

Takanami, I. (2003). Overexpression of CCR7 mRNA in nonsmall cell lung cancer: correlation with lymph node metastasis. Int J Cancer 105(2), 186-189.

Tang, L., Hu, H.D., Hu, P., Lan, Y.H., Peng, M.L., Chen, M., and Ren, H. (2007). Gene therapy with CX3CL1/Fractalkine induces antitumor immunity to regress effectively mouse hepatocellular carcinoma. Gene Ther 14(16), 1226-1234.

Tardáguila, M., Mira, E., García-Cabezas, M.A., Feijoo, A.M., Quintela-Fandino, M., Azcoitia, I., Lira, S.A., and Mañes, S. (2013). CX3CL1 Promotes Breast Cancer via Transactivation of the EGF Pathway. Cancer Res 73(14), 4461-4473

Tole, S., Durkan, A.M., Huang, Y.W., Liu, G.Y., Leung, A., Jones, L.L., Taylor, J.A., and Robinson, L.A. (2010). Thromboxane prostanoid receptor stimulation induces shedding of the transmembrane chemokine CX3CL1 yet enhances CX3CL1-dependent leukocyte adhesion. Am J Physiol Cell Physiol 298(6), C1469-1480.

Tong, N., Perry, S.W., Zhang, Q., James, H.J., Guo, H., Brooks, A., Bal, H., Kinnear, S.A., Fine, S., Epstein, L.G., et al. (2000). Neuronal fractalkine expression in HIV-1 encephalitis: roles for macrophage recruitment and neuroprotection in the central nervous system. J Immunol 164(3), 1333-1339.

Tsaur, I., Noack, A., Waaga-Gasser, A.M., Makarevic, J., Schmitt, L., Kurosch, M., Huesch, T., Wiesner, C., Wedel, S., Bartsch, G., et al. (2011). Chemokines involved in tumor promotion and dissemination in patients with renal cell cancer. Cancer Biomark 10(5), 195-204.

Tuo, J., Smith, B.C., Bojanowski, C.M., Meleth, A.D., Gery, I., Csaky, K.G., Chew, E.Y., and Chan, C.C. (2004). The involvement of sequence variation and expression of CX3CR1 in the pathogenesis of age-related macular degeneration. FASEB J 18(11), 1297-1299.

Vaday, G.G., Peehl, D.M., Kadam, P.A., and Lawrence, D.M. (2006). Expression of CCL5 (RANTES) and CCR5 in prostate cancer. Prostate 66(2), 124-134.

Varney, M.L., Singh, S., Li, A., Mayer-Ezell, R., Bond, R., and Singh, R.K. (2011). Small molecule antagonists for CXCR2 and CXCR1 inhibit human colon cancer liver metastases. Cancer Lett 300(2), 180-188.

Vicari, A.P., Treilleux, I., and Lebecque, S. (2004). Regulation of the trafficking of tumour-infiltrating dendritic cells by chemokines. Semin Cancer Biol 14(3), 161-169.

Viola, A., Contento, R.L., and Molon, B. (2006). T cells and their partners: The chemokine dating agency. Trends Immunol 27(9), 421-427.

Viola, A., Sarukhan, A., Bronte, V., and Molon, B. (2012). The pros and cons of chemokines in tumor immunology. Trends Immunol 33(10), 496-504.

Vitale, S., Cambien, B., Karimdjee, B.F., Barthel, R., Staccini, P., Luci, C., Breittmayer, V., Anjuere, F., Schmid-Alliana, A., and Schmid-Antomarchi, H. (2007). Tissue-specific differential antitumour effect of molecular forms of fractalkine in a mouse model of metastatic colon cancer. Gut 56(3), 365-372.

Volin, M.V., Woods, J.M., Amin, M.A., Connors, M.A., Harlow, L.A., and Koch, A.E. (2001). Fractalkine: a novel angiogenic chemokine in rheumatoid arthritis. Am J Pathol 159(4), 1521-1530.

von Kriegsheim, A., Baiocchi, D., Birtwistle, M., Sumpton, D., Bienvenut, W., Morrice, N., Yamada, K., Lamond, A., Kalna, G., Orton, R., et al. (2009). Cell fate decisions are specified by the dynamic ERK interactome. Nat Cell Biol 11(12), 1458-1464.

Wang, J., Dai, J., Jung, Y., Wei, C.L., Wang, Y., Havens, A.M., Hogg, P.J., Keller, E.T., Pienta, K.J., Nor, J.E., et al. (2007). A glycolytic mechanism regulating an angiogenic switch in prostate cancer. Cancer Res 67(1), 149-159.

Wang, J., Seethala, R.R., Zhang, Q., Gooding, W., van Waes, C., Hasegawa, H., and Ferris, R.L. (2008). Autocrine and paracrine chemokine receptor 7 activation in head and neck cancer: implications for therapy. J Natl Cancer Inst 100(7), 502-512.

Wang, J.P., Hu, W.M., Wang, K.S., Yu, J., Luo, B.H., Wu, C., Chen, Z.H., Luo, G.Q., Liu, Y.W., Liu, Q.L., et al. (2013). Expression of C-X-C chemokine receptor types 1/2 in patients with gastric carcinoma: Clinicopathological correlations and significance. Oncol Lett 5(2), 574-582.

White, G.E., Tan, T.C., John, A.E., Whatling, C., McPheat, W.L., and Greaves, D.R. (2009). Fractalkine has anti-apoptotic and proliferative effects on human vascular smooth muscle cells via epidermal growth factor receptor signalling. Cardiovasc Res 85(4), 825-835.

Wiley, H.E., Gonzalez, E.B., Maki, W., Wu, M.T., and Hwang, S.T. (2001). Expression of CC chemokine receptor-7 and regional lymph node metastasis of B16 murine melanoma. J Natl Cancer Inst 93(21), 1638-1643.

Xin, H., Kanehira, M., Mizuguchi, H., Hayakawa, T., Kikuchi, T., Nukiwa, T., and Saijo, Y. (2007). Targeted delivery of CX3CL1 to multiple lung tumors by mesenchymal stem cells. Stem Cells 25(7), 1618-1626.

Xin, H., Kikuchi, T., Andarini, S., Ohkouchi, S., Suzuki, T., Nukiwa, T., Huqun, Hagiwara, K., Honjo, T., and Saijo, Y. (2005). Antitumor immune response by CX3CL1 fractalkine gene transfer depends on both NK and T cells. Eur J Immunol 35(5), 1371-1380.

Yu, Y.R., Fong, A.M., Combadiere, C., Gao, J.L., Murphy, P.M., and Patel, D.D. (2007). Defective antitumor responses in CX3CR1-deficient mice. Int J Cancer 121(2), 316-322.

Zaitseva, M., Blauvelt, A., Lee, S., Lapham, C.K., Klaus-Kovtun, V., Mostowski, H., Manischewitz, J., and Golding, H. (1997). Expression and function of CCR5 and CXCR4 on human Langerhans cells and macrophages: implications for HIV primary infection. Nat Med 3(12), 1369-1375.

Zeelenberg, I.S., Ruuls-Van Stalle, L., and Roos, E. (2001). Retention of CXCR4 in the endoplasmic reticulum blocks dissemination of a T cell hybridoma. J Clin Invest 108(2), 269-277.

Zeng, Y., Huebener, N., Fest, S., Weixler, S., Schroeder, U., Gaedicke, G., Xiang, R., Schramm, A., Eggert, A., Reisfeld, R.A., et al. (2007). Fractalkine (CX3CL1)- and interleukin-2-enriched neuroblastoma microenvironment induces eradication of metastases mediated by T cells and natural killer cells. Cancer Res 67(5), 2331-2338.

Zhang, S., Youn, B.S., Gao, J.L., Murphy, P.M., and Kwon, B.S. (1999). Differential effects of leukotactin-1 and macrophage inflammatory protein-1 alpha on neutrophils mediated by CCR1. J Immunol 162(8), 4938-4942.

Zhao, P., De, A., Hu, Z., Li, J., Mulders, S.M., Sollewijn Gelpke, M.D., Duan, E.K., and Hsueh, A.J. (2008). Gonadotropin stimulation of ovarian fractalkine expression and fractalkine augmentation of progesterone biosynthesis by luteinizing granulosa cells. Endocrinology 149(6), 2782-2789.

Zhou, Y., Larsen, P.H., Hao, C., and Yong, V.W. (2002). CXCR4 is a major chemokine receptor on glioma cells and mediates their survival. J Biol Chem 277(51), 49481-49487.

Zlotnik, A., Burkhardt, A.M., and Homey, B. (2011). Homeostatic chemokine receptors and organ-specific metastasis. Nat Rev Immunol 11(9), 597-606.

Zlotnik, A., and Yoshie, O. (2000). Chemokines: a new classification system and their role in immunity. Immunity 12(2), 121-127.

Zlotnik, A., Yoshie, O., and Nomiyama, H. (2006). The chemokine and chemokine receptor superfamilies and their molecular evolution. Genome Biol 7(12), 243.

Zujovic, V., Benavides, J., Vige, X., Carter, C., and Taupin, V. (2000). Fractalkine modulates TNF-alpha secretion and neurotoxicity induced by microglial activation. Glia 29(4), 305-315.

Zujovic, V., Schussler, N., Jourdain, D., Duverger, D., and Taupin, V. (2001). In vivo neutralization of endogenous brain fractalkine increases hippocampal TNFalpha and 8-isoprostane production induced by intracerebroventricular injection of LPS. J Neuroimmunol 115(1-2), 135-143.

Road to Cancer via Cohesin Deregulation

Nenggang Zhang
Texas Children's Cancer Center
Department of Pediatrics
Baylor College of Medicine, USA

Debananda Pati
Texas Children's Cancer Center
Department of Pediatrics
Baylor College of Medicine, USA

1   Introduction

Cohesin is a multi-protein complex, which is conserved from yeast to human. It was initially shown to be essential for maintaining genomic stability by generating sister chromatid cohesion (SCC) and participating in homologous recombination-mediated DNA damage repair (DDR). In addition to its canonical functions in SCC and DDR, during the last decade, cohesin has also been found to regulate gene expression, DNA replication, and centrosome biogenesis, etc. In this chapter, we will review the cohesin-regulated cellular processes and discuss the significance of cohesin deregulation in the development of human cancers.

2   Roles of Cohesin

2.1   What Is Cohesin?

The cohesin complex consists of four core structural subunits, including α-kleisin (Rad21/Mcd1/Scc1), two structural maintenance of chromosomes (SMC) proteins (Smc1 and Smc3), and Scc3 *(Darwiche et al.*, 1999; Guacci *et al.*, 1997; Michaelis *et al.*, 1997; Vass *et al.*, 2003). In human somatic cells, there are two types of cohesin complexes– Rad21-Smc1-Smc3 plus one of the Scc3 orthologs, SA1 or SA2 (also known as stromal antigens, Stag1 and Stag2) (Table 1) (Hagstrom & Meyer, 2003; Losada *et al.*, 2000; Uhlmann, 2001). Both Smc1 and Smc3 are rod-shaped proteins containing ATP-binding cassette (ABC)-like ATPase motifs. They form intramolecular antiparallel coiled coils. Smc1 and Smc3 jointly form a hinge via the middle region of each molecule, creating a V-shaped heterodimer (Anderson *et al.*, 2002; Haering *et al.*, 2002; Lowe *et al.*, 2001) (Figure 1A). The N- and C-termini of each SMC molecule form an ATPase head domain at the distal end of the two coiled-coils arms (Haering *et al.*, 2002). Rad21 binds to the ATPase heads of Smc3 and Smc1 via its N- and C- terminus, respectively, resulting in the formation of a contiguous tripartite ring (Haering *et al.*, 2002) (Figure 1A). In meiotic cells, one or more cohesin subunits are replaced by their orthologs (Table 1).

   In addition to the four core subunits, numerous other proteins, including cohesin loaders (Scc2, Scc4), cohesin regulators (Pds5A, Pds5B, Sororin and Wapl), cohesin protectors (Sgol1, Sgol2), and cohesin modifiers (Esco1, Esco2 and HDAC8), also bind to or modify the cohesin complex (Losada *et al.*, 2005; Nishiyama *et al.*, 2010; Panizza *et al.*, 2000; Rankin *et al.*, 2005; Schmitz *et al.*, 2007; Watanabe & Kitajima, 2005; Zhang *et al.*, 2011) (Figure 1A).

   Several models have been proposed to depict how the cohesin complex associates with chromatin. Among them, the one-ring model and the two-ring handcuff model are supported by experimental data. The one-ring model suggests that one cohesin ring can hold two sister chromatids (Gruber *et al.*, 2003; Haering & Nasmyth, 2003; Nasmyth, 2005) or a looped back chromatin from one chromatid (Figure 1B). Handcuff model describes that the cohesin holo-complex consists of two Smc1-Smc3-Rad21 rings. Each ring embraces one chromatin, and the two rings are dimerized via the interaction of SA1/2 and/or other cohesin-associated proteins (Zhang *et al.*, 2008b; Zhang *et al.*, 2013; Zhang & Pati, 2009) (Figure 1C). The dimerization of two cohesin complexes that bind to the same chromatin at different regions can also loop the chromatin as shown in Figure 1C. Other alternative models, such as bracelet model and snap model, have also been suggested (Huang *et al.*, 2005; Nasmyth, 2005). The bracelet model proposes that Smc1 and Smc3 heterodimer can oligomerize to form filaments via the connection of Rad21. Such filaments could be used in a number of ways to mediate the tethering of sister chromatids. The snap model suggests that each Smc1 and Smc3 heterodimer can bind one chromatin and the tethering of the sister chromatids results from the dimerization of the Smc1/3 complexes.

	Generic Name	*S. cerevisiae*	*S. pombe*	*D. Melanogaster*	*H. sapiens* *M. musculus*	Function
Cohesin Complex	α-Kleisins	Scc1/Mcd1 Rec8	Rad21 Rec8	Rad21 C(2)M	Rad21 Rec8, Rad21L	Core subunit
	Smc proteins	Smc1	Psm1	Smc1	Smc1A, Smc1B	
		Smc3	Psm3	Smc3	Smc3	
	Scc3 orthologs	Scc3	Psc3 Rec11	SA	SA1/Stag1 SA2/Stag2 SA3/Stag3	
Cohesin Loading Complex	Scc2	Scc2	Mis4	Nipped-B	Scc2/Nipbl	Cohesin loading
	Scc4	Scc4	Ssl3	Scc4	Scc4/Mau2	
Cohesin Regulatory Complex	Pds5	Pds5	Pds5	Pds5	Pds5A Pds5B/AS3	Cohesion maintenance
	Sororin			Dalmatian	Sororin	Cohesion maintenance
	Wapl	Wpl1/Wapl/ Rad61	Wapl	Wapl	Wapal/Wapl	Cohesin removal
Cohesin Acetyltrans-ferases (CoATs)		Eco1/Ctf7	Eso1	Deco, San	Esco1, Esco2	Cohesion generation
Cohesin Protector	Shugosin	Sgo1	Sgo1, Sgo2	Mei-S332	Sgol1, Sgol2	Cohesin protection
Cohesin Deacetylases (CoDACs)		Hos1			HDAC8	Cohesin regeneration

Table 1: Cohesin subunits and its regulatory factors. Orthologous proteins are on the row. Proteins marked in red function specifically in meiosis.

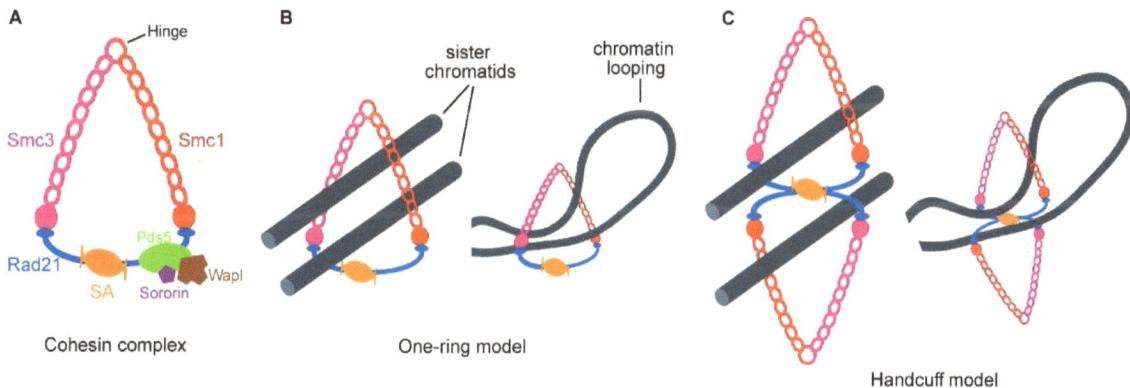

Figure 1: Cohesin complex and models supported by experimental data. (A). Cohesin is comprised of four core subunits Rad21, Smc1, Smc3, and a SA protein. Pds5, Wapl, and Sororin are cohesin-associate proteins. (B). One-ring model. (C). Handcuff model.

2.2   Cohesin Functions in Sister Chromatid Cohesion

In mammalian cells, cohesin complexes are loaded to chromatin at telophase by cohesin-loading complex that consists of Scc2 and Scc4 (Figure 2). After DNA is replicated in the S phase, the sister chromatids

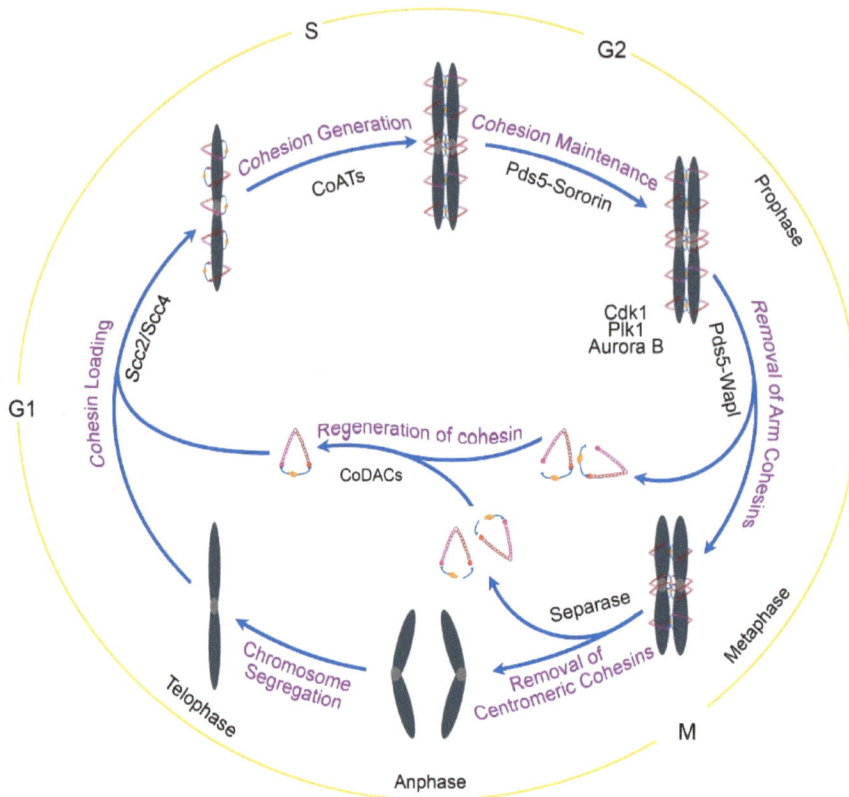

Figure 2: Cohesin cycle in sister chromatid cohesion and separation. Cohesins are loaded to the chromatins by loading complex Scc2-Scc4 at telophase in mammalian cells. During DNA replication at S phase, each cohesin ring embraces one of the sister chromatids. SCC is generated after the two cohesins are dimerized and Smc3 proteins are acetylated by CoATs. Pds5 and Sororin form a complex to maintain the SCC until prophase when Sororin is phosphorylated and destabilized. Formation of Pds5-Wapl complex facilitates the removal of cohesins on the chromosomal arms. The centromeric cohesins are removed by the activated Separase on the transition of metaphase and anaphase. The cohesins dissociated from chromosomes can be regenerated by Co-DACs that removes the acetyl groups from Smc3.

are held by the cohesin complex and SCC is generated after Smc3 is acetylated by cohesin acetyltransferases (CoATs) (Eco1/ctf7 in yeast or Esco1/2 in human) at K112 and K113 sites in yeast or K105 and K106 sites in human (Beckouet *et al.*, 2010; Ben-Shahar et al., 2008; Hou & Zou, 2005; Zhang *et al.*, 2008a). In vertebrates, Pds5, Sororin, and Wapl form a cohesin-regulatory complex, in which Sororin and Wapl compete to bind to an unidentified site on Pds5 (Nishiyama *et al.*, 2010; Zhang & Pati, 2012). The activity of the regulatory complex, either positively or negatively, depends on which protein binds to the site on Pds5. From S phase to prophase, Pds5 and Sororin form a positive regulatory complex and the SCC is maintained.

    When cells enter mitosis, the cohesin complexes on the sister chromatids start to be removed, which occurs in two steps (prophase removal of arm cohesin and anaphase removal of centromeric cohesin) in metazoans. Once the cell cycle progresses to prophase, Cdk1/cyclin B phosphorylates Sororin at

T159, which in turn functions as a docking protein to recruit Polo-like kinase 1 (Plk1) to phosphorylate cohesin complexes on chromosomal arms *(Gimenez-Abian et al., 2004; Sumara et al., 2000; Sumara et al.,* 2002; Zhang *et al.,* 2011). Additionally, phosphorylation of other sites on Sororin by protein kinases Cdk1, Plk1, Aurora B, etc. results in Sororin dissociation from the regulatory complex (Dreier *et al.,* 2011; Nishiyama *et al.,* 2010; Zhang *et al.,* 2011; Zhang *et al.,* 2012), which may facilitate the binding of Wapl to Pds5. The Pds5-Wapl complex acts as a negative regulator of SCC by removing the phosphorylated cohesin from the chromosomal arms. Majority of cohesins on chromosomal arms are removed at prophase step. A small population of cohesins on chromosomal arms and all cohesins on centromeres are protected by shugosin (Sgol1, Sgol2) at prophase. They dissociate from chromosomes after cohesin Rad21 is destroyed by an enzyme called Separase at anaphase step.

Cohesion-resolving enzyme Separase is a thiol protease. It is required to cleave cohesin Rad21 to set the sister chromatids apart at anaphase. Separase activity is tightly regulated by its inhibitory chaperone securin and by S1126 phosphorylation-dependent cyclin B binding (Ciosk *et al.,* 1998; Gorr *et al.,* 2005; Holland & Taylor, 2006; Stemmann *et al.,* 2001; Zou *et al.,* 1999). After sister chromatids align at the cell plate and their kinetochores are attached to the spindle microtubules, the spindle checkpoint is deactivated and anaphase-promoting complex-cdc20 (APC^{cdc20}) is activated on the metaphase-to-anaphase transition. Once the securin and cyclin B are ubiquitinated by APC^{cdc20} and degraded by proteasome, Separase is activated. The centromeric and any leftover arm cohesins are destroyed after Separase proteolytically cleaves the cohesin subunit Rad21 (Haering *et al.,* 2003; Hauf *et al.,* 2001). Consequently, the sister chromatids are free to be segregated to the two daughter cells. Although the dissociation of the cohesin complex from chromosomes takes place in two steps in metazoans (Waizenegger *et al.,* 2000), only one step occurs in yeast (i.e., all cohesins are removed by activated Separase at anaphase) (Uhlmann *et al.,* 1999; Uhlmann *et al.,* 2000). The unloaded cohesins are recycled after Smc3 proteins are deacetylated by cohesin deacetylases (CoDACs) (Hos1 in yeast and HDAC8 in human) (Borges *et al.,* 2010; Deardorff *et al.,* 2012; Xiong *et al.,* 2010) (Figure 2).

The major roles of cohesin in SCC are to keep sister chromatids together and to provide resistance when sister chromatids are pulled by microtubules through the kinetochores towards the opposing spindle poles, thus ensuring the accurate separation of sister chromatids during the transition from metaphase to anaphase (Nasmyth, 2001). Failure in the formation and maintenance of SCC results in premature chromosome segregation, which is thought to be a major pathway to aneuploidy (abnormal chromosomal number), a characteristic feature of most, if not all, human cancers (Panigrahi & Pati, 2009).

2.3   Cohesin in DNA Damage Repair and Cell Cycle Checkpoint Control

Cellular DNA damage induced by extracellular and intracellular DNA-damaging agents and events occurs frequently. Cells respond to this damage by activation of DNA-damage checkpoints that halt cell cycle progression until the damaged DNA is repaired by the DNA repair machinery. If the damage cannot be repaired properly, cells often undergo apoptosis. Eukaryote cells have two distinct mechanisms to repair DNA double-strand breaks (DSB), the non-homologous end-joining (NHEJ) pathway and the homologous recombination (HR) pathway. The NHEJ pathway re-ligates the two free ends of DNA DSB. This repair mechanism often leads to the loss of genetic information because it cannot recover the lost nucleotides or epigenetic modification at the DSB sites. To ensure conservation of the original sequence information, the HR pathway uses the sister chromatid as template to faithfully repair the damaged DNA. Which of these two pathways is selected to repair DNA DSBs depends on the phase of the cell cycle when the damage occurs (Rothkamm *et al.,* 2003). If DSBs happen in the G1 phase, the damage will be repaired by the NHEJ pathway because only the unreplicated DNA is present. If DSBs occur in the S phase, both NHEJ and HR pathways are operational; and in the G2-phase, the HR is mostly used.

The function of cohesin in repair of DSBs is evolutionarily conserved and can be traced back to its bacterial SMC protein ancestors (Graumann & Knust, 2009). The requirement of cohesin in DDR is conserved from yeast to humans (Atienza *et al.*, 2005; Birkenbihl & Subramani, 1992; Schar *et al.*, 2004; Sjogren & Nasmyth, 2001; Sonoda *et al.*, 2001). Rad21 was cloned originally by complementing the radiation sensitivity in fission yeast with a function in DNA-DSB repair, before its role in sister chromatid cohesion was identified (Birkenbihl *et al.*, 1992). In addition to the SCC generated in the S phase during DNA replication, additional cohesins must be recruited to a DNA-DSB site and new cohesion is created de novo in response to the damage for repair (Kim *et al.*, 2010). This newly created cohesion is called *damage-induced cohesion* (DI-cohesion). Besides cohesin itself, factors that are required to load cohesin onto chromatin, to establish cohesion, and to maintain cohesion are all needed for repair of the damaged DNA (Schmitz *et al.*, 2007; Sjogren *et al.*, 2001; Strom *et al.*, 2004; Strom *et al.*, 2007; Unal *et al.*, 2004; Unal *et al.*, 2007; Unal *et al.*, 2008). Defects in the cohesin-loading complex Scc2-Scc4, cohesin acetyl-transferase Eco1/Ctf7, or maintenance factor Sororin block the accumulation of cohesin at DSBs and prevent DDR, even though SCC generated at the S phase is intact. These observations suggest that the presence of cohesin on chromatin is not sufficient to mediate DNA repair and that instead additional cohesins that are capable of establishing SCC are required. The additional cohesion may help to structurally stabilize chromosomes for which the DNA backbone has been fragmented by DSBs. DI-Cohesin is also thought to provide the proximity between the damaged sister chromatid and the chromatid that is used as a template to allow HR to occur.

How does DSB cause de novo cohesion establishment? DSB in the G2 phase causes genome-wide DI-cohesion in both yeast and human cells (Kim *et al.*, 2010; Strom *et al.*, 2007; Unal *et al.*, 2007). DSB has been shown to activate Chk1 that phosphorylates Rad21/Scc1/Mcd1 at the conserved serine residue (S83) in yeast (Heidinger-Pauli *et al.*, 2008). S83 phosphorylation facilitates the acetylation of K84 and K210 residues in Rad21/Scc1/Mcd1 by Eco1. Acetylation of these sites antagonizes Wpl1's cohesin-removing function and results in the establishment of DI-cohesion (Heidinger-Pauli *et al.*, 2009). DI-cohesion is different from the SCC generated during the S phase, in which Smc3 is acetylated by Eco1 to counteract the anti-establishment activity of Wpl1 (Ben-Shahar *et al.*, 2008; Rowland *et al.*, 2009; Sutani *et al.*, 2009; Unal *et al.*, 2008; Zhang *et al.*, 2008a). Interestingly, the DNA damage-induced phosphorylation and acetylation on Rad21 in human cells have not been observed. Instead, the DNA damage-induced phosphorylation and acetylation on Smc3 were found to be important for the genome-wide DI-cohesion and DNA DSB repair (Kim *et al.*, 2010). This finding suggests that the biological process of DI-cohesion is conserved, but the molecular mechanisms are different between yeast and human cells.

In addition to the establishment of DI-cohesion, cohesin is required to activate checkpoints when DNA DSBs occur (Watrin & Peters, 2009). The components of the DNA damage checkpoints in human cells include sensors, signal transducers, and effectors (Finn *et al.*, 2012; Sancar *et al.*, 2004). The damage is first detected by sensors (AMT, ATR, MRE11, RAD50, NBS1, etc.) that, with the aid of mediators (Brca1, 53BP1, Mdc1, etc.), pass the signal to transducers (Chk1, Chk2), and finally activate the effectors (p53, Cdc25, etc.). Although the checkpoints of G1/S, intra-S, and the G2/M are distinct, most upstream components of checkpoints are shared and play more prominent roles in one checkpoint than in others. The effector components of the checkpoints, which block phase transition, determine the unique identities of the checkpoints. When DNA DSB occurs in the S and G2/M phase, cohesins are recruited to the damaged sites in a Mre11-Rad50-dependent manner (Kim *et al.*, 2002a) and cohesin subunits Smc1 (at S957 and S966 sites) and Smc3 (at S1083 site) are phosphorylated in an ATM- and NBS1-dependent way in human (Kim *et al.*, 2002b; Kitagawa *et al.*, 2004; Luo *et al.*, 2008; Yazdi *et al.*, 2002). The DNA DI-cohesins not only enforce the SCC but also facilitate the recruitment of checkpoint proteins to the DNA break sites (e.g., the mediator protein 53BP1 (Watrin *et al.*, 2009)), which is essential to activate the checkpoints. Although no SCC occurs in the G1 phase, cohesin is required for the phosphorylation and activation of Chk2, suggesting that the checkpoint function of cohesin is independent of its role in cohesion. This notion is supported by the finding that depletion of Sororin, a protein essential for the generation and maintenance of SCC, results in checkpoint activation but DSB repair failure (Watrin *et al.*, 2009). Scc2 is a component of the cohesin loading complex. In *C. elegans* with mutant Scc2, cohesin cannot be loaded to chromatin in meiosis. As a result, both DDR and checkpoint activation fail (Lightfoot *et al.*, 2011), indicating the importance of cohesin recruitment to the damaged chromatin. Although cohesin has been found to activate DNA checkpoints in higher eukaryotes, this pathway has not been confirmed in yeast (Dorsett & Strom, 2012). How cohesin functions in the checkpoint activation remains to be determined.

2.4 Cohesin Regulates Gene Expression

Besides being involved in SCC and DDR, cohesin also modulates gene transcription and development. Global gene expression is more sensitive to cohesin changes than SCC and DDR (Heidinger-Pauli *et al.*, 2010; Krantz *et al.*, 2004; Schaaf *et al.*, 2009; Tonkin *et al.*, 2004). Moderate reduction in the expression of Nipped-B, Smc1, or Pds5 in Drosophila (Dorsett *et al.*, 2005; Rollins *et al.*, 1999; Rollins *et al.*, 2004), Rad21 in zebrafish (Horsfield *et al.*, 2007), and Nipbl/Scc2, Pds5A or Pds5B in mouse (Kawauchi *et al.*, 2009; Zhang *et al.*, 2007; Zhang *et al.*, 2009) significantly affects gene expression and development without disrupting sister chromatid cohesion or segregation. Cohesin-regulated gene expression is independent of its role in cell division because it can influence gene expression in non-dividing cells *(Pauli et al.*, 2008; Schuldiner *et al.*, 2008; Seitan *et al.*, 2011). The expression of cohesin-regulated genes can be affected by the change of cohesin level within a few hours *(Kagey et al., 2010; Liu et al., 2009; Pauli et al.*, 2010; Schaaf *et al.*, 2009), suggesting that cohesin regulates gene expression directly and rapidly.

A series of recent studies have demonstrated that cohesin dynamically regulates allele-specific transcription by interacting with the boundary element CCCTC-binding factor (CTCF), tissue-specific transcription by interacting with tissue-specific transcription factors, and general progression of transcription by communicating with the basal transcription machinery (Liu *et al.*, 2009; Wendt *et al.*, 2008). Also, to effectuate proper transcription activation, cohesin loops chromatin to bring two distant regions together (Dorsett, 2011; Hadjur *et al.*, 2009; Merkenschlager & Odom, 2013). In budding yeast, the cohesin-loading complex is found mostly at the promoter region, but cohesin is located primarily between convergently transcribed genes (Glynn *et al.*, 2004; Kogut *et al.*, 2009; Lengronne *et al.*, 2004). The different locales of the loading complex and cohesin possibly result from cohesin sliding along the chromosome after it is loaded and pushed to the intergenic regions between converging transcription units by RNA polymerase (Glynn *et al.*, 2004; Lengronne *et al.*, 2004; Ocampo-Hafalla *et al.*, 2007). However, in Drosophila, cohesin and its loading factor Nipped-B co-localize at a subset of transcriptionally active genes and are excluded from silenced genes (Misulovin *et al.*, 2008). Most of the cohesin and Nipped-B bind to the promoter region, and some spread into the transcribed region of active genes. Similarly, cohesin and loading factor Nipbl/Scc2 have been found to bind to the promoters and enhancers of active genes in mammalian cells (Kagey *et al.*, 2010; Schmidt *et al.*, 2010). Although the pattern of cohesins binding to genes seems different among organisms, the common point that cohesins associate with transcriptionally active genes indicates a conserved cohesin-mediated, gene expression mechanism.

Cohesins have been found to co-localize with mediators (Kagey *et al.*, 2010), transcription factors (Faure *et al.*, 2012; Schmidt *et al.*, 2010), and CTCF (Wendt *et al.*, 2008) at promoters, enhancers, and insulators to regulate gene transcription at multiple levels. Cohesin is possible to associate genes topologically because depletion of the loading complex subunit Nipped-B or cohesin has equivalent effects on gene expression (Schaaf *et al.*, 2013). Cohesin-binding genes often have higher transcriptional activity and more efficient RNA polymerase II (Pol II) than those without cohesin. Nearly all extragenic enhancers are bound with cohesin. Depletion of cohesin frequently increases pausing and decreases gene body transcription on cohesin-binding genes (Schaaf *et al.*, 2013), implying that cohesin facilitates the transition of Pol II from pausing state to elongation state. In Drosophila and mammalian cells, a key transcriptional regulation is to pause the transcriptionally engaged RNA Pol II at several dozen nucleotides downstream of the promoter by the negative elongation factor (NELF) and the DRB-sensitivity inducing factor (DSIF) pausing complexes (Chien *et al.*, 2011; Faure *et al.*, 2012; Fay *et al.*, 2011; Nativio *et al.*, 2009). Release of the pause requires the phosphorylation of RNA Pol II, NELF, and DSIF by the P-TEFb complex (Peterlin & Price, 2006). This process is facilitated by the interaction of the promoter and the enhancer (Chien *et al.*, 2011; Seitan *et al.*, 2011). It is not clear how the promoter and the extragenic enhancer are brought together. One possibility is that dimerization of cohesins bound on the promoter and the enhancer facilitates the chromatin looping and the enhancer–promoter interactions (Figure 3).

In addition to mediating the promoter-enhancer interaction, cohesins also are recruited by CTCF to regulate gene expression (Parelho *et al.*, 2008; Rubio *et al.*, 2008; Stedman *et al.*, 2008; Wendt *et al.*, 2008). CTCF is a zinc finger DNA-binding protein with enhancer-blocking function and boundary-element activity (Gomes & Espinosa, 2010). Cohesin-CTCF-dependent chromatin insulator activity antagonizes the long-range enhancer functions in a manner of chromatin loop formation (Hadjur *et al.*, 2009) (Figure 3).

Besides directly regulating gene expression, cohesin can function indirectly. It has been shown that cohesin depletion reduces the levels of transcriptionally engaged Pol II at the promoters of most genes that do not bind cohesin (Schaaf *et al.*, 2013). The molecular basis for this type of regulation is possibly mediated by the transcriptional factors, such as Myc and p53, with their expression that is regulated by cohesins. In zebrafish, cohesin-regulated genes include pro-oncogene myca (c-Myc in human), tumor suppressor p53, and mdm2 (Rhodes *et al.*, 2010). Cohesin is found at transcription start sites of p53 and mdm2, expression of which is enhanced by the depletion of either Rad21 or CTCF. In contrast, loss of Rad21 decreases myca expression. Positive transcriptional regulation of the c-Myc gene by cohesin is evolutionarily conserved. Loss of cohesin or Nipped-B in Drosophila decreases the expression of both myc and its target genes (Rhodes *et al.*, 2010).

Although it is evident that cohesins are involved in gene transcription, how cohesins themselves are regulated during this process remains unclear. Do cohesins have only a passive role as a component of transcriptional factors or an active role in recruiting other factors and remodeling chromatin structure? Do cohesins associate with chromatin in the same fashion in gene expression regulation and SCC? It seems that cohesins are loaded to specific sites by cohesin-loading complex in order to function. However, it is not known whether cohesins are required to be unloaded after their missions are accomplished, and if so, how cohesins are removed.

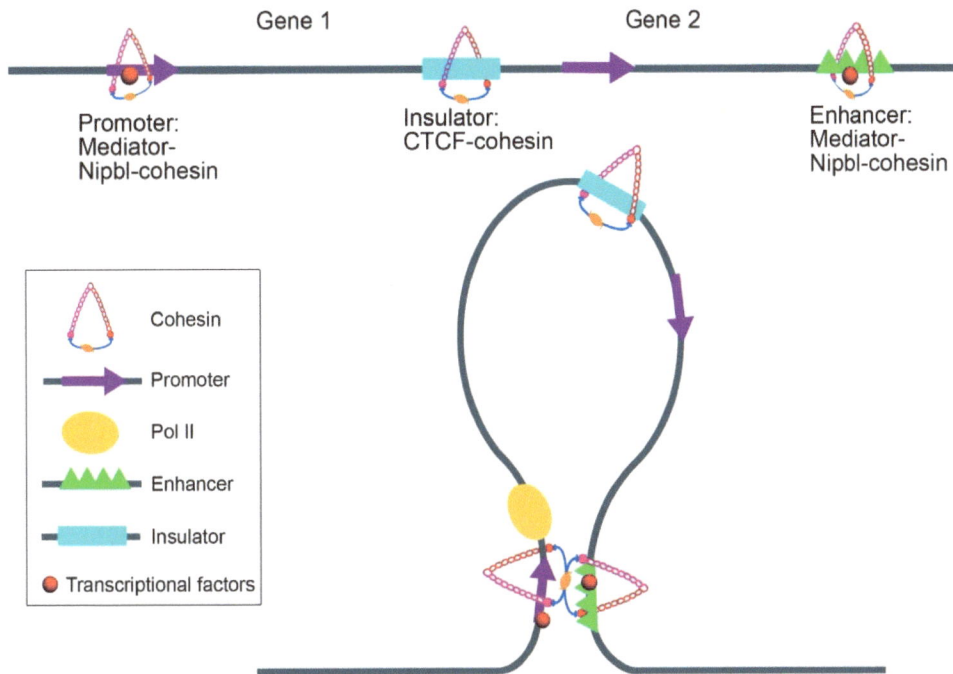

Figure 3: Cohesins regulate gene transcription. The upper panel shows two genes and cohesins associate with promoters, enhancers and insulators. The lower panel shows the long-range interaction of the promoter and the enhancer, which is possibly facilitated via cohesin dimerization. The influence of promoter-enhancer interaction on Gene 2 can be stopped by the cohesin-CTCF complex located before Gene 2.

2.5 Cohesin Regulates Centrosome Cycles

The centrosome plays a pivotal role in chromosome segregation during each cell cycle. It is comprised of two centrioles and the surrounding pericentriolar material in animal cells. The centrioles reside at the center of the centrosome and are important for the integrity and duplication of centrosomes. Similar to DNA replication, the duplication of centrioles is semi-conserved and is precisely regulated in order to coordinate centrosome activity with other cellular events, such as the chromosome cycle, and to ensure that each cell inherits one copy of centrosome (Figure 4). It is well known that the two engaged centrioles in each centrosome must disengage at the late M/early G1 phase before they are licensed to duplicate in the S phase (Tsou & Stearns, 2006). Centrosomes mature in the G2 phase, with mother and daughter centrioles engaged orthogonally (Kuriyama & Borisy, 1981) (Figure 4). When the cell cycle progresses to mitosis, the centrosomes are separated and move to the opposite poles of the cell. They determine the correct formation of spindle that pull the sister chromatids apart into the two daughter cells. The entire process from centriole disengagement and duplication to centrosome maturation and separation is called centrosome cycle (Figure 4).

Interestingly, as in the chromosome cycle, cohesin also regulates the centrosome cycle. Cohesin is required for the engagement of centrioles (Nakamura *et al.*, 2009; Schockel *et al.*, 2011; Tsou *et al.*, 2009).

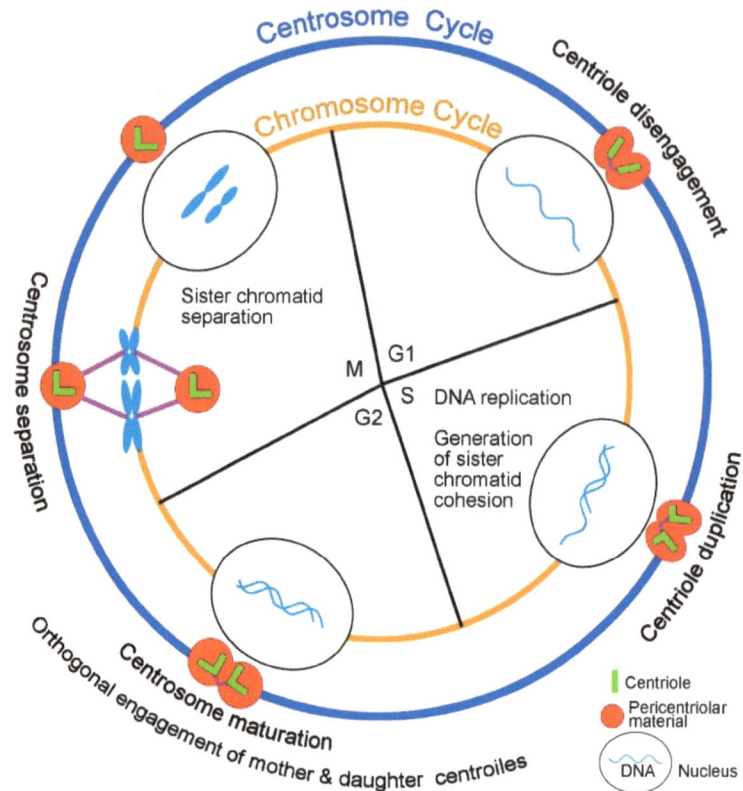

Figure 4: Centrosome cycle and chromosome cycle are coordinated in each cell cycle. Both centriole duplication and DNA replication are semi-conserved. Cohesin complex and its regulatory proteins function in both chromosome cycle and centrosome cycle.

Cohesin core subunits (Smc1, Smc3, Rad21) have been found in centrosomes (Beauchene *et al.*, 2010; Gimenez- Abian *et al.*, 2010; Guan *et al.*, 2008; Kong *et al.*, 2009; Nakamura *et al.*, 2009). Depletion of Rad21 not only causes the aberrant SCC (Losada *et al.*, 2005) but also the formation of multipolar spindles (Losada *et al.*, 2005; Nakamura *et al.*, 2009) and, importantly, centriole splitting (Beauchene *et al.*, 2010; Nakamura *et al.*, 2009). Cohesin protector Sgo1 and cohesion maintenance protein Sororin are also localized on centrosomes (Wang *et al.*, 2008; Zhang *et al.*, 2011). Ablation of Sgo1 leads to splitting centrioles and multiple spindles (Wang *et al.*, 2008). We have also observed similar results when Sororin was depleted (Zhang *et al* unpublished).

Two cohesin regulatory enzymes, Plk1 and Separase, have also been found to play a role in the centrosome cycle. Recent studies report that at the late G2 and early M phases (before the onset of anaphase) Plk1 regulates mitotic licensing of centriole duplication in the following S phase (Tsou *et al.*, 2009). Plk1 also promotes Separase-dependent centriole disengagement by phosphorylating Rad21, which is proteolytically cleaved by Separase in the late M phase (Schockel *et al.*, 2011). That Separase inhibitors, securin and cyclin B (Tsou *et al.*, 2006), and the depletion of Separase itself (Thein *et al.*, 2007) inhibits centriole disengagement underscores the importance of Separase in centrosome cycle. Cleavage of Rad21 (Nakamura *et al.*, 2009; Schockel *et al.*, 2011; Tsou *et al.*, 2009) and pericentrin (Lee & Rhee, 2012; Matsuo *et al.*, 2012) by Separase in centrosomes further confirms the requirement of Separase in centriole disengagement.

The function and regulation of cohesin in the centrosome cycle appear to mirror those in the chromosome cycle. However, the mechanism governing the function and regulation of cohesin in the centrosome cycle is less understood compared to that of the chromosome cycle. Many questions remain unanswered in this field. For example, how does cohesin topologically associate with centrioles to keep the two centrioles perpendicularly oriented? How does Plk1 phosphorylate cohesin and how is Plk1 activity modulated during the centrosome cycle? Centriole disengagement occurs during the late mitosis/early G1 phase (Beauchene *et al.*, 2010; Schockel *et al.*, 2011; Tsou *et al.*, 2009) when the sister chromatids have been separated by the activated Separase. What prevents the active Separase from disengaging centrioles is also not fully understood.

2.6 Deregulation of Cohesin and Its Regulatory Proteins in Cancer

2.6.1 Abnormal Expression of Cohesin in Cancer

The aberrant expressions of cohesin and cohesin-associated proteins are commonly found in human cancers (Xu *et al.*, 2011a). The overexpression of cohesin and its associated proteins has been found in a variety of tumors (Hagemann *et al.*, 2011). Rad21 is overexpressed in high-grade luminal, basal, and HER2 breast cancers, which confers poor prognosis and resistance to chemotherapy (Xu *et al.*, 2011b). SMC1 is overexpressed in a panel of triple-negative (HER2⁻, ER⁻, and PR⁻) breast cancer (TNBC) cell lines (Yadav *et al.*, 2013) and glioma cells (Ma *et al.*, 2013). The overexpression of Smc1 enhances cell migration and anchorage-independent growth and leads to the increase of vimentin (a mesenchymal marker) and the decrease of E-cadherin (a normal epithelial marker) (Yadav *et al.*, 2013). Reduction of the overexpressed cohesin can decrease cell growth and increase the cytotoxicity of chemotherapeutic drugs (Atienza *et al.*, 2005; Yadav *et al.*, 2013), suggesting that cohesin overexpression may contribute directly to tumor proliferation and resistance to DNA-damaging agents. In contrast, downregulation of cohesin has also been reported in cancer cells. Rad21 is underexpressed in high-metastatic-potential squamous cell carcinoma cells (Yamamoto *et al.*, 2006) and downregulation of the cohesion-protecting gene SGO1 has been linked to chromosomal instability with greater variation of centromeres in colorectal cancer (Iwaizumi *et al.*, 2009b).

2.6.2 Mutations of Cohesin in Cancer

In addition to the deregulation of cohesin expression, mutations of cohesin and its associated proteins have also been found in many cancers, including colorectal tumors (Barber *et al.*, 2008a), leukemias (Ding *et al.*, 2012; Walter *et al.*, 2009; Welch *et al.*, 2012), ovarian tumors (Cancer Genome Atlas Research Network, 2011; Gorringe *et al.*, 2009), Ewing's sarcomas, melanomas, and glioblastomas (Solomon *et al.*, 2011). Analyses of the data from Catalogue of Somatic Mutations in Cancer (COSMIC) database indicate that approximate 10% of human tumors have mutations in cohesin and cohesin-associated genes combined (Table 2). Most of these mutations are heterozygous missense mutations. Deletion, insertion, and mutations resulting in truncation or frameshift are rare. Most of the somatic mutations appear to be random. The collective mutational frequencies of cohesin and its associated proteins vary significantly among different cancer types, from 0 to 39% (Table 2). The mutation rate for a particular cohesin protein or its associated protein in a cancer type is low. The highest mutation rate is in STAG2 (9.43%) and ESPL1 (9.17%) in urinary tract carcinomas. Although these observations suggest that cohesin genes are essential, it also raises the question concerning how significant a particular mutation is to the development of cancer.

Cancer Type	% of Unique Mutated Samples														Sample Size	Total (%)
	RAD21	SMC1A	SMC3	STAG1 (SA1)	STAG2 (SA2)	PDS5A	PDS5B	WAPL	CDCA5 (Sororin)	NIPBL	MAU2 (Scc4)	ESCO1	ESCO2	ESPL1 (Separase)		
Breast	0.41	0.72	0.41	0.62	1.03	0.52	0.62	0.21	0.00	1.00	0.00	0.52	0.00	1.03	968-1005	7.1
Central nervous system	0.00	0.22	0.22	0.00	0.66	0.00	0.00	0.00	0.00	0.00	0.00	0.00	0.22	0.22	409-454	1.50
Endometrium	0.88	4.41	0.88	1.76	3.08	0.44	0.44	0.88	0.00	0.00	0.44	0.00	0.44	0.00	227	13.7
Hematopoietic & lymphoid	0.87	0.76	0.98	0.22	0.54	0.00	0.54	0.11	0.00	0.00	0.11	0.11	0.11	0.22	918	4.6
Kidney	0.00	0.00	1.66	0.65	1.91	0.83	1.10	1.10	0.00	2.56	0.83	0.00	0.00	0.91	362-459	11.6
Large intestine	2.11	0.35	1.76	2.46	1.75	2.20	1.05	1.76	0.35	3.54	0.00	2.46	1.76	2.11	273-311	23.7
Liver	0.00	0.00	0.00	0.00	0.00	0.00	0.00	0.00	0.00	1.41	0.00	0.00	0.00	0.00	71	1.4
Lung	1.30	0.71	0.96	1.66	2.25	1.32	0.84	1.44	0.24	1.78	0.84	1.56	0.60	1.77	835-846	17.3
Oesophagus	1.16	1.16	0.58	2.89	1.73	0.00	1.16	1.16	0.58	2.31	0.58	0.00	0.00	1.16	173	14.5
Ovary	0.50	1.00	0.33	0.67	0.67	0.00	1.00	0.50	0.00	2.00	0.00	0.00	0.00	0.50	601	7.2
Pancreas	0.00	0.00	0.30	0.00	0.00	0.00	0.30	0.00	0.00	0.60	0.00	0.00	0.00	0.00	330-331	1.2
Prostate	0.00	0.00	0.00	0.62	0.62	0.93	1.56	0.00	0.31	0.62	0.00	1.25	0.00	0.93	321	6.9
Skin	0.66	0.66	0.68	0.66	3.31	0.68	0.68	0.00	0.68	3.31	0.68	0.00	0.00	2.65	146-151	14.7
Upper aerodigestive tract	0.00	1.77	1.82	0.88	0.00	0.00	0.00	0.00	0.00	0.88	0.91	0.91	0.00	0.88	110-113	8.1
Urinary tract	0.96	2.88	1.96	1.92	9.43	1.96	0.98	1.96	2.94	2.88	0.00	0.98	0.98	9.17	102-109	39.0

Table 2: Frequency of somatic mutations in cohesin and its associated proteins in different cancers. The mutations include deletion, insertion and substitution. Protein name is shown in parentheses for those genes that protein name and gene name are not the same. Data were from the Catalogue of Somatic Mutations in Cancer (COSMIC) database (http://cancer.sanger.ac.uk/cancergenome/projects/cosmic/).

2.6.3 Mutations of Cohesin Core Subunits in Cancer

Further analyses of the COSMIC data indicate that each cohesin core subunit has two or more sites with mutations that are found in three or more tumor samples (Figure 5, Appendix 1). STAG2 is the most frequently mutated cohesin core subunit and has the most mutated sites found in three or more unique tumor samples (Figure 5, Appendix 1). Some of the sites are located on known functional domains. For example, a substitute mutation at R626 is located on the hinge domain of Smc1A. R184, R252, and R259 are located on the STAG domain of SA2 (Figure 5). The functional significance of these mutations is currently not known. However, the recurring mutations of a specific residue in multiple tumor samples suggest that the site is a potential hot spot. With more whole exomal sequencing of cancer samples, the potential hot spots will be identified. For instance, the mutations on STAG2 at R259, R305, R1012 and R1045 shown in Figure 5 have also been observed in myeloid neoplasms (Kon *et al.*, 2013). Functional study of these recurring mutations is expected to provide the functional information of these proteins and may also yield insight on the development of cancer.

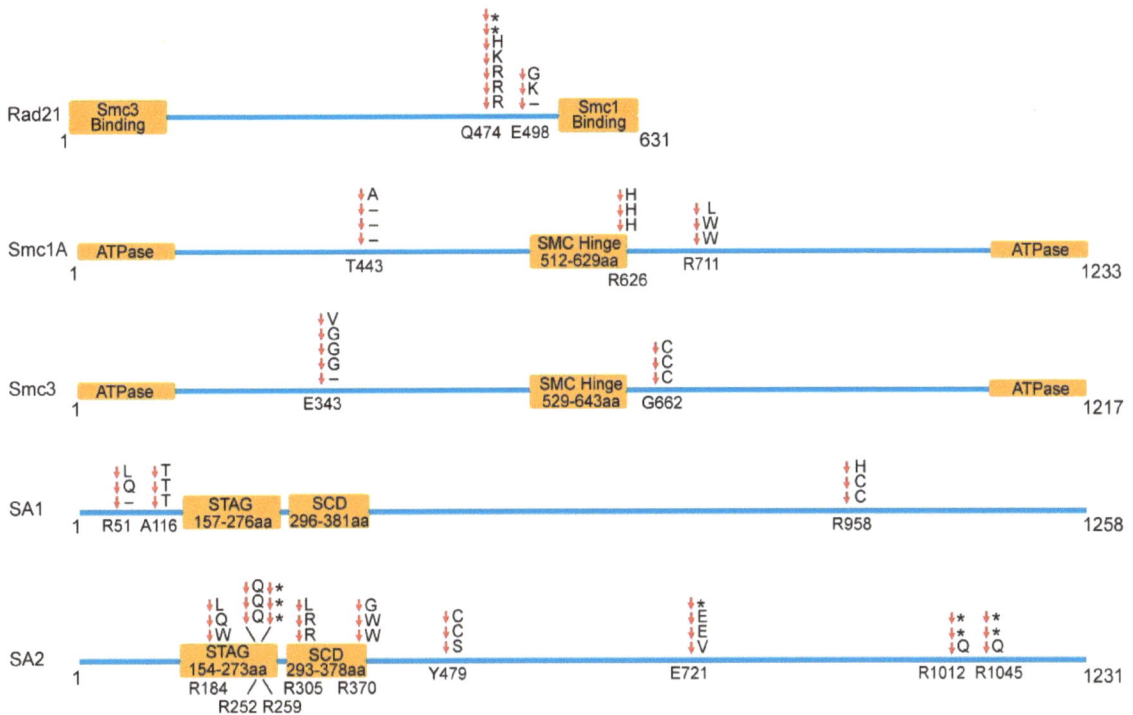

Figure 5: Illustration of the cohesin core subunits with mutations at a particular site found in three or more tumor samples. The mutations include missense mutation, nonsense mutation (*), and synonymous mutation (–). Data were from COSMIC database. See detail information on Appendix 1. Cohesin subunits are shown in blue and the conserved domains are shown in orange. The letters and numbers under the blue lines indicate the amino acid residual and its position. Each red arrow indicates the mutation site. The letter or symbol (*, -) beside the red arrow indicates the amino acid residual mutated to. SCD: stromalin conserved domain.

A detailed analysis of SA2 in tumors found that this protein is not expressed in 21% of Ewing's sarcomas, 19% of melanoma, and 19% of glioblastoma tumors (Solomon *et al.*, 2011). Deletions or truncating mutations are the probable reasons for the loss of SA2 in most of the samples. However, according to another study, compared to the matched normal tissues, SA2 is lost in 27% of gastric carcinomas, 23% of colorectal carcinomas, and 30% of prostate carcinomas (Kim *et al.*, 2012). Interestingly, no STAG2 somatic mutation was found in these cancers, suggesting loss of expression of STAG2 might be responsible to STAG2 inactivation (see below).

Tumor cells without STAG2 expression are viable, which is surprising given the importance of cohesin that is involved in chromosome segregation, DDR, and gene transcription. The viability of STAG2-deficient cells possibly contributes to the fact that STAG2 has a paralog, STAG1. Somatic cells use either STAG1 or STAG2 to form a cohesin complex. Although the function of these two types of cohesins has not been well-defined, STAG1-cohesin is found predominantly in telomeric regions and is responsible for the cohesion and replication of telomere (Canudas & Smith, 2009; Remeseiro *et al.*, 2012a). By contrast, STAG2-cohesin plays a role in the chromosomal arm and centromeric cohesion. Ablation of STAG2 leads to the loss of centromeric cohesion and aneuploidy (Canudas *et al.*, 2009; Solomon *et al.*, 2011).

Interestingly, mutation and loss of STAG2 but not STAG1 has been observed frequently in tumors (Solomon *et al.*, 2011; Welch *et al.*, 2012). This phenomenon could be explained by the fact that STAG2 is located on the X chromosome, which has only one copy in males and one active copy in females. Therefore, only one single somatic mutation is sufficient to result in the inactivation of STAG2. Loss of STAG2 resulting from the deletion of the region where STAG2 resides on X chromosome has been observed in many cancers (Gorringe *et al.*, 2009; Rocquain *et al.*, 2010; Solomon *et al.*, 2011; Walter *et al.*, 2009). Although SMC1A is also located on X chromosome, the cells are predicted not to be viable after loss of function of SMC1A because it is essential for the formation of the cohesin complex and no SMC1A orthologs occur in somatic cells.

One of the cohesin's roles is to regulate gene expression. Surprisingly, the gene expression profiles of STAG2-deficient and STAG2-proficient cells are almost identical (Solomon *et al.*, 2011), suggesting that STAG2 is not a major regulator of global gene expression in human cancer. Instead, STAG1-cohesin is more relevant to the regulation of gene transcription. Comparison of the genome-wide distribution of cohesin in wild-type and SA1-null mouse cells indicates that SA1 is largely responsible for cohesin accumulation at promoters and at sites bound by the insulator protein CTCF. Absence of SA1 dramatically reduces the accumulation of cohesin at promoters and CTCF sites and alters the gene expression (Remeseiro *et al.*, 2012b). Whether the gene expression profile altered by the reduction of STAG1 is related to the development of cancer remains unclear. However, heterozygous STAG1 animals have shorter lifespans and earlier onsets of tumorigenesis, possibly due to impaired replication of telomeres (Remeseiro *et al.*, 2012a).

2.6.4   Mutations of Cohesin Regulatory Proteins in Cancer

The function of cohesin is regulated by a number of cohesin regulatory proteins (Table 1). Mutations in these proteins can affect cohesin loading, removing, modification, and protection, etc. After analyzing the data from COSMIC database, we identified several cohesin regulatory proteins with a particular mutation found in three or more tumor samples, including PDS5B, SGOL2, ESCO2, and NIPBL (Figure 6, Appendix 2).

Pds5B/AS3/APRIN was originally identified as a mediator of androgen-induced proliferative arrest in prostate cells (Geck *et al.*, 1997; Geck *et al.*, 2000; Maffini *et al.*, 2002). It is one of the two Pds5 orthologs (Pds5A and Pds5B) in human. The function of Pds5 is to regulate the association of cohesin with sister chromatids, but the roles of Pds5A and Pds5B remain to be differentiated. Overexpression of Pds5B inhibits cell proliferation, while downregulation of Pds5B blocks the inhibitory effect of androgens on cell proliferation (Geck *et al.*, 2000). Its expression pattern and function is not only implicated in prostate cancer, but also in other cancers. For example, overexpression of Pds5B inhibits differentiation and proliferation and promotes apoptosis in P19 embryonal carcinoma cells (Zhou *et al.*, 2013). In addition, more than two third of esophageal squamous cell carcinomas (ESCC) lose heterozygosity of PDS5B locus, which is significantly correlated with higher pathological grade and leads to decrease of Pds5B gene expression in nearly half of the tumors (Zhang *et al.*, 2008c). Furthermore, PDS5B frameshift mutations were detected in one fifth of gastric cancers and colorectal cancers with high microsatellite instability. Those frameshift mutations often lead to the loss of PDS5B expression (Kim *et al.*, 2013). Downregulation of Pds5B can also result from epigenetic modifications, such as CpG methylation at promoter region. Low Pds5B expression is observed in about 65% of ER-negative breast tumors (Brough *et al.*, 2012). The correlation between Pds5B and ER expression possibly results from the fact that ER expression is positively regulated by cohesin (Prenzel *et al.*, 2012).

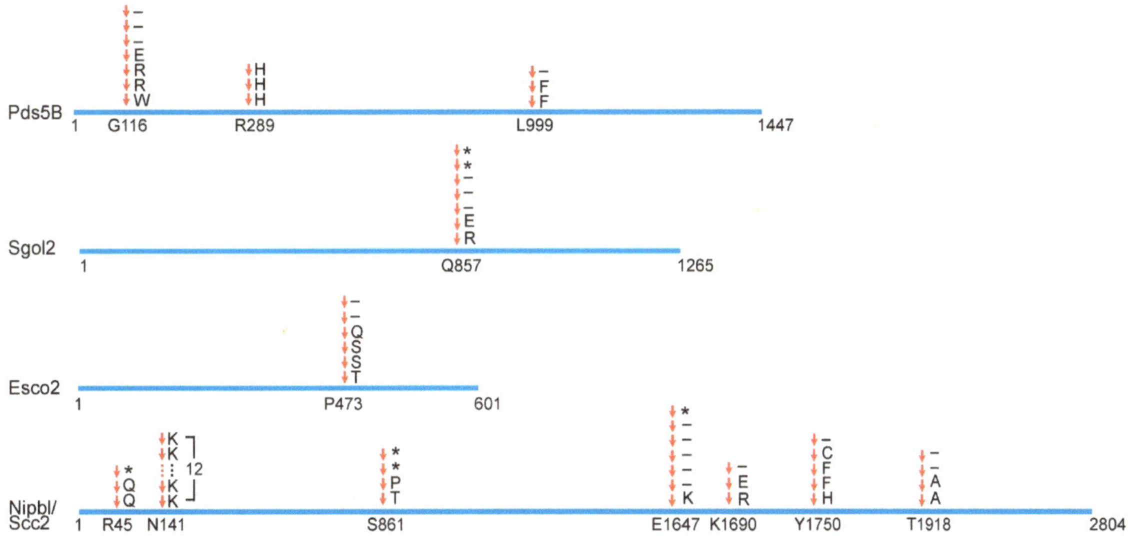

Figure 6: Illustration of cohesin regulatory proteins with mutations at a particular site found in three or more tumor samples. The mutations include missense mutation, nonsense mutation (*), and synonymous mutation (–). Data were from COSMIC database. See detail information on Appendix 2. The proteins are shown with blue lines. The letters and numbers under the blue lines indicate the amino acid residual and its position. Each red arrow indicates the mutation site. The letter or symbol (*, -) beside the red arrow indicates the amino acid residual mutated to.

As shown in Figure 6, there are three recurrent mutations in PDS5B at G116, R289, and L999. Most of these point mutations are missense/non-synonymous mutations whose functional significance remains to be defined. These data suggest that Pds5B is a putative tumor suppressor and often lost in cancer cells (Denes *et al.*, 2010).

Phosphorylation of cohesin by protein kinases facilitates the removal of cohesin from sister chromatids at mitosis. Shugosins (Sgol1, Sgol2) are centromeric cohesin protectors, which collaborate with protein phosphatase 2A (PP2A) to remove the phosphorylation on the centromeric cohesins and to protect the cohesins from cleavage by Separase (Tanno *et al.*, 2010; Xu *et al.*, 2009). Sgol1 is frequently downregulated in human colorectal cancers, and its downregulation is believed to cause chromosomal instability (Iwaizumi *et al.*, 2009a). A tumor-derived SGOL1 variant SGOL1-P1 transcript that skips exon 3 and results in a protein terminating within exon 4 causes abnormal mitosis and unstable chromatid cohesion (Kahyo *et al.*, 2011). Although currently very few studies have been reported regarding the deregulation of Sgol2 in tumors, the finding that Sgol2 was mutated at Q857 in multiple tumor samples with both nonsense and missense mutations (Figure 6) warrants further investigation into the significance of these mutations in tumorigenesis.

Esco1 and Esco2 are evolutionary conserved cohesin acetyltransferases. Mutations on Esco2 is the only gene known to cause Roberts syndrome (RBS) (Vega *et al.*, 2010), a human congenital disorder. Absence of Esco2 significantly reduces the acetylation of Smc3 and results in severe chromosome segregation defects and apoptosis (Whelan *et al.*, 2012). The mutation site on Esco2 at P473 (Figure 6) resides between the C2H2 zinc finger domain (389-411aa) and acetyltransferase domain (534-597aa). Mutation at P473 might result in the change of structural configuration, which possibly affects Esco2's localization or enzymatic activity or both. Consequently, it can lead to abnormal acetylation of cohesin.

Nipbl/Scc2 is a subunit of cohesin loading complex (Table 1). Mutations in NIPBL and two cohesin core subunits SMC1A and SMC3 result in developmental disorders, which etiologically account for about two third of individuals with Cornelia de Lange syndrome (CdLS) (Liu & Krantz, 2009). Mutations of NIPBL has been suggested as a possible cause of chromosome instability in human colorectal cancers (Barber *et al.*, 2008b). It is interesting to note that a large number (38) of point mutations occurred at seven different sites concentrating mostly in the N- and C-terminus of Nipl1 protein in a variety of tumors including breast, kidney, ovary and large intestine cancers (Figure 6, Appendix 2). These mutations include three truncated mutations at R45, S861 and 1647, 25 missense mutations and 10 non-synonymous mutations. These mutations are not overlapped with those found in CdLS patients (Gillis *et al.*, 2004), suggesting they may be tumor specific. Tamoxifen is an antagonist of the estrogen receptor and plays a very important role in breast cancer therapies. Silencing of cohesin-related genes NIPBL, RAD21and SMC3 causes tamoxifen resistance in breast cancer (Mendes-Pereira *et al.*, 2012). Considering the transcriptional regulation of ER by cohesin complex (Prenzel *et al.*, 2012), downregulation of NIPBL and/or cohesin might be a mechanism for some breast tumors to develop tamoxifen resistance.

The mechanisms that lead to the deregulated expression of cohesin and its regulatory proteins in human cancer are unclear. The gene-copy number variations results from both gains and losses of cohesin gene are one possible mechanism that causes aberrant cohesin gene expression. Gains at the RAD21, STAG1, and NIPBL loci and losses of ESCO2 and SMC1B loci have been reported in breast cancer (Xu *et al.*, 2011a). A significant correlation between cohesin component RAD21 expression and DNA copy number has been observed in grade III invasive breast ductal carcinomas (Xu *et al.*, 2011b). Complete loss or truncated protein expression due to nonsense mutation, deletion, or insertion is also found in cancers (Solomon *et al.*, 2011) (Appendix 1, 2). In addition, abnormal regulation of cohesin genes at transcriptional levels would also contribute to the deregulation of cohesin expression, which has not been reported.

3   Conclusion and Perspective

More than twenty genes encode cohesin and its regulatory partners. Each gene can be altered in multiple ways, which results in cohesin deregulation. Cohesins play essential roles in sister chromatid cohesion and segregation, centrosome biogenesis, DNA replication, DDR, gene transcriptional regulation, apoptosis, chromosomal remodeling, etc. Therefore, deregulation of cohesin can have profound consequence on the fate of cells (Figure 7). Cohesin and its regulatory proteins are mutated in approximately 10% of human cancers. The mutated cohesin can function differently from the normal protein, which may differentiate the cancer cells from the normal cells. Whether cohesin deregulation is the cause or the consequence of cancer has not been well-defined, but cohesin deregulation provides a target for cancer therapy. For example, synthetic genetic screen demonstrates that Smc1, Rad21, and Scc2 containing mutations similar to those identified in human tumors require a penal of proteins to mediate the replication fork progression and stability in both *S. cerevisiae* and *C. elegans* (McLellan *et al.*, 2012).

This finding reveals that one of the therapeutically targets for these cohesin-deregulated cancers is the replication fork. In human cells, poly-ADP ribose polymerases (PARPs) are required to repair stalled replication forks. Indeed, PARP inhibitors benzamide and olaparib significantly reduced the viability of

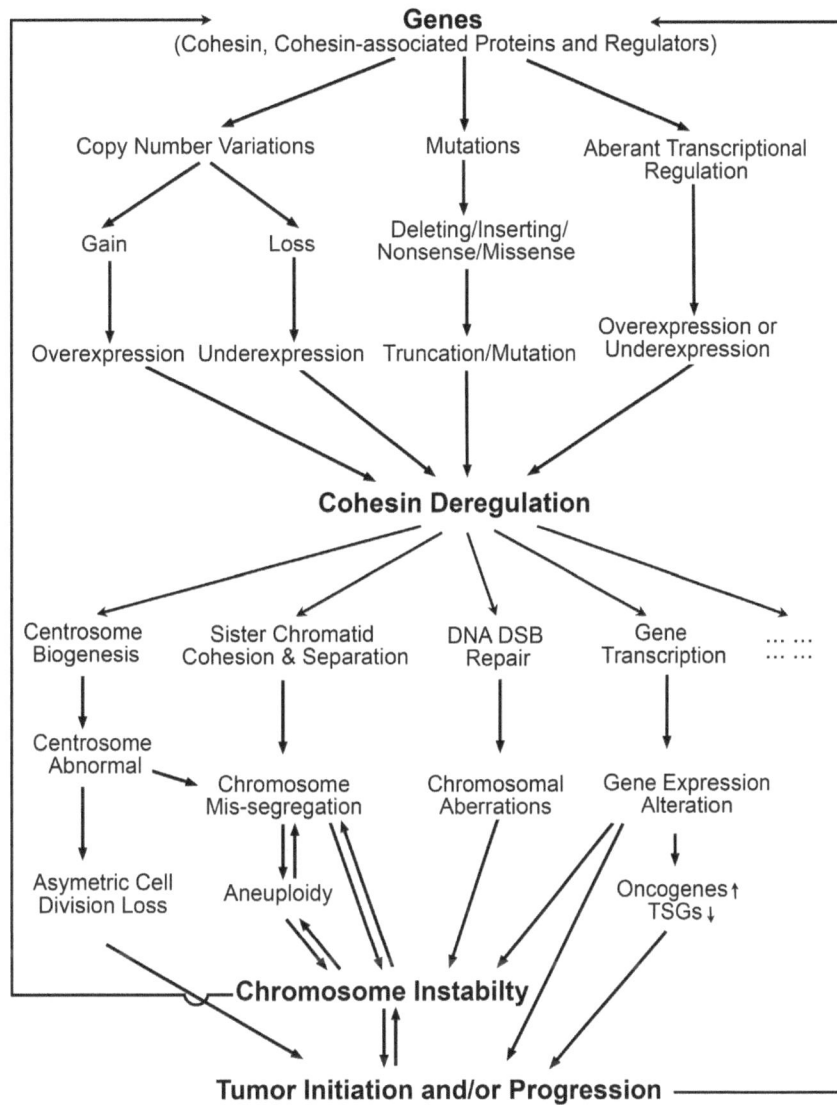

Figure 7: Pathways lead to cohesin deregulation and cancer. TSGs: tumor suppressor genes.

colon cancer-derived cell lines HT116 and HTB-38 in which cohesin subunit Rad21, Smc1, Smc3, SA1, SA2 or cohesin loading complex subunit Nipbl/Scc2 was depleted using siRNA (McLellan *et al.*, 2012).

Another example is that Pds5B interacts with Brca2, which is required for the normal response to DNA-damaging agents, the nuclear localization of RAD51 and BRCA2, and efficient homologous recombination (Brough *et al.*, 2012). Many cancers, including breast cancer, downregulate Pds5B expression. Disruption of Pds5B-Brca2 interaction due to downregulation of Pds5B provides an opportunity to treat the tumors with DNA-damaging chemotherapy. Clinical results show that in ER negative breast tumors, low Pds5B expression correlates with a statistically significant longer disease-free survival in patients treated with adjuvant DNA-damage drug anthracycline chemotherapy (Brough *et al.*, 2012). With decrease of the cost to sequence a whole genome and advance in understanding cohesin functions, identification of the deregulated cohesin genes and personalization of the therapy for each cancer patient become feasible.

Acknowledgement

We thank Dr. B. Lee Ligon at Baylor College of Medicine for editing this chapter.

Appendix

Protein / Gene	Mutation		Sample Name	Primary tissue	Histology	Zygosity	Somatic Status	Pumed ID
	Protein	cDNA						
RAD21	Q474*	1420C>T	TCGA-DC-6155-01	Large intestine	Carcinoma	Heterozygous	Reported	-
			NCI-H2009	Lung	Carcinoma	Heterozygous	Confirmed	-
	Q474R	1421A>G	TCGA-A6-6141-01	Large intestine	Carcinoma	Heterozygous	Unknown	-
			TCGA-F4-6570-01	Large intestine	Carcinoma	Heterozygous	Unknown	-
			TCGA-AZ-5403-01	Large intestine	Carcinoma	Heterozygous	Unknown	-
	Q474K	1420C>A	TCGA-EF-5830-01	Large intestine	Carcinoma	Heterozygous	Unknown	-
	Q474H	1422G>T	TCGA-CM-6674-01	Large intestine	Carcinoma	Heterozygous	Unknown	-
	E498G	1493A>G	TCGA-A6-6780-01	Large intestine	Carcinoma	Heterozygous	Unknown	-
	E498K	1492G>A	MZ7-mel	Skin	Malignant melanoma	Heterozygous	Confirmed	-
	E498E	1494A>G	TCGA-CM-6172-01	Large intestine	Carcinoma	Heterozygous	Unknown	-
SMC1A	T443A	1327A>G	TCGA-AA-3697-01	Large intestine	Carcinoma	Heterozygous	Unknown	-
	T443T	1329C>A	TCGA-AA-3713-01	Large intestine	Carcinoma	Heterozygous	Unknown	-
	T443T	1329C>T	TCGA-CM-5864-01	Large intestine	Carcinoma	Heterozygous	Unknown	-
	T443T	1329C>G	TCGA-25-1318-01	Ovary	Carcinoma	Heterozygous	Confirmed	21720365
	R626H	1877G>A	TCGA-24-1563-01	Ovary	Carcinoma	Heterozygous	Confirmed	21720365
			TCGA-AA-3713-01	Large intestine	Carcinoma	Heterozygous	Reported	-
			TCGA-AA-3662-01	Large intestine	Carcinoma	Heterozygous	Reported	-
	R711L	2132G>T	TCGA-AA-3673-01	Large intestine	Carcinoma	Unknown	Confirmed	22810696
	R711W	2131C>T	TCGA-AX-A2H5-01A-11D-A17D-09	Endometrium	Carcinoma	Unknown	Confirmed	-
			TCGA-A6-6780-01	Large intestine	Carcinoma	Heterozygous	Reported	-
SMC3	E343G	1028A>G	TCGA-A6-5661-01	Large intestine	Carcinoma	Heterozygous	Unknown	-
			TCGA-D5-6533-01	Large intestine	Carcinoma	Heterozygous	Unknown	-
			TCGA-AZ-5403-01	Large intestine	Carcinoma	Heterozygous	Unknown	-
	E343V	1028A>T	TCGA-24-1557-01	Ovary	Carcinoma	Heterozygous	Confirmed	21720365
	E343E	1029A>G	TCGA-G4-6588-01	Large intestine	Carcinoma	Heterozygous	Unknown	-
	G662C	1984G>T	H_GV-933124G-S_9043	Hematopoietic & lymphoid tissue	Hematopoietic neoplasm	Unknown	Confirmed	22237025
			933124	Hematopoietic & lymphoid tissue	Hematopoietic neoplasm	Unknown	Confirmed	22237025
			TCGA-AB-2993-03	Hematopoietic & lymphoid tissue	Hematopoietic neoplasm	Unknown	Confirmed	-
SA1/ STAG1	R51Q	152G>A	TCGA-25-1321-01	Ovary	Carcinoma	Heterozygous	Confirmed	21720365
	R51L	152G>T	TCGA-CM-6168-01	Large intestine	Carcinoma	Heterozygous	Unknown	-
	R51R	151C>A	TCGA-F4-6856-01	Large intestine	Carcinoma	Heterozygous	Unknown	-
	A116T	346G>A	LUAD-RT-S01702	Lung	Carcinoma	Unknown	Reported	22980975
			ESO-717	Oesophagus	Carcinoma	Unknown	Reported	23525077
			TCGA-AA-3518-01	Large intestine	Carcinoma	Unknown	Confirmed	-
	R958H	2873G>A	TCGA-A5-A0VQ-01A-11D-A10B-09	Endometrium	Carcinoma	Unknown	Confirmed	-
	R958C	2872C>T	TCGA-E2-A15O-01A-11D-A10Y-09	Breast	Carcinoma	Heterozygous	Reported	-
	R958C	2872C>T	TCGA-AG-A002-01	Large intestine	Carcinoma	Unknown	Confirmed	-
	R184W	550C>T	TCGA-20-0990-01	Ovary	Carcinoma	Heterozygous	Confirmed	21720365
	R184Q	551G>A	TCGA-AA-3496-01	Large intestine	Carcinoma	Heterozygous	Unknown	-
	R184L	551G>T	TCGA-CK-4948-01	Large intestine	Carcinoma	Heterozygous	Unknown	-

Protein/Gene	Protein	cDNA	Sample Name	Primary tissue	Histology	Zygosity	Somatic Status	Pumed ID
	R252Q	755G>A	ME002T	Skin	Malignant melanoma	Unknown	Unknown	22622578
			ESO-0176	Oesophagus	Carcinoma	Unknown	Unknown	23525077
			TCGA-E9-A1R0-01A-22D-A16D-09	Breast	Carcinoma	Heterozygous	Unknown	-
	R259*	775C>T	MD-144	Central nervous system	Primitive neuroectodermal tumour-medulloblastoma	Unknown	Confirmed	22820256
			MB_Exm17	Central nervous system	Primitive neuroectodermal tumour-medulloblastoma	Unknown	Reported	22832583
			MB_Exm17	Central nervous system	Primitive neuroectodermal tumour-medulloblastoma	Homozygous	Reported	-
SA2/STAG2	R305R	913C>A	TCGA-24-1563-01	Ovary	Carcinoma	Heterozygous	Confirmed	21720365
			TCGA-DM-A1DB-01	Large intestine	Carcinoma	Heterozygous	Reported	-
	R305L	914G>T	B89-4	Urinary tract	Carcinoma	Unknown	Confirmed	21822268
	R370W	1108C>T	LNCaP	Prostate	Carcinoma	Unknown	Confirmed	22722839
			TCGA-FD-A3NA-01A-11D-A21A-08	Urinary tract	Carcinoma	Unknown	Reported	-
	R370G	1108C>G	WA32	Prostate	Carcinoma	Unknown	Confirmed	22722839
	Y479S	1436A>C	CP66-MEL	Skin	Malignant melanoma	Homozygous	Confirmed	-
	Y479C	1436A>G	TCGA-G4-6317-01	Large intestine	Carcinoma	Heterozygous	Unknown	-
			TCGA-CM-6678-01	Large intestine	Carcinoma	Heterozygous	Unknown	-
	E721*	2161G>T	TCGA-A6-5666-01	Large intestine	Carcinoma	Heterozygous	Unknown	-
	E721E	2163A>G	TCGA-DY-A1DD-01	Large intestine	Carcinoma	Heterozygous	Unknown	-
			TCGA-G4-6586-01	Large intestine	Carcinoma	Heterozygous	Unknown	-
	E721V	2162A>T	TCGA-24-2267-01	Ovary	Carcinoma	Heterozygous	Confirmed	21720365
SA2/STAG2 (continued)	R1012*	3034C>T	MDS-19	Hematopoietic & lymphoid tissue	Hematopoietic neoplasm	Unknown	Confirmed	21909114
			TCGA-CF-A3MI-01A-11D-A20D-08	Urinary tract	Carcinoma	Unknown	Reported	-
	R1012Q	3035G>A	TCGA-AA-3510-01	Large intestine	Carcinoma	Heterozygous	Unknown	-
	R1045Q	3134G>A	587222	Large intestine	Carcinoma	Unknown	Confirmed	22770943
	R1045*	3133C>T	TCGA-A7-A0CH-01A-21W-A019-09	Breast	Carcinoma	Heterozygous	Reported	-
			TCGA-AB-2978-03	Hematopoietic & lymphoid tissue	Hematopoietic neoplasm	Unknown	Confirmed	-

Appendix 1: Mutations on cohesin core subunits are found in three or more tumor samples. The mutations include missense mutation, nonsense mutation (*), and synonymous mutation. Data were from COSMIC database. Somatic Status indicates the information on whether the sample was reported to be Confirmed Somatic (Confirmed), Previously Reported (Reported) or Variant of Unknown Origin (Unknown).

Protein/Gene	Mutation		Sample Name	Primary tissue	Histology	Zygosity	Somatic Status	Pumed ID
	Protein	cDNA						
	G116E	347G>A	TCGA-AZ-6600-01	Large intestine	Carcinoma	Heterozygous	Unknown	-
	G116G	348G>T	TCGA-D5-6537-01	Large intestine	Carcinoma	Heterozygous	Unknown	-
		348G>A	TCGA-CM-6680-01	Large intestine	Carcinoma	Heterozygous	Unknown	-
			TCGA-AZ-6601-01	Large intestine	Carcinoma	Heterozygous	Unknown	-
	G116R	346G>A	TCGA-CK-6751-01	Large intestine	Carcinoma	Heterozygous	Unknown	-
			TCGA-CK-6751-01	Large intestine	Carcinoma	Heterozygous	Unknown	-
	G116W	346G>T	TCGA-AA-3496-01	Large intestine	Carcinoma	Heterozygous	Unknown	-
PDS5B	R289H	866G>A	DLBCL-PatientD	Haematopoietic and lymphoid tissue	Lymphoid neoplasm	Unknown	Confirmed	21796119
			587226	Large intestine	Carcinoma	Unknown	Confirmed	22770943
			TCGA-AA-3492-01	Large intestine	Carcinoma	Heterozygous	Reported	-
	L999F	2997G>T	TCGA-24-1464-01	Ovary	Carcinoma	Heterozygous	Confirmed	21720365
			TCGA-CA-5797-01	Large intestine	Carcinoma	Heterozygous	Reported	-
	L999L	2997G>A	TCGA-A6-5664-01	Large intestine	Carcinoma	Heterozygous	Unknown	-
	Q857E	2569C>G	TCGA-25-2409-01	Ovary	Carcinoma	Heterozygous	Confirmed	21720365
	Q857Q	2571A>G	TCGA-A6-5659-01	Large intestine	Carcinoma	Heterozygous	Unknown	-
SGOL2			TCGA-AH-6549-01	Large intestine	Carcinoma	Heterozygous	Unknown	-
			TCGA-G4-6628-01	Large intestine	Carcinoma	Heterozygous	Unknown	-
	Q857R	2570A>G	TCGA-G4-6307-01	Large intestine	Carcinoma	Heterozygous	Unknown	-
	Q857*	2569C>T	TCGA-CM-6675-01	Large intestine	Carcinoma	Heterozygous	Unknown	-
			TCGA-CK-6748-01	Large intestine	Carcinoma	Heterozygous	Unknown	-
ESCO2	P473P	1419A>G	TCGA-CM-6164-01	Large intestine	Carcinoma	Heterozygous	Unknown	-
			TCGA-CA-6717-01	Large intestine	Carcinoma	Heterozygous	Unknown	-
	P473Q	1418C>A	TCGA-CM-5349-01	Large intestine	Carcinoma	Heterozygous	Unknown	-

Gene	AA mutation	DNA mutation	Sample	Tissue	Histology	Zygosity	Somatic Status	PubMed
NIPBL	P473S	1417C>T	Br27P	Central nervous system	Glioma	Heterozygous	Confirmed	18772396
			TCGA-CL-5918-01	Large intestine	Carcinoma	Heterozygous	Reported	-
	P473T	1417C>A	TCGA-DC-5337-01	Large intestine	Carcinoma	Heterozygous	Unknown	-
	R45Q	134G>A	TCGA-AG-A002-01	Large intestine	Carcinoma	Unknown	Confirmed	
			TCGA-AZ-4315-01	Large intestine	Carcinoma	Heterozygous	Reported	
	R45*	133C>T	ESO-859	Oesophagus	Carcinoma	Unknown	Unknown	23525077
	N141K	423T>A	RC-2	Kidney	Carcinoma	Unknown	Unknown	22385958
			RC-3	Kidney	Carcinoma	Unknown	Unknown	22385958
			RC-4	Kidney	Carcinoma	Unknown	Unknown	22385958
			RC-5	Kidney	Carcinoma	Unknown	Unknown	22385958
			RC-7	Kidney	Carcinoma	Unknown	Unknown	22385958
			RC-8	Kidney	Carcinoma	Unknown	Unknown	22385958
			RC-9	Kidney	Carcinoma	Unknown	Unknown	22385958
			RC-10	Kidney	Carcinoma	Unknown	Unknown	22385958
			RC-12	Kidney	Carcinoma	Unknown	Unknown	22385958
			RC-16	Kidney	Carcinoma	Unknown	Unknown	22385958
			RC-18	Kidney	Carcinoma	Unknown	Unknown	22385958
			RC-19	Kidney	Carcinoma	Unknown	Unknown	22385958
	S861P	2581T>C	TCGA-A6-5659-01	Large intestine	Carcinoma	Heterozygous	Unknown	
	S861T	2581T>A	TCGA-D5-6920-01	Large intestine	Carcinoma	Heterozygous	Unknown	
	S861*	2582C>A	TCGA-13-1496-01	Ovary	Carcinoma	Heterozygous	Confirmed	21720365
		2582C>G	TCGA-CM-6162-01	Large intestine	Carcinoma	Heterozygous	Unknown	
	E1647E	4941A>G	TCGA-AA-3712-01	Large intestine	Carcinoma	Heterozygous	Unknown	
			TCGA-AZ-6605-01	Large intestine	Carcinoma	Heterozygous	Unknown	
			TCGA-EI-6507-01	Large intestine	Carcinoma	Heterozygous	Unknown	
			TCGA-DM-A1D7-01	Large intestine	Carcinoma	Heterozygous	Unknown	
			TCGA-CM-6678-01	Large intestine	Carcinoma	Heterozygous	Unknown	
	E1647K	4939G>A	HCC1008	Breast	Carcinoma	Heterozygous	Confirmed	16959974
	E1647*	4939G>T	TCGA-AZ-6601-01	Large intestine	Carcinoma	Heterozygous	Unknown	
	K1690E	5068A>G	TCGA-G4-6315-01	Large intestine	Carcinoma	Heterozygous	Unknown	
			TCGA-A6-5660-01	Large intestine	Carcinoma	Heterozygous	Unknown	
	K1690K	5070A>G	TCGA-CM-6168-01	Large intestine	Carcinoma	Heterozygous	Unknown	
	K1690R	5069A>G	TCGA-13-0924-01	Ovary	Carcinoma	Heterozygous	Confirmed	21720365
	Y1750C	5249A>G	TCGA-AZ-6600-01	Large intestine	Carcinoma	Heterozygous	Unknown	
	Y1750F	5249A>T	TCGA-DM-A28F-01	Large intestine	Carcinoma	Heterozygous	Unknown	
			TCGA-AA-3663-01	Large intestine	Carcinoma	Heterozygous	Unknown	
	Y1750H	5248T>C	TCGA-AZ-4616-01	Large intestine	Carcinoma	Heterozygous	Unknown	
	Y1750Y	5250T>C	PD2198a	Kidney	Carcinoma	Heterozygous	Confirmed	20054297
	T1918A	5752A>G	TCGA-13-1507-01	Ovary	Carcinoma	Heterozygous	Confirmed	21720365
			TCGA-D5-6539-01	Large intestine	Carcinoma	Heterozygous	Reported	
	T1918T	5754T>C	TCGA-DM-A28E-01	Large intestine	Carcinoma	Heterozygous	Unknown	
			TCGA-A6-6781-01	Large intestine	Carcinoma	Heterozygous	Unknown	

Appendix 2: Mutations on cohesin regulatory proteins are found in three or more tumor samples. The Data were from COSMIC database. The mutations include missense mutation, nonsense mutation (*), and synonymous mutation. Data were from COSMIC database. Somatic Status indicates the information on whether the sample was reported to be confirmed somatic (Confirmed), previously reported (Reported) or variant of unknown origin (Unknown).

References

Anderson, D. E., Losada, A., Erickson, H. P., & Hirano, T. (2002). Condensin and cohesin display different arm conformations with characteristic hinge angles. J Cell Biol, 156, 419-424.

Atienza, J. M., Roth, R. B., Rosette, C., Smylie, K. J., Kammerer, S., Rehbock, J., et al. (2005). Suppression of RAD21 gene expression decreases cell growth and enhances cytotoxicity of etoposide and bleomycin in human breast cancer cells. Mol Cancer Ther, 4, 361-368.

Barber, T. D., McManus, K., Yuen, K. W., Reis, M., Parmigiani, G., Shen, D., et al. (2008b). Chromatid cohesion defects may underlie chromosome instability in human colorectal cancers. Proc Natl Acad Sci U S A, 105, 3443-3448.

Barber, T. D., McManus, K., Yuen, K. W., Reis, M., Parmigiani, G., Shen, D., et al. (2008a). Chromatid cohesion defects may underlie chromosome instability in human colorectal cancers. Proc Natl Acad Sci U S A, 105, 3443-3448.

Beauchene, N. A., az-Martinez, L. A., Furniss, K., Hsu, W. S., Tsai, H. J., Chamberlain, C., et al. (2010). Rad21 is required for centrosome integrity in human cells independently of its role in chromosome cohesion. Cell Cycle, 9, 1774-1780.

Beckouet, F., Hu, B., Roig, M. B., Sutani, T., Komata, M., Uluocak, P., et al. (2010). An Smc3 acetylation cycle is essential for establishment of sister chromatid cohesion. Mol Cell, 39, 689-699.

Ben-Shahar, T. R., Heeger, S., Lehane, C., East, P., Flynn, H., Skehel, M., et al. (2008). Eco1-dependent cohesin acetylation during establishment of sister chromatid cohesion. Science, 321, 563-566.

Birkenbihl, R. P. & Subramani, S. (1992). Cloning and characterization of rad21 an essential gene of Schizosaccharomyces pombe involved in DNA double-strand-break repair. Nucleic Acids Res, 20, 6605-6611.

Borges, V., Lehane, C., Lopez-Serra, L., Flynn, H., Skehel, M., Rolef Ben-Shahar, T., et al. (2010). Hos1 deacetylates Smc3 to close the cohesin acetylation cycle. Mol Cell, 39, 677-688.

Brough, R., Bajrami, I., Vatcheva, R., Natrajan, R., Reis-Filho, J. S., Lord, C. J., et al. (2012). APRIN is a cell cycle specific BRCA2-interacting protein required for genome integrity and a predictor of outcome after chemotherapy in breast cancer. EMBO J, 31, 1160-1176.

Cancer Genome Atlas Research Network (2011). Integrated genomic analyses of ovarian carcinoma. Nature, 474, 609-615.

Canudas, S. & Smith, S. (2009). Differential regulation of telomere and centromere cohesion by the Scc3 homologues SA1 and SA2, respectively, in human cells. J Cell Biol, 187, 165-173.

Chien, R., Zeng, W., Kawauchi, S., Bender, M. A., Santos, R., Gregson, H. C., et al. (2011). Cohesin mediates chromatin interactions that regulate mammalian beta-globin expression. J Biol Chem, 286, 17870-17878.

Ciosk, R., Zachariae, W., Michaelis, C., Shevchenko, A., Mann, M., & Nasmyth, K. (1998). An ESP1/PDS1 complex regulates loss of sister chromatid cohesion at the metaphase to anaphase transition in yeast. Cell, 93, 1067-1076.

Darwiche, N., Freeman, L. A., & Strunnikov, A. (1999). Characterization of the components of the putative mammalian sister chromatid cohesion complex. Gene, 233, 39-47.

Deardorff, M. A., Bando, M., Nakato, R., Watrin, E., Itoh, T., Minamino, M., et al. (2012). HDAC8 mutations in Cornelia de Lange syndrome affect the cohesin acetylation cycle. Nature, 489, 313-317.

Denes, V., Pilichowska, M., Makarovskiy, A., Carpinito, G., & Geck, P. (2010). Loss of a cohesin-linked suppressor APRIN (Pds5b) disrupts stem cell programs in embryonal carcinoma: an emerging cohesin role in tumor suppression. Oncogene, 29, 3446-3452.

Ding, L., Ley, T. J., Larson, D. E., Miller, C. A., Koboldt, D. C., Welch, J. S., et al. (2012). Clonal evolution in relapsed acute myeloid leukaemia revealed by whole-genome sequencing. Nature, 481, 506-510.

Dorsett, D. (2011). Cohesin: genomic insights into controlling gene transcription and development. Curr Opin Genet Dev, 21, 199-206.

Dorsett, D., Eissenberg, J. C., Misulovin, Z., Martens, A., Redding, B., & McKim, K. (2005). Effects of sister chromatid cohesion proteins on cut gene expression during wing development in Drosophila. Development, 132, 4743-4753.

Dorsett, D. & Strom, L. (2012). The ancient and evolving roles of cohesin in gene expression and DNA repair. Curr Biol, 22, R240-R250.

Dreier, M. R., Bekier, M. E., & Taylor, W. R. (2011). Regulation of sororin by Cdk1-mediated phosphorylation. J Cell Sci, 124, 2976-2987.

Faure, A. J., Schmidt, D., Watt, S., Schwalie, P. C., Wilson, M. D., Xu, H., et al. (2012). Cohesin regulates tissue-specific expression by stabilizing highly occupied cis-regulatory modules. Genome Res, 22, 2163-2175.

Fay, A., Misulovin, Z., Li, J., Schaaf, C. A., Gause, M., Gilmour, D. S., et al. (2011). Cohesin selectively binds and regulates genes with paused RNA polymerase. Curr Biol, 21, 1624-1634.

Finn, K., Lowndes, N. F., & Grenon, M. (2012). Eukaryotic DNA damage checkpoint activation in response to double-strand breaks. Cell Mol Life Sci, 69, 1447-1473.

Geck, P., Maffini, M. V., Szelei, J., Sonnenschein, C., & Soto, A. M. (2000). Androgen-induced proliferative quiescence in prostate cancer cells: the role of AS3 as its mediator. Proc Natl Acad Sci U S A, 97, 10185-10190.

Geck, P., Szelei, J., Jimenez, J., Lin, T. M., Sonnenschein, C., & Soto, A. M. (1997). Expression of novel genes linked to the androgen-induced, proliferative shutoff in prostate cancer cells. J Steroid Biochem Mol Biol, 63, 211-218.

Gillis, L. A., McCallum, J., Kaur, M., Descipio, C., Yaeger, D., Mariani, A., et al. (2004). NIPBL mutational analysis in 120 individuals with Cornelia de Lange syndrome and evaluation of genotype-phenotype correlations. Am J Hum Genet, 75, 610-623.

Gimenez-Abian, J. F., az-Martinez, L. A., Beauchene, N. A., Hsu, W. S., Tsai, H. J., & Clarke, D. J. (2010). Determinants of Rad21 localization at the centrosome in human cells. Cell Cycle, 9, 1759-1763.

Gimenez-Abian, J. F., Sumara, I., Hirota, T., Hauf, S., Gerlich, D., de la, T. C., et al. (2004). Regulation of sister chromatid cohesion between chromosome arms. Curr Biol, 14, 1187-1193.

Glynn, E. F., Megee, P. C., Yu, H. G., Mistrot, C., Unal, E., Koshland, D. E., et al. (2004). Genome-wide mapping of the cohesin complex in the yeast Saccharomyces cerevisiae. PLoS Biol, 2, E259.

Gomes, N. P. & Espinosa, J. M. (2010). Gene-specific repression of the p53 target gene PUMA via intragenic CTCF-Cohesin binding. Genes Dev, 24, 1022-1034.

Gorr, I. H., Boos, D., & Stemmann, O. (2005). Mutual inhibition of separase and Cdk1 by two-step complex formation. Mol Cell, 19, 135-141.

Gorringe, K. L., Ramakrishna, M., Williams, L. H., Sridhar, A., Boyle, S. E., Bearfoot, J. L., et al. (2009). Are there any more ovarian tumor suppressor genes? A new perspective using ultra high-resolution copy number and loss of heterozygosity analysis. Genes Chromosomes Cancer, 48, 931-942.

Graumann, P. L. & Knust, T. (2009). Dynamics of the bacterial SMC complex and SMC-like proteins involved in DNA repair. Chromosome Res, 17, 265-275.

Gruber, S., Haering, C. H., & Nasmyth, K. (2003). Chromosomal cohesin forms a ring. Cell, 112, 765-777.

Guacci, V., Koshland, D., & Strunnikov, A. (1997). A direct link between sister chromatid cohesion and chromosome condensation revealed through the analysis of MCD1 in S. cerevisiae. Cell, 91, 47-57.

Guan, J., Ekwurtzel, E., Kvist, U., & Yuan, L. (2008). Cohesin protein SMC1 is a centrosomal protein. Biochem Biophys Res Commun, 372, 761-764.

Hadjur, S., Williams, L. M., Ryan, N. K., Cobb, B. S., Sexton, T., Fraser, P., et al. (2009). Cohesins form chromosomal cis-interactions at the developmentally regulated IFNG locus. Nature, 460, 410-413.

Haering, C. H., Lowe, J., Hochwagen, A., & Nasmyth, K. (2002). Molecular architecture of SMC proteins and the yeast cohesin complex. Mol Cell, 9, 773-788.

Haering, C. H. & Nasmyth, K. (2003). Building and breaking bridges between sister chromatids. Bioessays, 25, 1178-1191.

Hagemann, C., Weigelin, B., Schommer, S., Schulze, M., Al-Jomah, N., Anacker, J., et al. (2011). The cohesin-interacting protein, precocious dissociation of sisters 5A/sister chromatid cohesion protein 112, is up-regulated in human astrocytic tumors. Int J Mol Med, 27, 39-51.

Hagstrom, K. A. & Meyer, B. J. (2003). Condensin and cohesin: more than chromosome compactor and glue. Nat Rev Genet, 4, 520-534.

Hauf, S., Waizenegger, I. C., & Peters, J. M. (2001). Cohesin cleavage by separase required for anaphase and cytokinesis in human cells. Science, 293, 1320-1323.

Heidinger-Pauli, J. M., Mert, O., Davenport, C., Guacci, V., & Koshland, D. (2010). Systematic reduction of cohesin differentially affects chromosome segregation, condensation, and DNA repair. Curr Biol, 20, 957-963.

Heidinger-Pauli, J. M., Unal, E., Guacci, V., & Koshland, D. (2008). The kleisin subunit of cohesin dictates damage-induced cohesion. Mol Cell, 31, 47-56.

Heidinger-Pauli, J. M., Unal, E., & Koshland, D. (2009). Distinct targets of the Eco1 acetyltransferase modulate cohesion in S phase and in response to DNA damage. Mol Cell, 34, 311-321.

Holland, A. J. & Taylor, S. S. (2006). Cyclin-B1-mediated inhibition of excess separase is required for timely chromosome disjunction. J Cell Sci, 119, 3325-3336.

Horsfield, J. A., Anagnostou, S. H., Hu, J. K., Cho, K. H., Geisler, R., Lieschke, G., et al. (2007). Cohesin-dependent regulation of Runx genes. Development, 134, 2639-2649.

Hou, F. & Zou, H. (2005). Two human orthologues of Eco1/Ctf7 acetyltransferases are both required for proper sister-chromatid cohesion. Mol Biol Cell, 16, 3908-3918.

Huang, C. E., Milutinovich, M., & Koshland, D. (2005). Rings, bracelet or snaps: fashionable alternatives for Smc complexes. Philos Trans R Soc Lond B Biol Sci, 360, 537-542.

Iwaizumi, M., Shinmura, K., Mori, H., Yamada, H., Suzuki, M., Kitayama, Y., et al. (2009b). Human Sgo1 downregulation leads to chromosomal instability in colorectal cancer. Gut, 58, 249-260.

Iwaizumi, M., Shinmura, K., Mori, H., Yamada, H., Suzuki, M., Kitayama, Y., et al. (2009a). Human Sgo1 downregulation leads to chromosomal instability in colorectal cancer. Gut, 58, 249-260.

Kagey, M. H., Newman, J. J., Bilodeau, S., Zhan, Y., Orlando, D. A., van Berkum, N. L., et al. (2010). Mediator and cohesin connect gene expression and chromatin architecture. Nature, 467, 430-435.

Kahyo, T., Iwaizumi, M., Shinmura, K., Matsuura, S., Nakamura, T., Watanabe, Y., et al. (2011). A novel tumor-derived SGOL1 variant causes abnormal mitosis and unstable chromatid cohesion. Oncogene, 30, 4453-4463.

Kawauchi, S., Calof, A. L., Santos, R., Lopez-Burks, M. E., Young, C. M., Hoang, M. P., et al. (2009). Multiple organ system defects and transcriptional dysregulation in the Nipbl(+/-) mouse, a model of Cornelia de Lange Syndrome. PLoS Genet, 5, e1000650.

Kim, B. J., Li, Y., Zhang, J., Xi, Y., Li, Y., Yang, T., et al. (2010). Genome-wide reinforcement of cohesin binding at pre-existing cohesin sites in response to ionizing radiation in human cells. J Biol Chem, 285, 22784-22792.

Kim, J. S., Krasieva, T. B., LaMorte, V., Taylor, A. M., & Yokomori, K. (2002a). Specific recruitment of human cohesin to laser-induced DNA damage. J Biol Chem, 277, 45149-45153.

Kim, M. S., An, C. H., Yoo, N. J., & Lee, S. H. (2013). Frameshift mutations of chromosome cohesion-related genes SGOL1 and PDS5B in gastric and colorectal cancers with high microsatellite instability. Hum Pathol, 44, 2234-2240.

Kim, M. S., Kim, S. S., Je, E. M., Yoo, N. J., & Lee, S. H. (2012). Mutational and expressional analyses of STAG2 gene in solid cancers. Neoplasma, 59, 524-529.

Kim, S. T., Xu, B., & Kastan, M. B. (2002b). Involvement of the cohesin protein, Smc1, in Atm-dependent and independent responses to DNA damage. Genes Dev, 16, 560-570.

Kitagawa, R., Bakkenist, C. J., McKinnon, P. J., & Kastan, M. B. (2004). Phosphorylation of SMC1 is a critical downstream event in the ATM-NBS1-BRCA1 pathway. Genes Dev, 18, 1423-1438.

Kogut, I., Wang, J., Guacci, V., Mistry, R. K., & Megee, P. C. (2009). The Scc2/Scc4 cohesin loader determines the distribution of cohesin on budding yeast chromosomes. Genes Dev, 23, 2345-2357.

Kon, A., Shih, L. Y., Minamino, M., Sanada, M., Shiraishi, Y., Nagata, Y., et al. (2013). Recurrent mutations in multiple components of the cohesin complex in myeloid neoplasms. Nat Genet, 45, 1232-1237.

Kong, X., Ball, A. R., Jr., Sonoda, E., Feng, J., Takeda, S., Fukagawa, T., et al. (2009). Cohesin associates with spindle poles in a mitosis-specific manner and functions in spindle assembly in vertebrate cells. Mol Biol Cell, 20, 1289-1301.

Krantz, I. D., McCallum, J., Descipio, C., Kaur, M., Gillis, L. A., Yaeger, D., et al. (2004). Cornelia de Lange syndrome is caused by mutations in NIPBL, the human homolog of Drosophila melanogaster Nipped-B. Nat Genet, 36, 631-635.

Kuriyama, R. & Borisy, G. G. (1981). Centriole cycle in Chinese hamster ovary cells as determined by whole-mount electron microscopy. J Cell Biol, 91, 814-821.

Lee, K. & Rhee, K. (2012). Separase-dependent cleavage of pericentrin B is necessary and sufficient for centriole disengagement during mitosis. Cell Cycle, 11, 2476-2485.

Lengronne, A., Katou, Y., Mori, S., Yokobayashi, S., Kelly, G. P., Itoh, T., et al. (2004). Cohesin relocation from sites of chromosomal loading to places of convergent transcription. Nature, 430, 573-578.

Lightfoot, J., Testori, S., Barroso, C., & Martinez-Perez, E. (2011). Loading of meiotic cohesin by SCC-2 is required for early processing of DSBs and for the DNA damage checkpoint. Curr Biol, 21, 1421-1430.

Liu, J. & Krantz, I. D. (2009). Cornelia de Lange syndrome, cohesin, and beyond. Clin Genet, 76, 303-314.

Liu, J., Zhang, Z., Bando, M., Itoh, T., Deardorff, M. A., Clark, D., et al. (2009). Transcriptional dysregulation in NIPBL and cohesin mutant human cells. PLoS Biol, 7, e1000119.

Losada, A., Yokochi, T., & Hirano, T. (2005). Functional contribution of Pds5 to cohesin-mediated cohesion in human cells and Xenopus egg extracts. J Cell Sci, 118, 2133-2141.

Losada, A., Yokochi, T., Kobayashi, R., & Hirano, T. (2000). Identification and characterization of SA/Scc3p subunits in the Xenopus and human cohesin complexes. J Cell Biol, 150, 405-416.

Lowe, J., Cordell, S. C., & van den, E. F. (2001). Crystal structure of the SMC head domain: an ABC ATPase with 900 residues antiparallel coiled-coil inserted. J Mol Biol, 306, 25-35.

Luo, H., Li, Y., Mu, J. J., Zhang, J., Tonaka, T., Hamamori, Y., et al. (2008). Regulation of intra-S phase checkpoint by ionizing radiation (IR)-dependent and IR-independent phosphorylation of SMC3. J Biol Chem, 283, 19176-19183.

Ma, Z., Lin, M., Li, K., Fu, Y., Liu, X., Yang, D., et al. (2013). Knocking down SMC1A inhibits growth and leads to G2/M arrest in human glioma cells. Int J Clin Exp Pathol, 6, 862-869.

Maffini, M. V., Geck, P., Powell, C. E., Sonnenschein, C., & Soto, A. M. (2002). Mechanism of androgen action on cell proliferation: AS3 protein as a mediator of proliferative arrest in the rat prostate. Endocrinology, 143, 2708-2714.

Matsuo, K., Ohsumi, K., Iwabuchi, M., Kawamata, T., Ono, Y., & Takahashi, M. (2012). Kendrin is a novel substrate for separase involved in the licensing of centriole duplication. Curr Biol, 22, 915-921.

McLellan, J. L., O'Neil, N. J., Barrett, I., Ferree, E., van Pel, D. M., Ushey, K., et al. (2012). Synthetic lethality of cohesins with PARPs and replication fork mediators. PLoS Genet, 8, e1002574.

Mendes-Pereira, A. M., Sims, D., Dexter, T., Fenwick, K., Assiotis, I., Kozarewa, I., et al. (2012). Genome-wide functional screen identifies a compendium of genes affecting sensitivity to tamoxifen. Proc Natl Acad Sci U S A, 109, 2730-2735.

Merkenschlager, M. & Odom, D. T. (2013). CTCF and cohesin: linking gene regulatory elements with their targets. Cell, 152, 1285-1297.

Michaelis, C., Ciosk, R., & Nasmyth, K. (1997). Cohesins: chromosomal proteins that prevent premature separation of sister chromatids. Cell, 91, 35-45.

Misulovin, Z., Schwartz, Y. B., Li, X. Y., Kahn, T. G., Gause, M., MacArthur, S., et al. (2008). Association of cohesin and Nipped-B with transcriptionally active regions of the Drosophila melanogaster genome. Chromosoma, 117, 89-102.

Nakamura, A., Arai, H., & Fujita, N. (2009). Centrosomal Aki1 and cohesin function in separase-regulated centriole disengagement. J Cell Biol, 187, 607-614.

Nasmyth, K. (2001). Disseminating the genome: joining, resolving, and separating sister chromatids during mitosis and meiosis. Annu Rev Genet, 35, 673-745.

Nasmyth, K. (2005). How might cohesin hold sister chromatids together? Philos Trans R Soc Lond B Biol Sci, 360, 483-496.

Nativio, R., Wendt, K. S., Ito, Y., Huddleston, J. E., Uribe-Lewis, S., Woodfine, K., et al. (2009). Cohesin is required for higher-order chromatin conformation at the imprinted IGF2-H19 locus. PLoS Genet, 5, e1000739.

Nishiyama, T., Ladurner, R., Schmitz, J., Kreidl, E., Schleiffer, A., Bhaskara, V., et al. (2010). Sororin mediates sister chromatid cohesion by antagonizing Wapl. Cell, 143, 737-749.

Ocampo-Hafalla, M. T., Katou, Y., Shirahige, K., & Uhlmann, F. (2007). Displacement and re-accumulation of centromeric cohesin during transient pre-anaphase centromere splitting. Chromosoma, 116, 531-544.

Panigrahi, A. K. & Pati, D. (2009). Road to the crossroads of life and death: Linking sister chromatid cohesion and separation to aneuploidy, apoptosis and cancer. Crit Rev Oncol Hematol, 72, 181-193.

Panizza, S., Tanaka, T., Hochwagen, A., Eisenhaber, F., & Nasmyth, K. (2000). Pds5 cooperates with cohesin in maintaining sister chromatid cohesion. Curr Biol, 10, 1557-1564.

Parelho, V., Hadjur, S., Spivakov, M., Leleu, M., Sauer, S., Gregson, H. C., et al. (2008). Cohesins functionally associate with CTCF on mammalian chromosome arms. Cell, 132, 422-433.

Pauli, A., Althoff, F., Oliveira, R. A., Heidmann, S., Schuldiner, O., Lehner, C. F., et al. (2008). Cell-type-specific TEV protease cleavage reveals cohesin functions in Drosophila neurons. Dev Cell, 14, 239-251.

Pauli, A., van Bemmel, J. G., Oliveira, R. A., Itoh, T., Shirahige, K., van, S. B., et al. (2010). A direct role for cohesin in gene regulation and ecdysone response in Drosophila salivary glands. Curr Biol, 20, 1787-1798.

Peterlin, B. M. & Price, D. H. (2006). Controlling the elongation phase of transcription with P-TEFb. Mol Cell, 23, 297-305.

Prenzel, T., Kramer, F., Bedi, U., Nagarajan, S., Beissbarth, T., & Johnsen, S. A. (2012). Cohesin is required for expression of the estrogen receptor-alpha (ESR1) gene. Epigenetics Chromatin, 5, 13.

Rankin, S., Ayad, N. G., & Kirschner, M. W. (2005). Sororin, a substrate of the anaphase-promoting complex, is required for sister chromatid cohesion in vertebrates. Mol Cell, 18, 185-200.

Remeseiro, S., Cuadrado, A., Carretero, M., Martinez, P., Drosopoulos, W. C., Canamero, M., et al. (2012a). Cohesin-SA1 deficiency drives aneuploidy and tumourigenesis in mice due to impaired replication of telomeres. EMBO J, 31, 2076-2089.

Remeseiro, S., Cuadrado, A., Gomez-Lopez, G., Pisano, D. G., & Losada, A. (2012b). A unique role of cohesin-SA1 in gene regulation and development. EMBO J, 31, 2090-2102.

Rhodes, J. M., Bentley, F. K., Print, C. G., Dorsett, D., Misulovin, Z., Dickinson, E. J., et al. (2010). Positive regulation of c-Myc by cohesin is direct, and evolutionarily conserved. Dev Biol, 344, 637-649.

Rocquain, J., Gelsi-Boyer, V., Adelaide, J., Murati, A., Carbuccia, N., Vey, N., et al. (2010). Alteration of cohesin genes in myeloid diseases. Am J Hematol, 85, 717-719.

Rollins, R. A., Korom, M., Aulner, N., Martens, A., & Dorsett, D. (2004). Drosophila nipped-B protein supports sister chromatid cohesion and opposes the stromalin/Scc3 cohesion factor to facilitate long-range activation of the cut gene. Mol Cell Biol, 24, 3100-3111.

Rollins, R. A., Morcillo, P., & Dorsett, D. (1999). Nipped-B, a Drosophila homologue of chromosomal adherins, participates in activation by remote enhancers in the cut and Ultrabithorax genes. Genetics, 152, 577-593.

Rothkamm, K., Kruger, I., Thompson, L. H., & Lobrich, M. (2003). Pathways of DNA double-strand break repair during the mammalian cell cycle. Mol Cell Biol, 23, 5706-5715.

Rowland, B. D., Roig, M. B., Nishino, T., Kurze, A., Uluocak, P., Mishra, A., et al. (2009). Building sister chromatid cohesion: smc3 acetylation counteracts an antiestablishment activity. Mol Cell, 33, 763-774.

Rubio, E. D., Reiss, D. J., Welcsh, P. L., Disteche, C. M., Filippova, G. N., Baliga, N. S., et al. (2008). CTCF physically links cohesin to chromatin. Proc Natl Acad Sci U S A, 105, 8309-8314.

Sancar, A., Lindsey-Boltz, L. A., Unsal-Kacmaz, K., & Linn, S. (2004). Molecular mechanisms of mammalian DNA repair and the DNA damage checkpoints. Annu Rev Biochem, 73, 39-85.

Schaaf, C. A., Kwak, H., Koenig, A., Misulovin, Z., Gohara, D. W., Watson, A., et al. (2013). Genome-wide control of RNA polymerase II activity by cohesin. PLoS Genet, 9, e1003382.

Schaaf, C. A., Misulovin, Z., Sahota, G., Siddiqui, A. M., Schwartz, Y. B., Kahn, T. G., et al. (2009). Regulation of the Drosophila Enhancer of split and invected-engrailed gene complexes by sister chromatid cohesion proteins. PLoS ONE, 4, e6202.

Schar, P., Fasi, M., & Jessberger, R. (2004). SMC1 coordinates DNA double-strand break repair pathways. Nucleic Acids Res, 32, 3921-3929.

Schmidt, D., Schwalie, P. C., Ross-Innes, C. S., Hurtado, A., Brown, G. D., Carroll, J. S., et al. (2010). A CTCF-independent role for cohesin in tissue-specific transcription. Genome Res, 20, 578-588.

Schmitz, J., Watrin, E., Lenart, P., Mechtler, K., & Peters, J. M. (2007). Sororin is required for stable binding of cohesin to chromatin and for sister chromatid cohesion in interphase. Curr Biol, 17, 630-636.

Schockel, L., Mockel, M., Mayer, B., Boos, D., & Stemmann, O. (2011). Cleavage of cohesin rings coordinates the separation of centrioles and chromatids. Nat Cell Biol, 13, 966-972.

Schuldiner, O., Berdnik, D., Levy, J. M., Wu, J. S., Luginbuhl, D., Gontang, A. C., et al. (2008). piggyBac-based mosaic screen identifies a postmitotic function for cohesin in regulating developmental axon pruning. Dev Cell, 14, 227-238.

Seitan, V. C., Hao, B., Tachibana-Konwalski, K., Lavagnolli, T., Mira-Bontenbal, H., Brown, K. E., et al. (2011). A role for cohesin in T-cell-receptor rearrangement and thymocyte differentiation. Nature, 476, 467-471.

Sjogren, C. & Nasmyth, K. (2001). Sister chromatid cohesion is required for postreplicative double-strand break repair in Saccharomyces cerevisiae. Curr Biol, 11, 991-995.

Solomon, D. A., Kim, T., az-Martinez, L. A., Fair, J., Elkahloun, A. G., Harris, B. T., et al. (2011). Mutational inactivation of STAG2 causes aneuploidy in human cancer. Science, 333, 1039-1043.

Sonoda, E., Matsusaka, T., Morrison, C., Vagnarelli, P., Hoshi, O., Ushiki, T., et al. (2001). Scc1/Rad21/Mcd1 is required for sister chromatid cohesion and kinetochore function in vertebrate cells. Dev Cell, 1, 759-770.

Stedman, W., Kang, H., Lin, S., Kissil, J. L., Bartolomei, M. S., & Lieberman, P. M. (2008). Cohesins localize with CTCF at the KSHV latency control region and at cellular c-myc and H19/Igf2 insulators. EMBO J, 27, 654-666.

Stemmann, O., Zou, H., Gerber, S. A., Gygi, S. P., & Kirschner, M. W. (2001). Dual inhibition of sister chromatid separation at metaphase. Cell, 107, 715-726.

Strom, L., Karlsson, C., Lindroos, H. B., Wedahl, S., Katou, Y., Shirahige, K., et al. (2007). Postreplicative formation of cohesion is required for repair and induced by a single DNA break. Science, 317, 242-245.

Strom, L., Lindroos, H. B., Shirahige, K., & Sjogren, C. (2004). Postreplicative recruitment of cohesin to double-strand breaks is required for DNA repair. Mol Cell, 16, 1003-1015.

Sumara, I., Vorlaufer, E., Gieffers, C., Peters, B. H., & Peters, J. M. (2000). Characterization of vertebrate cohesin complexes and their regulation in prophase. J Cell Biol, 151, 749-762.

Sumara, I., Vorlaufer, E., Stukenberg, P. T., Kelm, O., Redemann, N., Nigg, E. A., et al. (2002). The dissociation of cohesin from chromosomes in prophase is regulated by Polo-like kinase. Mol Cell, 9, 515-525.

Sutani, T., Kawaguchi, T., Kanno, R., Itoh, T., & Shirahige, K. (2009). Budding yeast Wpl1(Rad61)-Pds5 complex counteracts sister chromatid cohesion-establishing reaction. Curr Biol, 19, 492-497.

Tanno, Y., Kitajima, T. S., Honda, T., Ando, Y., Ishiguro, K., & Watanabe, Y. (2010). Phosphorylation of mammalian Sgo2 by Aurora B recruits PP2A and MCAK to centromeres. Genes Dev, 24, 2169-2179.

Thein, K. H., Kleylein-Sohn, J., Nigg, E. A., & Gruneberg, U. (2007). Astrin is required for the maintenance of sister chromatid cohesion and centrosome integrity. J Cell Biol, 178, 345-354.

Tonkin, E. T., Wang, T. J., Lisgo, S., Bamshad, M. J., & Strachan, T. (2004). NIPBL, encoding a homolog of fungal Scc2-type sister chromatid cohesion proteins and fly Nipped-B, is mutated in Cornelia de Lange syndrome. Nat Genet, 36, 636-641.

Tsou, M. F. & Stearns, T. (2006). Mechanism limiting centrosome duplication to once per cell cycle. Nature, 442, 947-951.

Tsou, M. F., Wang, W. J., George, K. A., Uryu, K., Stearns, T., & Jallepalli, P. V. (2009). Polo kinase and separase regulate the mitotic licensing of centriole duplication in human cells. Dev Cell, 17, 344-354.

Uhlmann, F. (2001). Chromosome cohesion and segregation in mitosis and meiosis. Curr Opin Cell Biol, 13, 754-761.

Uhlmann, F., Lottspeich, F., & Nasmyth, K. (1999). Sister-chromatid separation at anaphase onset is promoted by cleavage of the cohesin subunit Scc1. Nature, 400, 37-42.

Uhlmann, F., Wernic, D., Poupart, M. A., Koonin, E. V., & Nasmyth, K. (2000). Cleavage of cohesin by the CD clan protease separin triggers anaphase in yeast. Cell, 103, 375-386.

Unal, E., Heidinger-Pauli, J. M., Kim, W., Guacci, V., Onn, I., Gygi, S. P., et al. (2008). A molecular determinant for the establishment of sister chromatid cohesion. Science, 321, 566-569.

Unal, E., Heidinger-Pauli, J. M., & Koshland, D. (2007). DNA double-strand breaks trigger genome-wide sister-chromatid cohesion through Eco1 (Ctf7). Science, 317, 245-248.

Unal, E., rbel-Eden, A., Sattler, U., Shroff, R., Lichten, M., Haber, J. E., et al. (2004). DNA damage response pathway uses histone modification to assemble a double-strand break-specific cohesin domain. Mol Cell, 16, 991-1002.

Vass, S., Cotterill, S., Valdeolmillos, A. M., Barbero, J. L., Lin, E., Warren, W. D., et al. (2003). Depletion of drad21/scc1 in Drosophila cells leads to instability of the cohesin complex and disruption of mitotic progression. Curr Biol, 13, 208-218.

Vega, H., Trainer, A. H., Gordillo, M., Crosier, M., Kayserili, H., Skovby, F., et al. (2010). Phenotypic variability in 49 cases of ESCO2 mutations, including novel missense and codon deletion in the acetyltransferase domain, correlates with ESCO2 expression and establishes the clinical criteria for Roberts syndrome. J Med Genet, 47, 30-37.

Waizenegger, I. C., Hauf, S., Meinke, A., & Peters, J. M. (2000). Two distinct pathways remove mammalian cohesin from chromosome arms in prophase and from centromeres in anaphase. Cell, 103, 399-410.

Walter, M. J., Payton, J. E., Ries, R. E., Shannon, W. D., Deshmukh, H., Zhao, Y., et al. (2009). Acquired copy number alterations in adult acute myeloid leukemia genomes. Proc Natl Acad Sci U S A, 106, 12950-12955.

Wang, X., Yang, Y., Duan, Q., Jiang, N., Huang, Y., Darzynkiewicz, Z., et al. (2008). sSgo1, a major splice variant of Sgo1, functions in centriole cohesion where it is regulated by Plk1. Dev Cell, 14, 331-341.

Watanabe, Y. & Kitajima, T. S. (2005). Shugoshin protects cohesin complexes at centromeres. Philos Trans R Soc Lond B Biol Sci, 360, 515-21, discussion.

Watrin, E. & Peters, J. M. (2009). The cohesin complex is required for the DNA damage-induced G2/M checkpoint in mammalian cells. EMBO J, 28, 2625-2635.

Welch, J. S., Ley, T. J., Link, D. C., Miller, C. A., Larson, D. E., Koboldt, D. C., et al. (2012). The origin and evolution of mutations in acute myeloid leukemia. Cell, 150, 264-278.

Wendt, K. S., Yoshida, K., Itoh, T., Bando, M., Koch, B., Schirghuber, E., et al. (2008). Cohesin mediates transcriptional insulation by CCCTC-binding factor. Nature, 451, 796-801.

Whelan, G., Kreidl, E., Peters, J. M., & Eichele, G. (2012). The non-redundant function of cohesin acetyltransferase Esco2: some answers and new questions. Nucleus, 3, 330-334.

Xiong, B., Lu, S., & Gerton, J. L. (2010). Hos1 is a lysine deacetylase for the Smc3 subunit of cohesin. Curr Biol, 20, 1660-1665.

Xu, H., Tomaszewski, J. M., & McKay, M. J. (2011a). Can corruption of chromosome cohesion create a conduit to cancer? Nat Rev Cancer, 11, 199-210.

Xu, H., Yan, M., Patra, J., Natrajan, R., Yan, Y., Swagemakers, S., et al. (2011b). Enhanced RAD21 cohesin expression confers poor prognosis and resistance to chemotherapy in high grade luminal, basal and HER2 breast cancers. Breast Cancer Res, 13, R9.

Xu, Z., Cetin, B., Anger, M., Cho, U. S., Helmhart, W., Nasmyth, K., et al. (2009). Structure and function of the PP2A-shugoshin interaction. Mol Cell, 35, 426-441.

Yadav, S., Sehrawat, A., Eroglu, Z., Somlo, G., Hickey, R., Yadav, S., et al. (2013). Role of SMC1 in Overcoming Drug Resistance in Triple Negative Breast Cancer. PLoS ONE, 8, e64338.

Yamamoto, G., Irie, T., Aida, T., Nagoshi, Y., Tsuchiya, R., & Tachikawa, T. (2006). Correlation of invasion and metastasis of cancer cells, and expression of the RAD21 gene in oral squamous cell carcinoma. Virchows Arch, 448, 435-441.

Yazdi, P. T., Wang, Y., Zhao, S., Patel, N., Lee, E. Y., & Qin, J. (2002). SMC1 is a downstream effector in the ATM/NBS1 branch of the human S-phase checkpoint. Genes Dev, 16, 571-582.

Zhang, B., Chang, J., Fu, M., Huang, J., Kashyap, R., Salavaggione, E., et al. (2009). Dosage effects of cohesin regulatory factor PDS5 on mammalian development: implications for cohesinopathies. PLoS ONE, 4, e5232.

Zhang, B., Jain, S., Song, H., Fu, M., Heuckeroth, R. O., Erlich, J. M., et al. (2007). Mice lacking sister chromatid cohesion protein PDS5B exhibit developmental abnormalities reminiscent of Cornelia de Lange syndrome. Development, 134, 3191-3201.

Zhang, J., Shi, X., Li, Y., Kim, B. J., Jia, J., Huang, Z., et al. (2008a). Acetylation of Smc3 by Eco1 is required for S phase sister chromatid cohesion in both human and yeast. Mol Cell, 31, 143-151.

Zhang, N., Jiang, Y., Mao, Q., Demeler, B., Tao.Y.J., & Pati, D. (2013). Characterization of the interaction between the cohesin subunits Rad21 and SA1/2. PLoS ONE, 8, e69458.

Zhang, N., Kuznetsov, S. G., Sharan, S. K., Li, K., Rao, P. H., & Pati, D. (2008b). A handcuff model for the cohesin complex. J Cell Biol, 183, 1019-1031.

Zhang, N., Panigrahi, A. K., Mao, Q., & Pati, D. (2011). Interaction of Sororin with polo-like kinase 1 mediates the resolution of chromosomal arm cohesion. J Biol Chem, 286, 41826-41837.

Zhang, N. & Pati, D. (2009). Handcuff for sisters: a new model for sister chromatid cohesion. Cell Cycle, 8, 399-402.

Zhang, N. & Pati, D. (2012). Sororin is a master regulator of sister chromatid cohesion and separation. Cell Cycle, 11, 2073-2083.

Zhang, Y., Huang, X., Qi, J., Yan, C., Xu, X., Han, Y., et al. (2008c). Correlation of genomic and expression alterations of AS3 with esophageal squamous cell carcinoma. J Genet Genomics, 35, 267-271.

Zhou, X., Kong, X., Xu, W., & Chen, J. (2013). Overexpression of APRIN inhibits differentiation and proliferation and promotes apoptosis in P19 embryonal carcinoma cells. Mol Biol Rep, 40, 491-495.

Zou, H., McGarry, T. J., Bernal, T., & Kirschner, M. W. (1999). Identification of a vertebrate sister-chromatid separation inhibitor involved in transformation and tumorigenesis. Science, 285, 418-422.

Relevance of Molecular Biomarkers for Differential Diagnostics of Thyroid Cancer

Artūrs Ābols, Kristīne Ducena, Aija Linē
Latvian Biomedical Research and Study center
University of Latvia, Rīga, Latvia

Valdis Pīrāgs
Pauls Stradiņš Clinical University Hospital
University of Latvia, Rīga, Latvia

1   Diagnostics of Thyroid Cancer

Thyroid nodular disease is a common clinical finding. The prevalence of palpable nodules ranges from 3 to 7% in the general population, with an incidence of approximately 1 case in 1000 individuals per year (Gharib, Papini, & Paschke, 2008; Ries LAG, Melbert D, & Krapcho M, 2007; Parkin, Bray, Ferlay, & Pisani, 2005). Asymptomatic thyroid nodules are detected up to 65% on ultrasound and ~50% in pathologic examination of autopsy studies in North America. Although only less than 5% of the palpable nodules are malignant lesions, however thyroid cancers are the most common malignancy of endocrine organs.

The etiology of thyroid tumors is multifactorial, including environmental, genetic and endogen hormonal factors. Iodine deficiency is the major environmental factor, contributing the development of both endemic and sporadic nontoxic nodular goiter. The evidence of genetic predisposition is best established for medullary carcinoma and approximately 25% of these tumors are involved in multiple endocrine neoplasia syndromes: MEN 2A, MEN 2B and familial medullary carcinoma (FMTC).

Thyroid tumors may manifest in patients with well-known hereditary genetic syndromes like familial adenomatous polyposis (FAP) and Cowden disease and as well as in cases of rare genetic syndromes, including Carney complex, Werner syndrome, Peutz-Jegers syndrome and MEN1 syndrome (Charkes, 2006; Charkes, 1998).

The role of endogenous hormonal factors is based on evidence of significant prevalence of thyroid tumors in woman. Some studies have found that the increased risk of thyroid cancer is associated with use of estrogen containing oral hormonal contraceptives. This hypothesis is supported by the fact that estrogens interact with the mitogen-activated protein kinase (*MAPK*) signaling pathways which play a significant role in proliferation and differentiation of thyroid cancer (Chen, Vlantis, Zeng, & van Hasselt, 2008; Manole, Schildknecht, Gosnell, Adams, & Derwahl, 2001).

The examination of patient with newly discovered thyroid nodules starts with complete evaluation of the history of disease and the basic physical examination, including inspection of regional lymph nodes. The clinical risk factors indicating for thyroid malignancy include history of head and neck irradiation in the childhood, total body irradiation for bone marrow transplantation, family history of thyroid carcinoma or genetic syndromes, including Cowden's syndrome, Carney complex, familial polyposis, MEN 2 syndrome, Werner's syndrome, as well as exposure to ionizing radiation in childhood or adolescence and a rapid growth of a nodule. Physical symptoms suggesting for the thyroid malignancy include a firm consistence of a nodule, hoarseness, vocal cord paralysis, lateral cervical lymphadenopathy, fixation of the nodule to surrounding tissue (Gharib *et al.*, 2008; Hegedus, 2010).

1.1   Serum Thyrotropin Measurement

Serum thyrotropin (TSH) measurement is the most informative laboratory test. Patients with normal or elevated TSH level should undergo ultrasound imaging, but those with the suppressed TSH level additionally should perform radionucleotide scan, as it likely may be a signal of toxic adenoma *(Boelaert et al.*, 2006; Gharib *et al.*, 2008; Hegedus, 2010).

Several studies also show that TSH can serve as a thyroid tumor marker. For example, Bolaert and colleagues demonstrated that the risk of malignancy increases if the patient's TSH is >0,9 mIU/I. Binary regression analyses demonstrate that patients whose TSH is between 1,0 – 1,7 mIU/I have a greater risk to develop thyroid cancer than patients whose TSH is lower than 0,4 mIU/I, but the risk is even greater if the patient's TSH is between 1,8 – 5,5 mIU/I (Boelaert *et al.*, 2006).

However, some reports accent limitations of the use of TSH for malignancy risk evaluation. For example, patients with a nodular goiter referred for thyroid surgery do not represent the average population. It should be noted that the level of TSH differs among various racial and ethnic groups as well as during the aging process. For example, Caucasians show a higher overall concentration of TSH, while older people (>80 years) show a higher level of TSH compared with individuals aged 20 – 29. These data lead one to surmise that TSH *per se,* increases the possibility of tumor development in thyroid nodules as patients get older (Jin, Machekano, & McHenry, 2010).

1.2   Evaluation of Thyroid Nodules with Ultrasonography

High resolution ultrasonography (US) is the most commonly used imaging method for evaluation of thyroid nodules. US allow detecting small non palpable nodules, although the malignancy risk is the same comparing with the palpable nodules of the same size. Nearly 17-67% of randomly selected population has thyroid nodules at US and majority of them does not cause serious health problems (Hegedus, Bonnema, & Bennedbaek, 2003; AACE/AME, 2006; Hegedus, 2010).

Guideline accepted US features associated with thyroid malignancy include: microcalcifications, marked hypoechogenity, irregular or blurred margins, nodule taller than wide, absence of halo and increased intra-nodular vascularity (Frates *et al.*, 2005; Hoang, Lee, Lee, Johnson, & Farrell, 2007; Kim *et al.*, 2008; Peccin *et al.*, 2002).

Microcalcifications are psammoma bodies, ~10-100μm round laminar crystalline calcific deposits and in US they appear like punctuate hyperechoic foci without acoustic shadowing (Hoang *et al.*, 2007). It is the most specific US feature of malignancy, with a specificity of 85.8-95% and a positive predictive value of 41.8-94,2 in the large population studies. Microcalcifications are found in 29-59% of all primary thyroid carcinomas, mostly in the cases of papillary thyroid carcinoma (Frates *et al.*, 2005; Hong *et al.*, 2010; Kim *et al.*, 2008; AACE/AME, 2006).

Capelli C *et al.* analyzed US of 7445 nodules (diameter 6-100mm) from the period of 1991 till 2004 and verified that presence of microcalcifications is highly associated with the presence of thyroid cancer in surgery material comparing with the benign findings (72,2 vs. 28,7%, p<0,001). Coarse or macrocalcifications are more specific to benign thyroid nodules, especially with long duration of disease (Cappelli *et al.*, 2007), although can appear together with microcalcifications in papillary thyroid carcinomas, and more often in the cases of medullary thyroid tumors (Hoang *et al.*, 2007; Takashima *et al.*, 1995).

Marked hypoechogenicity of the nodule comparing with the surrounding normal thyroid parenchyma is very suggestive for malignancy. Malignant thyroid nodules typically appear like solid hypoechoic formations and combination of microcalcifications and marked hypoechogenicity have sensitivity as high as 87%, but low specificity (15.6%-27%) and positive predictive value for malignancy. In a large retrospective study Moon *et al.* analyzing more than 8000 patients, hypoechogenicity was found in 33, 7% of all benign nodules and 46,1% of malignant nodules (Moon *et al.*, 2008). Most of the studies emphasize that exactly marked hypoechogenicity is highly suggestive for malignancy than hypoechogenicity assessed comparing with surrounding thyroid tissue (Frates *et al.*, 2005; Hoang *et al.*, 2007; Kim *et al.*, 2008; AACE/AME, 2006).

Thyroid nodule is defined as irregular in the cases if >50 % of the border is not clearly demarcated. The average reported sensitivity for this US feature is very wide (7%-97%) and the specificity ranges from 15-59%. A large population study of Capelli *et al* demonstrated **irregular or blurred margins** in

52,8% cases of malignant nodules comparing with 18,8% of cases in benign ones (P<0,001) (Cappelli *et al.*, 2007).

Shape taller than a wide is also well-known US predictor of malignancy. Capelli *et al* found if a nodule with shape taller than wide (anteroposterior/transverse diameter ratio ≥1, A/T ≥1) together with two other specific US features (microcalcifications, blurred margins, hypoechoic pattern) is the best model for predicting malignancy. In this study A/T ≥1 was significantly more frequent in malignant lesion than in benign nodules (76% vs 40%, p<0,001), but the combination with another two US features demonstrates high diagnostic value (sensitivity of 99%, specificity 57%, PPV 6,0%, NPV 99%, missed carcinoma 0,9%) (Cappelli *et al.*, 2006; Cappelli *et al.*, 2005).

A halo zone is a hypoechoic rim around a thyroid nodule and is very characteristic to benign nodules with the specificity up to 95%, although 20-24% of all PTC have a partial or distinct halo zone (Frates *et al.*, 2005; Hoang *et al.*, 2007; Kim *et al.*, 2008; AACE/AME, 2006). Some studies emphasize, that halo is absent more than half of benign nodules (Hoang *et al.*, 2007; Propper, Skolnick, Weinstein, & Dekker, 1980).

Increased intranodular vascularity of the nodule, detected by using color Doppler, is well known predictor of thyroid malignancy comparing with benign nodules that present peripheral vascular pattern.(AACE/AME, 2006; Alexander, 2008; Frates *et al.*, 2005; Peccin *et al.*, 2002). Study of Frates *et al.* confirmed that solid hypervascular nodules possess higher malignancy risk (Frates, Benson, Doubilet, Cibas, & Marqusee, 2003). Also Papini *et al.* reported intranodal vascular pattern in 74,2% of malignant nodules and it serves as an individual risk factor (Papini *et al.*, 2002). Capelli *et al* found intranodal vascularity in 61.6% of malignant nodules and also associated it with increased cancer risk. In the opposite, completely vascular nodules rarely are malignant(Cappelli *et al.*, 2007).

Local invasion and lymph node metastases are highly specific to malignancy. Extracapsular invasion has been demonstrated in 36% of thyroid malignancies in postoperative histological analyses (Alexander, 2008; Hoang *et al.*, 2007; Papini *et al.*, 2002). It is known that differentiated thyroid carcinoma (mainly papillary) involves cervical lymph nodes in 20-50% of patients and may be present even when the primary tumor is small and intrathyroidal. Metastases in regional lymph nodes correlate with the further prognosis and recurrence of the disease (Frates *et al.*, 2005; Hoang *et al.*, 2007; Kim *et al.*, 2008; Peccin *et al.*, 2002; AACE/AME, 2006).

Some studies are aimed to evaluate US malignancy features especially for non-palpable nodules. Study of Papini *et al.* has evaluated the risk of malignancy of small non-palpable thyroid nodules with diameter 8-15mm and they found that cancer prevalence was similar both in nodules greater or smaller than 10mm (9.1 vs. 7.0%) This study demonstrated that significant majority of cancers appeared at US as hypoechoic structures (87% of cases) and the independent US risk features of malignancy in US were irregular or blurred margins (77,4%), increased intranodular vascularity (74,2%) and microcalcifications (29%) (Papini *et al.*, 2002). The study of Kim *et al* evaluated 1325 non-palpable thyroid nodules in 1009 patients from which FNA cytology revealed 823 benign, 154 indeterminate, 198 nondiagnostic and 150 malignant nodules. 58 malignant nodules and 82 benign nodules were included for the further analysis, were 3 radiologists analyzes the echogenity, shape, margins, calcifications, degree of cystic changes and the size of nodules. Results showed that marked hypoechogenicity, an irregular shape, a taller than shape, a well-defined speculated margin, microcalcification and entirely solid nature were significant predictors for malignancy (p<0,05), whereas a cutoff value of 1 cm in longest diameter was not significant (p<0,184) (Kim *et al.*, 2008).

US findings like size of nodule, interval growth of nodule and number of nodules are not helpful for predicting or excluding thyroid malignancy (Hoang *et al.*, 2007; Jun, Chow, & Jeffrey, 2005).

Considering that US is commonly used diagnostic tool for assessing thyroid malignancy, sensitivity, specificity, positive and negative predictive values ranges widely in reported studies. Park *et al* described average inter observer variability and concluded that the sensitivity, specificity, PPV and NPP were 65,3%-81,9%, 60,7%-68,9%, 69,7%-73,8% and 66,6-75,5%, respectively (Park *et al.*, 2010). Choi SH evaluated four radiologists with more than 5 years' experience in thyroid US, analyzing 204 thyroid nodules (89 benign and 115 malignant). Echogenity, calcifications, composition, margins, shape and vascularity were analyzed with the final assessment. Inter and intra-observer variability were detected with Cohen's kappa statistics and accuracy was calculated. Overall sensitivity, specificity, PPV, NPV and diagnostic accuracy were 88,2%, 78,7%, 76,2%, 98,6% and 82,8% for malignancy risk and conclusions were done with high accuracy in final assessment (Choi, Kim, Kwak, Kim, & Son, 2010). The study of Hong YJ evaluated the PPV of suspicious sonographic features and the results demonstrated that PPV for microcalcifications were 38,6%, for irregular margins 28,2%, for marked hypoechogenicity 49.4%, for nodule taller than wide 59,8% and concluded that three US features: microcalcifications, marked hypoechogenicity and a shape taller than wide are the best predictors of malignancy (Hong *et al.*, 2010). One of the reasons for wide inter-observer variability could be explained by fact that thyroid US is done by different specialists with different US experience. Interesting study of Kim at al reported inter-observer variability in the interpretation of US findings of thyroid nodules and authors concluded that final agreements between five academic faculty radiologists were fair-to-good, but poor-to-fair between four residents of radiology (Kim, Kwak, Kim, Choi, & Moon, 2012). Finally, although inter-observer variability can differ between studies, the majority of reported findings suggests that microcalcifications, irregular or blurred margins, marked hypoechogenicity, increased nodal vascularity and abnormal neck lymphadenopathy are associated with higher malignancy risk (Alexander, 2008; Choi *et al.*, 2010; Frates *et al.*, 2005; Hoang *et al.*, 2007; Hong *et al.*, 2010; Kim *et al.*, 2012; Kim *et al.*, 2008; Peccin *et al.*, 2002; AACE/AME, 2006).

1.3   Ultrasound Elastography

As mentioned above, palpation is a basic clinical examination method of thyroid nodules. Benign nodules are usually firm on physical examination; however malignant nodules turn to be much harder. Ultrasound elastography provides direct information corresponding to a hardness of nodule. It is a dynamic technique which estimates the tissue stiffness by measuring the degree of distortion under the application of external force and is based on the evidence that softer nodules have a greater elastic strain comparing with harder nodules of no strain. Using a numeric score system (graded 1-5), US elastography has been successfully used for differentiation benign nodules from malignant (Alexander, 2008; Rago, Santini, Scutari, Pinchera, & Vitti, 2007; Rago *et al.*, 2010). Study of Rago T *et al.* evaluated 92 patients who underwent thyroid surgery due to compressive symptoms of suspicion of malignancy on FNA cytology. The results showed scores 1 and 2 were found in 49 cases (all benign nodules), score 3 in 13 cases (12 benign, one malignant) and scores 4 and 5 in 30 cases (all carcinomas) with a conclusion that elasticity scores 4-5 were highly predictive for malignancy (p<0.0001) with a sensitivity of 97%, specificity of 100%, PPV of 100% and NPV of 98%. Another study of Rago T et al. included 176 patients with indeterminate or non-diagnostic cytology on FNA and a total of 195 nodules were evaluated and elasticity was scored as 1 (high), 2 (intermediate) and 3 (low). Results demonstrated that in indeterminate lesions, score 1 was highly associated with benign nodule (103 cases, 102 benign, 1 carcinoma, p<0.0001), score 2 was found in

14 cases (8 benign nodules and 6 carcinomas) and score 3 was found in 25 cases (1 benign, 24 carcinomas). In cases of non-diagnostic cytology, score 1 was found in 40 cases (39 benign lesions, 1 cancer), score 2 in four nodules (3 benign, 1 carcinoma) and score 3 in 9 nodules (six carcinomas, three benign nodules) with conclusion that US elastography is a useful tool in cases of indeterminate and non-diagnostic cytology for selecting candidates with potential need of thyroid surgery (Rago *et al.*, 2010). The study of Hong Y *et al.* included 90 patients with thyroid nodules who were referred for surgery and 145 nodules were evaluated by B-mode US, colour Doppler ultrasound and US elastography and tissue stiffness was scored from 1 (low stiffness) to 6 (high stiffness). Results showed that on real-time US elastography, 86 of 96 benign nodules (90%) had a score 1-3, while 43 of 49 malignant nodules (88%) had a score 4-6 (p<0.001), with sensitivity of 88%, specificity of 90%, a PPV of 81% and a NPV of 93% with conclusion that US elastography is a useful imaging technique for differential diagnosis of thyroid cancer (Hong *et al.*, 2009). As US beam is unable to cross calcified structures, the main limitations for US elastography are nodules having calcified shells or rims, partially or completely pure cystic nodules and in cases of multinodular goiter. Recently a new shear wave elastography (SWE) that estimates tissue stiffness in real time and user independent has been developed. The quantitative information is expressed as an elasticity index (EI) and expressed in kilopascal (kPa) on continuous scale without applying external force (Hegedus, 2010; Sebag *et al.*, 2010). The study of Sebag *et al* assessed the efficiency of SWE and compared it with high resolution US, evaluating 146 nodules from 93 patients, from those 29 nodules (19.9%) were malignant. Mean (±SD) EI was 150±95kPa in malignant nodules vs. 36±30 kPa in benign nodules (p<0.001), PPV 80%, sensitivity 85,2%, specificity 83.97%. Comparing with US score, reported sensitivity was 51.9%, specificity 97%, but in combination of US +SWE, sensitivity raised to 81%, specificity 97% (Sebag *et al.*, 2010).

In summary, although conventional US and US elastography are highly predictive, still all thyroid guidelines recommend to do FNA as universal agreement for assessing malignancy risk of thyroid nodules (Hegedus, 2010).

1.4   Cytological Evaluation of FNA

Fine-needle aspiration (FNA) currently is the most widely used preoperative method for evaluation of thyroid nodules. FNA is cost effective, minimally invasive and safe procedure, although it has limitations for certain types of tumors.

In October 2007, The National Cancer Institute (NCI) reviewed the algorithms for the use of FNA in the management of thyroid nodules and summarized the indications of FNA, pre-FNA requirements, diagnostic terminology, post FNA testing and treatment options (Baloch *et al.*, 2008; Kim *et al.*, 2008; Layfield, Cibas, Gharib, & Mandel, 2009).

FNA with following cytopathology is recommended for most of patients with normal or elevated TSH level and thyroid nodules>1-1,5 cm, detected by palpation or thyroid US, unless they are simple or separated cysts with no solid elements. The functioning thyroid nodules do not require FNA in the absence of significant clinical or US findings. The same indications for FNA are also related for incidentally found thyroid nodules. The American Association of Clinical Endocrinologists recommended FNA even for nodules smaller than 10mm for patients with suspicious clinical or US features of malignancy. Traditionally, one of the main indications for FNA was the presence of a solitary nodule (Baloch *et al.*, 2008; Kim *et al.*, 2008; Layfield *et al.*, 2009).

In the recent years, the large clinical observations indicate that patients with the multiple nodules have the same malignancy risk as a solitary nodule. It means that the presence of suspicious US features is the main indication for performing FNA, so all the nodules >1cm, with microcalcifications, marked hypoechogenity, irregular or microlobulated margins, intranodal vascularity, a shape taller than wide and extracapsular invasion should undergo FNA (Baloch *et al.*, 2008; Kim *et al.*, 2008; Layfield *et al.*, 2009).

Pre-FNA requirements include informed consent form and the discussion of procedure with patient, including the information about potential risks and complications (slight local pain and minor hematoma). The techniques for FNA are widely described in the literature. Traditionally, for US guided FNA the patient is placed in a supine position with the neck slightly extended. A local anesthesia with 1-2 ml of 1% lidocaine hydrochloride solution is injected at the predeterminate site of biopsy. Commonly available25-27 gauge needles are used together with injection syringe, with the exceptions of cysts with viscous contents when the larger needle sizes (22-23 gauges) are needed (Hamburger, Husain, Nishiyama, Nunez, & Solomon, 1989; Kelly *et al.*, 2006; Wang, 2006; Baloch *et al.*, 2008).

It is strongly recommended that aspiration should be performed at least twice from the suspicious nodule, each from the different area of the nodule. The FNA specimen is directly smeared on glass slides for air dried or alcohol fixed preparations, stained by Romanowsky or Papanicolaou techniques, respectively. Papanicolaou staining is the most commonly used for the cytological analysis, demonstrating the clearest description of nuclear changes of the thyroid cells (Baloch *et al.*, 2008; Hamburger *et al.*, 1989; Kelly *et al.*, 2006; Layfield *et al.*, 2009; Wang, 2006).

FNA sample is considered adequate for the interpretation, if the sample contains a minimum of 6 clusters of at least 10 follicular epithelial cells on two or more slides. Aspirates are considered as non-diagnostic, if the material is poorly fixed, prepared and stained or contains only cyst fluid or peripheral blood cells.

Different cytological classification systems are used in the clinical practice depending from the professional societies. The most commonly used is Bethesda System, containing of six following categories (Baloch *et al.*, 2008; Kim *et al.*, 2008; Layfield *et al.*, 2009):

- Benign – low risk of malignancy, <1%. The category includes adenomatoid nodules (with the variable amount of colloid or increased number of follicular epithelial cells), chronic lymphocytic thyroiditis, non-neoplastic nodular goiter.

- Atypia of undetermined significance (AUS) or follicular lesion of undetermined significance (FLUS), the risk of malignancy 5-15%. Very marked variability in use; the cytological findings are not convincingly benign, but the cellular atypia is insufficient for the diagnosis of malignancy. The main clinical dilemma: repeat FNA/clinical follow up or lobectomy.

- Follicular neoplasm or suspicious for follicular neoplasm (FN/SFN) and Hürtle cell neoplasm or suspicious for Hürtle cell neoplasm, low to intermediate risk of malignancy 20-30%. The majority of studies demonstrate that up to 20% of follicular neoplasms are found to be malignant in postoperative histology and risk of malignancy is >20% for Hürtle cell neoplasms.

- Suspicious for malignancy (SMN). The category mostly includes cases suspicious for papillary carcinoma and in the majority of cases (50-75%) follicular variant of PTC is founded. The category also applies to the cases suspicious for medullary carcinoma (cases when FNA sample is insufficient to perform confirmatory immunohistochemical staining for calcitonin), suspicious for other primary or secondary malignancies and suspicious for anaplastic carcinoma (total necrosis of lesion cells).

- Malignant. The FNA specimen confirms the diagnosis of papillary, medullary, anaplastic or metastatic carcinoma. This category is associated with the false –positive rate of less than 1%.

- Nondiagnostic or unsatisfactory. The FNA specimen of too few cells for diagnosis or is poorly fixed or contains excessive peripheral blood cells.

Despite high diagnostic accuracy of FNA, it has limitations, especially for diagnosis of follicular lesions. Currently a follicular adenoma cannot be distinguished from follicular carcinoma in FNA cytology and patients with follicular neoplasm still undergo diagnostic surgery for this reason (Alexander, 2008; Deveci, Deveci, LiVolsi, & Baloch, 2006; McHenry & Phitayakorn, 2011; Prasad *et al.*, 2005; Scognamiglio, Hyjek, Kao, & Chen, 2006; Bussolati, Gugliotta, Volante, Pace, & Papotti, 1997). The ratio of follicular adenoma to carcinoma in surgical specimens is approximately 5 to 1. The differential diagnosis of follicular adenoma usually includes dominant hyperplastic nodule, follicular carcinoma and encapsulated follicular variant of papillary carcinoma. The main histological difference is capsular or vascular invasion, however, a slight vascular invasion can be found in benign follicular tumors as well. In addition, both tumor types are characterized by various degrees of cellular atypia and vascular invasion and some studies report that minimally invasive follicular carcinoma is a less aggressive tumor with a similar risk of prognosis as benign follicular adenoma. Invasive follicular carcinoma has vascular invasion beyond the tumor capsule and it is associated with a worse prognosis. FNA cytology from patients both with follicular adenoma and follicular carcinoma reveals abundant follicular epithelial cells, microfollicle formation and typically very little or no colloid. A group of patients with follicular tumors have FNA cytology with follicular cells with abnormal architecture and atypia and according to the Bethesda classification system, they are categorized as „atypia of undetermined significance" or „follicular lesion of undetermined significance", with the 5-15% malignancy risk (Prasad *et al.*, 2005; Scognamiglio *et al.*, 2006; Serra & Asa, 2008; van Heerden *et al.*, 1992; Sanders & Silverman, 1998).

In addition, up to 30% of FNA is classified as indeterminate, but only 10-15 % of them prove to be malignant in post-operative histological evaluation and the large majority of patients with indeterminate or atypical cytology undergo thyroid surgery as a diagnostic procedure. The indeterminate categories include: Atypia of undeterminate significance/follicular lesion of undetermined significance (AUS/FLUS), follicular (Hurtle) neoplasms and cases suspicious for carcinoma. Some uncertainties still exist, concerning necessity to repeat FNA in indeterminate cases. Some centers suggest that a larger sample provides better analysis of cellular processes, while others debate that a benign finding in repeated aspiration may provide false assurance of benignity. AACE/AME guidelines consider surgical excision as the best management and argue that repeat biopsy is not helpful and even lead to confusion, while ATA guidelines suggest using molecular markers and a radioiodine scan, to exclude thyroid hyperfunction, in cases of suspicious cytology. Many controversies exist regarding the amount of surgery in indeterminate cases. AACE/AME guidelines recommend thyroid surgery, without specifying the extent or surgery, while ATA suggest lobectomy for a solitary indeterminate nodule, whereas ETA recommends lobectomy for solitary nodule and a near-total thyroidectomy for multinodular goiter (Alexander, 2008; Baloch, Sack, Yu, Livolsi, & Gupta, 1998).

In conclusion - cytological evaluation of FNA is currently the major diagnostic tool, however large proportion of patients with nodules with indeterminate cytology would benefit from the application of molecular biomarkers that could improve the diagnostic accuracy and would avoid unnecessary surgery.

2   Molecular Biomarkers of Thyroid Cancer

An ideal molecular biomarker or a panel of biomarkers should differentiate thyroid nodules into subtypes or at least discriminate benign from malignant nodule in any lesion that is considered as suspicious or indeterminate to improve thyroid cancer diagnosis and treatment. The assay should be reproducible, cost-effective and simple to apply. In past decades there has been a great effort to identify such molecular biomarkers that would meet these requirements. The development of the high throuput technologies have provided us with many new potential candidates that are very promising. Here we try to give an insight into the various types of molecular biomarkers, discuss their diagnostic value and the possibilities to exploit them as auxiliary biomarkers for improving FNA accuracy or serum biomarkers for developing non-invasive diagnostic tools (see Table 1).

2.1   Somatic Mutation Biomarkers

So far, the greatest attention has been paid to detecting the cancer-associated somatic mutations in FNA biopsies. One of the most studied somatic point mutation in thyroid cancer is *BRAF* (V-raf murine sarcoma viral oncogene homolog B1) V600E mutation that leads to the constitutive activation of *BRAF* kinase and stimulation of MAPK pathway that is tumorigenic for thyroid cells (Knauf *et al.*, 2005). This mutation is most common genetic alteration in PTC. *BRAF* V600E mutation is present in 40–50% of classical PTC tissues, 20–25% of FVPTC tissues but only 1,4% of FTC tissues (Chiosea *et al.*, 2009; Kebebew *et al.*, 2007). A number of investigators have evaluated a *BRAF* mutation analysis in FNA. For example, Jo and colleagues prospectively evaluated *BRAF* V600E mutational analysis in 101 patient thyroid nodule FNAB samples (43 benign, 30 malignant, 24 indeterminate or suspicious, 4 nondiagnostic) by applying pyrosequencing. Thyroidectomy was performed in 54 patients with malignant/indeterminate nodules. 22 malignant, 7 indeterminate nodules and one patient with a nondiagnostic nodule was *BRAF* positive. All *BRAF* positive nodules, including the one nondiagnostic and seven indeterminate nodules, were PTC on final histopathology, yielding a sensitivity, specificity and NPV for PTC of 75%, 100% and 85,9% respectively. However in different studies these data varies in sensitivity from 42 to 84%, in specificity 97-100% and in NPV 17,9 - 86% (Bentz, Miller, Holden, Rowe, & Bentz, 2009; Jo *et al.*, 2009; Kim *et al.*, 2008; Marchetti *et al.*, 2009; Nam *et al.*, 2010). These different results could be explained with different size of sample groups, sample heterogeneity and different methods that were applied to detect *BRAF* V600E mutation.

There is also data that mutations in *RAS* (Rat sarcoma) gene family (*H-RAS, N-RAS* and *K-RAS*) that stimulate both the MAPK and phosphatidylinositol-3-kinase (*PI3K*)/*Akt* pathways is found in 20-40% of thyroid cancer and mostly in FTC and FVPTC (follicular variant of papillary thyroid cancer) (Xing, 2010). However these mutations are also present in 20-40% of FA (follicular adenoma) and other benign nodules, but there is some evidence that *RAS* - mutated FA may be precursors of FTC (Alexander, 2008; Esapa, Johnson, Kendall-Taylor, Lennard, & Harris, 1999; Namba, Rubin, & Fagin, 1990).

The most common chromosomal rearrangements in thyroid cancer are the intrachromosomal rearrangements, *RET/PTC1* and *RET/PTC3*. Fusion of proto-oncogene *RET* with *RFG/ELE1* gene leads to the production of hybrid gene *RET/PTC* (Rearranged in Transformation/Papillary Thyroid Carcinomas) that encodes for tyrosine kinase with increased activity that also constitutively activates *MAPK* pathway. This translocation is present in approximately 50% of PTC and also in benign nodules, but its prevalence is highly variable due to genetic heterogeneity of population that differs between geographical location (Nikiforov, 2002; Tallini & Asa, 2001), so this marker alone cannot be used as marker for malignancy. In

Study design, substrate and sample size	Method	Biomarkers	Diagnostic value/outcome	Reference
Prospective analysis of 967 consecutive thyroid FNA samples (AUS/FLUS - 653, FN/SFN - 247, SMC - 67) from 729 patients. Histologically confirmed was 513 FNA samples (AUS/FLUS - 32 malignant; 184 - benign; FN/SFN - 58 malignant; 152 - benign; SMC - 28 malignant; 23 benign)	PCR assay	BRAF V600E, NRAS, HRAS, KRAS, RET/PTC1, RET/PTC3, PAX8/PPAR γ	AUS/FLUS Sn - 63%, Sp - 99%, PPV - 88%, NPV - 94%; FN/SFN Sn - 57%, Sp - 97%; PPV - 87%; NPV - 86%; SMC Sn - 68%, Sp - 96%, PPV - 95%; NPV - 72%.	(Nikiforov et al., 2011)
Prospective analysis of 156 FNAB samples from patients undergoing thyroidectomy and results were compared with the definite histological outcome comprising 7 FTC, 11 PTC, 40 FA, 53 adenomatous nodules, 45 surrounding normal thyroid tissues	qRT-PCR	ADM3/TFF3 and ADM3/ACTB	Distinction of FA and malignant follicular neoplasia with NPV - 94% and PPV - 86%.	(Karger et al., 2012)
Multicenter prospective analysis of 4812 FNA (577 were indeterminate) from 3789 patients involving 49 clinical sites as reference using results of blinded histopathological review from 413 resected nodules with indeterminate cytology. After sample inclusion criteria were met, gene expression panel where used to test 265 indeterminate nodules	Human exon microarrays	167 gene expression panel	Performance of the data set of indeterminate nodules where following: Sn - 92%; Sp - 52%; PPV - 47%; NPV - 93%.	(Alexander et al., 2012)
Testing of 7 microRNA panel in 62 FNAB samples. Based on cytological analysis 13 patients had operation (4malignant, 8 atypical cytology) and histopathological analysis revealed 8 malignant (7 PTC and 1 FTC) nodules and 5 hyperplastic nodules	qRT-PCR	miR-187, miR-221, miR-222, miR-146b, miR-155, miR-224, and miR-197	Overall performance of the data set resulted in 100% specificity, 94% sensitivity and accuracy of 95%.	(Nikiforova et al., 2008)
Four microRNA expression panel that where established in training set of 60 FNAB that had histopathological diagnosis and analyzed in 68 FNAB vali-	qRT-PCR	miRNA - 146b; 221; 187 and 30d	For the validation sample set authors obtained a diagnostic accuracy of 85,3%, sensitivity of 88.9%, specificity of 78,3%, PPV of 89%, and NPV	(Shen et al., 2012)

dation set (24 benign nodules and 44 malignant nodules (FVPTC=3; FTC=8; PTC=33).			of 78%. For the 30 atypia cases in the validation sample set they obtained a diagnostic accuracy of 73,3%, sensitivity of 63,6%, specificity of 78,9%, PPV of 64%, and NPV of 79%.	
Multicenter, prospective protein expression analysis in 150 FNAB with corresponding operation specimen for histopathological evaluation, where 42 % was AUS, FN, and SM-PTC.	ICC	CK19 and HBME-1	Results for indeterminate cytological cases favored malignant or benign disease with sensitivity, specificity, NPV and PPV of 100%, 85,2%, 100%, and 86,2%, respectively.	(Cochand-Priollet et al., 2011)
Circulating thyrotropin receptor which is derived from circulating thyroid cancer cells was measured by qRT-PCR from blood drawn preoperatively in 526 patients undergoing thyroid surgery, postoperatively in 418 patients undergoing differentiated thyroid cancer follow-up and in 151 patients monitored for known benign nodule	qRT-PCR	TSHR mRNA	Combination of diagnostic ultrasound, thyroid nodule FNA cytological diagnosis of follicular neoplasm and a TSHR mRNA diagnostic performance was: sensitivity of 97%; specificity of 88 %; PPV of 88% and NPV of 95% for predicting thyroid cancer.	(Milas et al., 2010)
Promoter methylation of 24 tumor suppressor genes in 11 - PTC, 2 - FTC, 5 normal thyroid and 3 hyperthyroid samples	MS-MLPA assay and MSP for NIS gene	CASP8, RASSF1and NIS	In the normal samples, CASP8, RASSF1 and NIS were methylated in 5/5, 4/5 and 1/5 respectively. In the hyperthyroid samples, CASP8, RASSF1 and NIS were methylated in 3/3, 2/3 and 1/3 respectively. In the thyroid cancers, CASP8, RASSF1, and NIS were methylated in 9/13, 10/13, and 7/13 respectively.	(Stephen et al., 2011)
3 identified in serum miRNA validation in 245 samples (106 patients with PTC, 95 patients with benign nodules and 44 healthy controls)	Serum miR-NA identification by Solexa followed by qRT-PCR validation	let-7e, miR-151-5p, miR-222	AUC of 0,917 (Sn - 87,8% and Sp - 88,4%) and an AUC of 0,897 (Sn - 86,8% and Sp - 79,5%) in separation the PTC group from the benign and healthy control groups.	(Yu et al., 2012)

Table 1: Recent studies investigating new biomarkers for differential diagnostics of thyroid nodules

contrast to *RET/PTC* rearrangement PAX8/PPAR gamma fusion results from an interchromosomal translocation where paired box 8 (*PAX8*) gene from chromosome 2q13 encoding a transcription factor that has a role in thyroid development, joins with the gene encoding peroxisome proliferator activated receptor γ (*PPARγ*) from chromosome 3p25, (Eberhardt, Grebe, McIver, & Reddi, 2010). *PAX8/PPARγ* is found in 30–40% of conventional-type follicular carcinomas and in a small fraction of follicular adenomas and occasionally in the follicular variant of papillary carcinoma (Nikiforova, Biddinger, Caudill, Kroll, & Nikiforov, 2002).

Initial studies centered mostly on the detection of a single mutation, while more recent studies have analyzed various combinations or panels of mutations (Cantara *et al.*, 2010; Ohori *et al.*, 2010). Non-overlapping constitutive activating mutations of *RET, RAS*, and *BRAF* - which are principle initiators of thyroid cancer by stimulating *MAPK* and (*PI3K*)/*Akt* pathways, and *PAX8/PPARγ* fusion are present in 70% of thyroid cancer (Bhaijee & Nikiforov, 2011)

Yuri E. Nikiforov and group in the end of 2011 published a research where they prospective analyzed *BRAF* V600E, *NRAS* codon 61, *HRAS* codon 61, and *KRAS* codons 12/13 point mutations and *RET/PTC1*, *RET/PTC3*, and *PAX8/PPARγ* rearrangements in 967 consecutive thyroid FNA samples (AUS/FLUS - 653 samples, FN/SFN - 247 samples, and SMC - 67 samples) from 729 patients, that to our knowledge is the biggest patient cohort with indeterminate cytology where somatic mutations were analyzed till now. The detection of any mutation in FNA sample conferred the risk of histologic malignancy. 479 patients underwent thyroidectomy, which provided a histopathological diagnosis for 513 FNA samples. Among the histologically confirmed 513 FNA samples (32 malignant and 184 benign nodules in the AUS/FLUS group; 58 malignant and 152 benign nodules in the FN/SFN group; 28 malignant and 23 benign nodules in the SMC group), 61 *RAS*, 17 *BRAF* V600E, one *RET/PTC*, and four *PAX8/PPARγ* mutations were identified. The correlation of mutational analysis in FNA samples and histopathological outcome in specific groups of indeterminate cytology was the following: AUS/FLUS Sn - 63%, Sp - 99%, PPV - 88%, NPV - 94%; FN/SFN Sn - 57%, Sp - 97%; PPV - 87%; NPV - 86%; SMC Sn - 68%, Sp - 96%, PPV - 95%; NPV - 72% (Nikiforov et al., 2011). This study shows that diagnostic panel of mutation is more accurate than single mutation diagnostic tests and can be successfully used for treatment decisions in cases with indeterminate FNA cytology.

2.2   Gene Expression Biomarkers

Gene expression profiling using cDNA microarrays or serial analysis of gene expression (SAGE) has revealed several hundreds of genes that are differentially expressed between malignant and benign thyroid nodules (Barden *et al.*, 2003; Finley, Arora, Zhu, Gallagher, & Fahey, III, 2004; Finley, Lubitz, Wei, Zhu, & Fahey, III, 2005). A number of them, including *LGALS3, FN1*(fibronectin1) and others that have been shown to be functionally involved in the carcinogenic process, have been validated by qRT-PCR and confirmed at protein level by immunohistochemistry (Alexander, 2008; Finley, Zhu, Barden, & Fahey, III, 2004; Jarzab *et al.*, 2005). However, several studies have demonstrated that none of these genes individually has sufficient sensitivity and specificity to be exploited as an independent diagnostic biomarker (Cerutti *et al.*, 2004; Cerutti *et al.*, 2007) and there is a great diversity of the results comparing individual genes between studies. Possible source of variability, especially in FNA samples, could be contributed to different number of thyroid follicular cells and adjacent cell population (for example red blood cells, lymphocytes and macrophages) in the sample, variability of RNA quality and the method for normalization of qRT-PCR data. One of the possible ways to acquire higher accuracy would be multiplexing the assay by including a panel of relevant genes. There are many reports which propose gene expression combinations for differential diagnostics of thyroid cancer, but only few of them has been confirmed by other scientists. However majority of these panels contain at least one of the three genes - *FN1*, *LGALS3* and *TFF3* that are often reported as differentiated expressed genes in thyroid cancer (da Silveira Mitteldorf, de Sousa-Canavez, Leite, Massumoto, & Camara-Lopes, 2011; Ducena *et al.*, 2011; Huang *et al.*, 2001; Takano, Miyauchi, Yoshida, Kuma, & Amino, 2005). For example, *FN1, GALE, MET* and *QPCT* are significantly overexpressed in PTC and can discriminate PTC in FNAB cases with indeterminate/suspicious cytology (da Silveira Mitteldorf *et al.*, 2011). *LGALS3* is statistically significant overexpressed in thyroid cancer, but *TFF3* expression is downregulated, and *TFF3* and *LGALS3* expression ratio could discriminate FTC from FA with 72,4% sensitivity and 83,3% specificity (or 80% and 91.5%, when the pathologically questionable cases were excluded) (Takano *et al.*, 2005) or malignant nodules from benign with sensitivity 72,7% and specificity 85,3% (Ducena *et al.*, 2011), but these combinations needs to be tested in FNAB.

Recently, a group from Germany in prospective study analyzed the expression of 6 genes (*ADM3/HGD1/LGALS3/PLAB/TFF3/TG*) in 156 FNAB samples from patients undergoing thyroidectomy by applying qRT-PCR (Karger *et al.*, 2012). The results of molecular diagnostics were compared with the definite histological outcome comprising 7 FTC, 11 PTC, 40 FA, 53 adenomatous nodules and 45 surrounding normal thyroid tissues. Significant expression differences were found for *TFF3, HGD1, ADM3* and *LGALS3* in FNAB of thyroid cancer compared with benign thyroid nodules and normal thyroid. Two FNAB marker gene combinations *ADM3/TFF3* and *ADM3/ACTB* allowed the distinction of FA and malignant follicular neoplasia with NPV up to 94% and PPV up to 86%. There were previously reported that these six gene combination per sample allowed correct prediction of benign nodule in 150 thyroid nodule operation specimen (20 FTC, 20 PTC, 6 AC, 52 benign thyroid nodules, and 52 normal thyroid tissues) with sensitivity of 91%, a specificity of 100%, PPV of 100% and NPV of 94% (Karger *et al.*, 2012; Krause *et al.*, 2008). The authors of the study proposed these promising biomarker combinations for multicenter FNAB studies to improve FNAB especially in FTC and FVPTC cases, which is almost impossible to differentiate from FA in cytological evaluation of FNAB.

Alexander EK *et al* recently reported a large, prospective multicenter validation study of a gene expression classifier developed by *Veracyte*. In this study, the classifier, which is based on the measurement of the expression levels of 167 genes, was applied to classify 265 indeterminate FNA biopsies. These specimens were selected from 4812 fine-needle aspirates collected at 49 clinical sites and had corresponding histopathological specimens that were subjected to central, blinded review. The gene expression classifier correctly identified 78 of the 85 malignant samples and 93 of the 180 benign samples, yielding a: Sn - 92%; Sp - 52%; PPV - 47%; NPV - 93%. Due to the very high negative predictive value, the classifier is best suited to identify benign, rather than malignant nodules. 7 malignant samples (6 PTC, 1 Hürthle cell carcinoma) were misclassified as benign. The authors showed that all 6 PTC samples had error in sample collection or cellular heterogeneity of the nodule because there was low follicular cell content. In conclusion the authors summarize that this gene expression panel can be used to identify subpopulation of patients with low risk of cancer in a population of patients that otherwise had an operation because of the indeterminate cytology in FNAB (Alexander *et al.*, 2012; Chudova *et al.*, 2010).

2.3   miRNA as Biomarkers

MicroRNA (miRNA or miR) are small ~22 nucleotides long non-coding RNA that regulates gene expression usually on posttranscriptional level by binding mRNA 3' UTR which leads to transcriptional repression or mRNA degradation. One miRNA can regulates even several hundreds of protein coding genes and one protein coding gene can be targeted by several microRNAs. They are involved in all cell processes and can act as oncogenes or tumor-suppressor genes (Hussain, 2012). Deregulated microRNA have been reported almost in every type of thyroid cancer, moreover miRNA expression signature differs between thyroid nodule subtypes (Alexander, 2008; Nikiforova, Chiosea, & Nikiforov, 2009; Vriens *et al.*, 2012). Weber with group compared FTC and FA by miRNA microarray analysis and found that *microRNA-197* and *microRNA- 346* were differentially expressed between these two groups with a accuracy of 87% (Weber, Teresi, Broelsch, Frilling, & Eng, 2006). While *microRNA-146b; 221; 222* are significantly overexpressed in PTC compared to other thyroid cancer and nodule subtypes (p<0,02) (Chen, Kitabayashi, Zhou, Fahey, III, & Scognamiglio, 2008). *MicroRNA-146b; 221* overexpression and *microRNA-34b; 130b* down regulation correlates with PTC aggressiveness and can be used as prognostic biomarkers (Yip *et al.*, 2011). *MicroRNA-17-92* cluster that contains seven miRNAs (*microRNA-17-3p; 17-5p; 18a; 19a; 19b; 20a, and 92-1*) are overexpressed in AC cell lines and AC lesions compared to adjacent normal thyroid tissues and plays an important role in AC development and could be also a novel target for AC treatment (Takakura *et al.*, 2008). MicroRNA differs even between hereditary MTC and sporadic MTC, for example, *microRNA-183* and *375* are overexpressed (P=0.001; 0.031) and *microRNA-9** is under-expressed (P=0.011) in sporadic MTC versus hereditary MTC. Also overexpression of *microRNA-183 and 375* in MTC predicts lateral lymph node metastases (P=0.001; P=0.001) (Abraham *et al.*, 2011). While there is convincing evidence that microRNA expression signature clearly differs between thyroid nodule subtypes only a few studies till now have tested these microRNAs in FNAB. One of the first study, where seven microRNA (*microRNA-187; 221; 222; 146b; 155; 224; 197*) where tested in 62 FNAB samples was published in 2008. Based on cytological analysis 13 patients had operation (4malignant, 8 atypical cytology) and histopathological analysis revealed 8 malignant (7 PTC and 1 FTC) nodules and 5 hyperplastic nodules. These 7 microRNA were analyzed in all FNA samples without knowing the surgical pathology diagnosis for all samples. Among them all 8 malignant and one hyperplastic FNAB samples revealed more than 2-fold change overexpression of one to six microRNA. 46 of 49 samples from patients that didn't have operation revealed no up-regulation of any of these microRNA and overall performance of the data set resulted in 100% specificity, 94% sensitivity and accuracy of 95% (Nikiforova, Tseng, Steward, Diorio, & Nikiforov, 2008). In more recent study Rulong Shen established four microRNA expression panel (*microRNA - 146b; 221; 187* and *30d*) in training set of 60 FNAB that had histopathological diagnosis and tested it in 68 FNAB validation set (24 benign nodules and 44 malignant nodules - FVPTC=3; FTC=8; PTC=33). For the validation sample set they obtained a diagnostic accuracy of 85,3%, sensitivity of 88,9%, specificity of 78,3%, PPV of 89%, and NPV of 78%. For the 30 atypia cases in the validation sample set they obtained a diagnostic accuracy of 73,3%, sensitivity of 63,6%, specificity of 78,9%, PPV of 64%, and NPV of 79%, however the authors conclude that this microRNA expression panel is subject for inaccurate results in FTC in indeterminate FNAB cases (Shen *et al.*, 2012). These two studies show that microRNA amplification in FNAB samples is feasible and that *microRNA - 146b; 221; 187* can be potentially used in microRNA expression panel to identify PTC in FNAB with indeterminate cytology. Although promising as diagnostic markers further studies that include many more tumor or indeterminate FNA samples as well as different combinations of microRNA are needed.

2.4   Protein Based Biomarkers

Protein-based assays probably may have most practical potential for clinical use than PCR-based assays since most clinical laboratories are familiar with immunocytochemistry (ICC) (Griffith, Chiu, Gown,

Jones, & Wiseman, 2008). On the other hand, tremendous variability in specimen processing and interobserver interpretation of results often prevents easy and fast introduction of a protein marker into widespread clinical practice.

Till now the most studied immunohistochemistry panels include Galectin-3 (Gal-3), *HBME-1*, and *CK19* (Griffith, Chiu, Gown, Jones, & Wiseman, 2008; Saleh *et al.*, 2009). Gal-3 encoded by *LGALS3* gene is a carbohydrate-binding lectin with an affinity for galactosides. It has diverse functions that include cell growth and cycle regulation, tumorigenesis, and apoptosis (Liu & Rabinovich, 2005). It is one of the most studied yet controversial markers in thyroid malignancy (Bartolazzi *et al.*, 2008). One of the largest prospective multicenter studies was performed by the Italian Thyroid Cancer study group. Immunocytochemistry of Gal-3 in cellblocks of 544 patients with indeterminate cytology revealed sensitivity of 78% and specificity of 93%. However researchers concluded that although immunocytochemistry for Gal-3 could not replace FNA cytology, but it could serve as a complimentary method and/or be a part of a diagnostic panel (Bartolazzi *et al.*, 2008). Hector Battifora mesothelial cell (*HBME*)-1 monoclonal antibody recognizes an antigen on the microvilli of mesothelioma cells (Sheibani, Esteban, Bailey, Battifora, & Weiss, 1992). The same antigen has also been identified in well differentiated thyroid cancer. In several recently published studies in FNA samples with indeterminate or suspicious cytology *HBME-1* immunocytochemistry had a sensitivity of 79–87% and a specificity of 83–96% (Raggio *et al.*, 2010; Torregrossa *et al.*, 2010). *CK19* has been found to be upregulated in malignant thyroid cells. Positive *CK19* staining is present in FNA samples from PTC and has been found to be useful in differentiating suspicious thyroid cytological specimens (Khurana, Truong, LiVolsi, & Baloch, 2003). Recent was published a study where *CK19* and *HBME-1* was tested in 150 FNAB with corresponding operation specimen for histopathological evaluation, by applying liquid based cytology. ICC results were defined as non-contributory, favoring benign, favoring malignant, or indeterminate. In 48 cases ICC was helpful for discriminating benign nodules from malignant with cytology of AUS, FN, and SM-PTC (42% of these lesions). Six (4%) ICC results were false positive (rather malignant than benign) but none were false negative (rather benign than malignant). Results for indeterminate cytological cases favored malignant or benign disease with sensitivity, specificity, NPV and PPV of 100%, 85,2%, 100%, and 86,2%, respectively. In conclusions authors proposed that immunocytochemistry of thyroid FNA with CK 19 and HBME1 antibodies can reduce the false-positive and false-negative results of single morphological analyses thus improving diagnostic accuracy and reducing the need for surgical controls (Cochand-Priollet *et al.*, 2011).

2.5 Epigenetic Biomarkers

An increasing body of evidence suggests that epigenetic changes play important roles in thyroid tumor genesis, as a result of their effects on tumor-cell differentiation and proliferation. Epigenetic alterations are changes around a gene that alter gene expression without affecting the nucleotide sequence of the gene and play a fundamental role in the regulation of human gene expression. Two epigenetic mechanisms are commonly used by cells to regulate gene expression - DNA methylation and histone modifications (Bird, 2002; Yoo & Jones, 2006). Epigenetic changes in tumorpromoting, tumor-suppressor and thyroid-specific genes contribute to the deregulation of thyrocyte growth and different aspects of tumorigenesis, such as apoptosis, motility and invasiveness (Xing *et al.*, 2003). For example Xing with colleges showed that hypermethylation of *RAS* association domain family member 1 (*RASSF1*), a known tumor suppressor gene, are found in 75% (9 of 12) of FTC as well as in a smaller percentage of benign adenomas (44%), and PTC (20%), these data indicates that this epigenetic silencing possibly occurs early in thyroid tumorigenesis (Xing *et al.*, 2004).

In one of the most recent study Stephen and colleges examined aberrant promoter methylation in 24 tumor suppressor genes in 21 patient samples (11 - PTC, 2 - FTC, 5 normal thyroid and 3 hyperthyroid samples) by applying methylation specific multiplex ligation-dependent probe amplification (MS-MLPA) assay and in the *NIS* gene using methylation-specific PCR (MSP). The most frequently methylated genes were *CASP8* (17/21), *RASSF1* (16/21) and *NIS* (9/21), however these genes where methylated in the normal samples - 5/5, 4/5 and 1/5 respectively and in the hyperthyroid samples 3/3, 2/3 and 1/3 respectively. In the thyroid cancers *CASP8* was methylated in 9/13, *RASSF1* in 10/13 and *NIS* were methylated in 7/13. *CASP8, RASSF1* and *NIS* were also methylated in 3/11, 4/11 and 3/11 normal thyroid tissue matched with thyroid cancer cases. The authors conclude that aberrant methylation of *CASP8, RASSF1,* and *NIS* probably is an early change in thyroid tumorigenesis (Stephen *et al.*, 2011). However further confirmation and validation of these findings in larger patient cohorts and FNA is needed to support these gene methylations as early makers of thyroid tumorigenesis.

2.6   Peripheral Blood Biomarkers

All of the studies to identify pre-operative molecular biomarkers described above have been based on material obtained from thyroid nodule FNA. Another way to diagnose malignant nodule preoperatively is to identify thyroid cancer specific molecular biomarkers in blood. Since thyroglobulin, no new blood tests for differentiated thyroid cancer have been introduced into routine clinical practice. A unique analysis of follicular thyroid nodules in 2004 has been described based on blood sample collection and measurement of circulating thyrotropin receptor (*TSHR*) mRNA which is derived from circulating thyroid cancer cells (Chinnappa *et al.*, 2004). Recently there was published a study were *TSHR* mRNA was measured by qRT-PCR in blood drawn perioperatively in 526 patients undergoing thyroid surgery, postoperatively in 418 patients undergoing differentiated thyroid cancer follow-up and in 151 patients monitored for known benign nodule. In patients with malignant or suspicious cytology, preoperative evaluated *TSHR* mRNA had 96% of differentiated thyroid cancer diagnosed on histopathology, whereas 95% of patients with undetectable mRNA and benign thyroid sonography had benign nodules. Elevated *TSHR* mRNA levels became undetectable in all patients with differentiated thyroid cancer on the first postoperative day, except five patients who manifested persistent or recurrent cervical disease within the year. Authors report that utilizing a preoperative combination of diagnostic ultrasound, thyroid nodule FNA cytological diagnosis of follicular neoplasm and a *TSHR* mRNA diagnostic performance is sensitivity of 97%; specificity of 88 %; PPV of 88% and NPV of 95% for predicting thyroid cancer (Milas *et al.*, 2010). However, the above publications have occurred at a single institution and an expanded clinical experience from other institutions is needed to verify this algorithmic approach.

In recent years several studies have demonstrated that miRNAs are released into the blood from cancer cells and exist there in a remarkably stable form thus suggesting that circulating miRNA may be used as minimal-invasive biomarkers (Chen *et al.*, 2012; Mitchell *et al.*, 2008). Since that, numerous studies have attempted to identify cell-free miRNAs with the diagnostic relevance in the blood from patients with different types of cancer. However, to the best of our knowledge, only one of these studies was focused on the thyroid cancer. Yu and colleges from China have determined serum miRNA expression profiles using Solexa sequencing followed by qRT-PCR validation in 245 samples (106 patients with PTC, 95 patients with benign nodules and 44 healthy controls). A panel of miRNA was evaluated in the sera of patients with PTC or benign nodules. This resulted in the identification of three microRNAs (*let-7e, miR-151-5p, and miR-222*) whose expression levels were significantly increased in the sera from PTC patients relative to patients with benign nodules and healthy donors. Serum *let-7e, miR-151-5p, and miR-*

222 levels correlated with certain clinicopathological variables, such as nodal status, tumor size, multifocal lesion status and metastasis. Furthermore, this study showed that expression of serum *miR-151-5p* and *miR-222* in a subset of PTC patients decreased significantly after tumor excision (Yu *et al.*, 2012). Taken together, this study demonstrated the feasibility of detecting thyroid cancer-associated microRNAs in the blood of patients; however the diagnostic value of circulating microRNAs remains to be determined.

3   Conclusions

In summary, until now there were no diagnostic tools that could help the clinicians in decision-making and management of cytological indeterminate thyroid nodules. Currently, the first auxiliary biomarkers assays that can improve FNA accuracy are being introduced into some clinics and the experience gained by their exploitation will be helpful for improving the guidelines for the management of thyroid nodules. In parallel, a number of novel biomarkers with remarkably high sensitivity and specificity have been identified, however they have to undergo thorough validation in prospective, multi-centre studies before considering for the exploitation in routine clinical practice. So far, fewer studies have succeeded in the identification of reliable biomarkers in patients' blood. However, the discovery of cancer-associated miRNAs in the blood of patients with thyroid cancer give rise to new hope that profiling microRNAs in the serum might lead to the identification of microRNA profiles that could be exploited for the development of non-invasive diagnostic assays. Currently, some molecular test panels are available which can aid in the decision making process for the management in cytological indeterminate FNAB cases. However in near future prospective, multi - canter validation studies of these and new developed biomarker tests should help to clinician in decision making and treatment management of cytological indeterminate thyroid nodules. But still the potential introduction of molecular markers as an adjunct to cytology diagnosis needs to take in account for inter- and intraobserver differences in cytological diagnoses as well as differences in inter- and intraobserver pathological evaluation.

Acknowledgement

This work was supported by European Regional Development Fund 2010/0196/2DP/2.1.1.2./10/APIA/ VIAA/004.

Abbreviations

3' UTR - three prime untranslated region
AACE - American Association of Clinical Endocrinologists
AC - anaplastic thyroid cancer
ACTB - actin, beta
ADM3 - adrenomedullin 3
ATA - American Thyroid Association
AUC - Area Under the Curve
AUS - Atypia of undetermined significance

BRAF - V-raf murine sarcoma viral oncogene homolog B1

CASP8 - caspase 8

CK19 - cytokeratin-19

EI - elasticity index

ETA - European Thyroid Association

FA - follicular adenoma

FAP - familial adenomatous polyposis

FLUS - follicular lesion of undetermined significance

FMTC - familial medullary carcinoma

FN/SFN - follicular neoplasm or suspicious for follicular neoplasm

FN1 - fibronectin 1

FNA – fine-needle aspiration FNAB

FTC- follicular thyroid cancer

FVPTC - follicular variant of papillary thyroid cancer

GALE - UDP-galactose-4-epimerase

HBME-1- Hector Battifora mesothelial cell - 1

ICC - immunocytochemistry

LGALS3 - lectin, galactoside-binding, soluble, 3

MAPK - mitogen-activated protein kinase

MEN syndromes – multiple endocrine neoplasia syndromes

MET - hepatocyte growth factor receptor

miRNA or miR - microRNA

mRNS - messengerRNA11

MS-MLPA - methylation specific multiplex ligation-dependent probe amplification

MSP - methylation-specific PCR

MTC- medullary thyroid cancer

NCI - The National Cancer Institute

NIS - sodium/iodide symporter

NPV – negative predictive value

PAX8 - paired box 8

PLAB - growth differentiation factor 15

PPARγ - peroxisome proliferatoractivated receptor γ

PPV – positive predictive value

PTC – papillary thyroid cancer

QPCT - glutaminyl-peptide cyclotransferase

qRT-PCR - quantitive reverse transcription polymerase chain reaction

RAS - Rat sarcoma

RASSF1 - RAS association domain family member 1

RET/PTC - Rearranged in Transformation/Papillary Thyroid Carcinomas

SMN - Suspicious malignancy of nodule

Sn - Sensitivity

Sp - Specificity

SWE - shear wave elastography

TFF3 - trefoil factor 3

TG - thyroglobulin
TSH - Serum thyrotropin measurement
TSH – thyroid stimulating hormone
TSHR - thyrotropin receptor
US- ultrasonography

References

AACE/AME. (2006). Task Force on Thyroid Nodules: American Association of Clinical Endocrinologists and Associazione Medici Endocrinologi medical guidelines for clinical practice for the diagnosis and managment of thyroid nodules. Ref Type: Generic

Abraham, D., Jackson, N., Gundara, J. S., Zhao, J., Gill, A. J., Delbridge, L. et al. (2011). MicroRNA profiling of sporadic and hereditary medullary thyroid cancer identifies predictors of nodal metastasis, prognosis, and potential therapeutic targets. Clin.Cancer Res., 17, 4772-4781.

Alexander, E. K. (2008). Approach to the patient with a cytologically indeterminate thyroid nodule. J.Clin.Endocrinol.Metab, 93, 4175-4182.

Alexander, E. K., Kennedy, G. C., Baloch, Z. W., Cibas, E. S., Chudova, D., Diggans, J. et al. (2012). Preoperative diagnosis of benign thyroid nodules with indeterminate cytology. N.Engl.J.Med., 367, 705-715.

Baloch, Z. W., Cibas, E. S., Clark, D. P., Layfield, L. J., Ljung, B. M., Pitman, M. B. et al. (2008). The National Cancer Institute Thyroid fine needle aspiration state of the science conference: a summation. Cytojournal., 5, 6.

Baloch, Z. W., Sack, M. J., Yu, G. H., Livolsi, V. A., & Gupta, P. K. (1998). Fine-needle aspiration of thyroid: an institutional experience. Thyroid, 8, 565-569.

Barden, C. B., Shister, K. W., Zhu, B., Guiter, G., Greenblatt, D. Y., Zeiger, M. A. et al. (2003). Classification of follicular thyroid tumors by molecular signature: results of gene profiling. Clin.Cancer Res., 9, 1792-1800.

Bartolazzi, A., Orlandi, F., Saggiorato, E., Volante, M., Arecco, F., Rossetto, R. et al. (2008). Galectin-3-expression analysis in the surgical selection of follicular thyroid nodules with indeterminate fine-needle aspiration cytology: a prospective multicentre study. Lancet Oncol., 9, 543-549.

Bentz, B. G., Miller, B. T., Holden, J. A., Rowe, L. R., & Bentz, J. S. (2009). B-RAF V600E mutational analysis of fine needle aspirates correlates with diagnosis of thyroid nodules. Otolaryngol.Head Neck Surg., 140, 709-714.

Bhaijee, F. & Nikiforov, Y. E. (2011). Molecular analysis of thyroid tumors. Endocr.Pathol., 22, 126-133.

Bird, A. (2002). DNA methylation patterns and epigenetic memory. Genes Dev., 16, 6-21.

Boelaert, K., Horacek, J., Holder, R. L., Watkinson, J. C., Sheppard, M. C., & Franklyn, J. A. (2006). Serum thyrotropin concentration as a novel predictor of malignancy in thyroid nodules investigated by fine-needle aspiration. J.Clin.Endocrinol.Metab, 91, 4295-4301.

Bussolati, G., Gugliotta, P., Volante, M., Pace, M., & Papotti, M. (1997). Retrieved endogenous biotin: a novel marker and a potential pitfall in diagnostic immunohistochemistry. Histopathology, 31, 400-407.

Cantara, S., Capezzone, M., Marchisotta, S., Capuano, S., Busonero, G., Toti, P. et al. (2010). Impact of proto-oncogene mutation detection in cytological specimens from thyroid nodules improves the diagnostic accuracy of cytology. J.Clin.Endocrinol.Metab, 95, 1365-1369.

Cappelli, C., Castellano, M., Pirola, I., Cumetti, D., Agosti, B., Gandossi, E. et al. (2007). The predictive value of ultrasound findings in the management of thyroid nodules. QJM., 100, 29-35.

Cappelli, C., Castellano, M., Pirola, I., Gandossi, E., De, M. E., Cumetti, D. et al. (2006). Thyroid nodule shape suggests malignancy. Eur.J.Endocrinol., 155, 27-31.

Cappelli, C., Pirola, I., Cumetti, D., Micheletti, L., Tironi, A., Gandossi, E. et al. (2005). Is the anteroposterior and transverse diameter ratio of nonpalpable thyroid nodules a sonographic criteria for recommending fine-needle aspiration cytology? Clin.Endocrinol.(Oxf), 63, 689-693.

Cerutti, J. M., Delcelo, R., Amadei, M. J., Nakabashi, C., Maciel, R. M., Peterson, B. et al. (2004). A preoperative diagnostic test that distinguishes benign from malignant thyroid carcinoma based on gene expression. J.Clin.Invest, 113, 1234-1242.

Cerutti, J. M., Oler, G., Michaluart, P., Jr., Delcelo, R., Beaty, R. M., Shoemaker, J. et al. (2007). Molecular profiling of matched samples identifies biomarkers of papillary thyroid carcinoma lymph node metastasis. Cancer Res., 67, 7885-7892.

Charkes, N. D. (1998). On the prevalence of familial nonmedullary thyroid cancer. Thyroid, 8, 857-858.

Charkes, N. D. (2006). On the prevalence of familial nonmedullary thyroid cancer in multiply affected kindreds. Thyroid, 16, 181-186.

Chen, G. G., Vlantis, A. C., Zeng, Q., & van Hasselt, C. A. (2008). Regulation of cell growth by estrogen signaling and potential targets in thyroid cancer. Curr.Cancer Drug Targets., 8, 367-377.

Chen, X., Hu, Z., Wang, W., Ba, Y., Ma, L., Zhang, C. et al. (2012). Identification of ten serum microRNAs from a genome-wide serum microRNA expression profile as novel noninvasive biomarkers for nonsmall cell lung cancer diagnosis. Int.J.Cancer, 130, 1620-1628.

Chen, Y. T., Kitabayashi, N., Zhou, X. K., Fahey, T. J., III, & Scognamiglio, T. (2008). MicroRNA analysis as a potential diagnostic tool for papillary thyroid carcinoma. Mod.Pathol., 21, 1139-1146.

Chinnappa, P., Taguba, L., Arciaga, R., Faiman, C., Siperstein, A., Mehta, A. E. et al. (2004). Detection of thyrotropin-receptor messenger ribonucleic acid (mRNA) and thyroglobulin mRNA transcripts in peripheral blood of patients with thyroid disease: sensitive and specific markers for thyroid cancer. J.Clin.Endocrinol.Metab, 89, 3705-3709.

Chiosea, S., Nikiforova, M., Zuo, H., Ogilvie, J., Gandhi, M., Seethala, R. R. et al. (2009). A novel complex BRAF mutation detected in a solid variant of papillary thyroid carcinoma. Endocr.Pathol., 20, 122-126.

Choi, S. H., Kim, E. K., Kwak, J. Y., Kim, M. J., & Son, E. J. (2010). Interobserver and intraobserver variations in ultrasound assessment of thyroid nodules. Thyroid, 20, 167-172.

Chudova, D., Wilde, J. I., Wang, E. T., Wang, H., Rabbee, N., Egidio, C. M. et al. (2010). Molecular classification of thyroid nodules using high-dimensionality genomic data. J.Clin.Endocrinol.Metab, 95, 5296-5304.

Cochand-Priollet, B., Dahan, H., Laloi-Michelin, M., Polivka, M., Saada, M., Herman, P. et al. (2011). Immunocytochemistry with cytokeratin 19 and anti-human mesothelial cell antibody (HBME1) increases the diagnostic accuracy of thyroid fine-needle aspirations: preliminary report of 150 liquid-based fine-needle aspirations with histological control. Thyroid, 21, 1067-1073.

da Silveira Mitteldorf, C. A., de Sousa-Canavez, J. M., Leite, K. R., Massumoto, C., & Camara-Lopes, L. H. (2011). FN1, GALE, MET, and QPCT overexpression in papillary thyroid carcinoma: molecular analysis using frozen tissue and routine fine-needle aspiration biopsy samples. Diagn.Cytopathol., 39, 556-561.

Deveci, M. S., Deveci, G., LiVolsi, V. A., & Baloch, Z. W. (2006). Fine-needle aspiration of follicular lesions of the thyroid. Diagnosis and follow-Up. Cytojournal., 3, 9.

Ducena, K., Abols, A., Vilmanis, J., Narbuts, Z., Tars, J., Andrejeva, D. et al. (2011). Validity of multiplex biomarker model of 6 genes for the differential diagnosis of thyroid nodules. Thyroid Res., 4, 11.

Eberhardt, N. L., Grebe, S. K., McIver, B., & Reddi, H. V. (2010). The role of the PAX8/PPARgamma fusion oncogene in the pathogenesis of follicular thyroid cancer. Mol.Cell Endocrinol., 321, 50-56.

Esapa, C. T., Johnson, S. J., Kendall-Taylor, P., Lennard, T. W., & Harris, P. E. (1999). Prevalence of Ras mutations in thyroid neoplasia. Clin.Endocrinol.(Oxf), 50, 529-535.

Finley, D. J., Arora, N., Zhu, B., Gallagher, L., & Fahey, T. J., III (2004). Molecular profiling distinguishes papillary carcinoma from benign thyroid nodules. J.Clin.Endocrinol.Metab, 89, 3214-3223.

Finley, D. J., Lubitz, C. C., Wei, C., Zhu, B., & Fahey, T. J., III (2005). Advancing the molecular diagnosis of thyroid nodules: defining benign lesions by molecular profiling. Thyroid, 15, 562-568.

Finley, D. J., Zhu, B., Barden, C. B., & Fahey, T. J., III (2004). Discrimination of benign and malignant thyroid nodules by molecular profiling. Ann.Surg., 240, 425-436.

Frates, M. C., Benson, C. B., Charboneau, J. W., Cibas, E. S., Clark, O. H., Coleman, B. G. et al. (2005). Management of thyroid nodules detected at US: Society of Radiologists in Ultrasound consensus conference statement. Radiology, 237, 794-800.

Frates, M. C., Benson, C. B., Doubilet, P. M., Cibas, E. S., & Marqusee, E. (2003). Can color Doppler sonography aid in the prediction of malignancy of thyroid nodules? J.Ultrasound Med., 22, 127-131.

Gharib, H., Papini, E., & Paschke, R. (2008). Thyroid nodules: a review of current guidelines, practices, and prospects. Eur.J.Endocrinol., 159, 493-505.

Griffith, O. L., Chiu, C. G., Gown, A. M., Jones, S. J., & Wiseman, S. M. (2008). Biomarker panel diagnosis of thyroid cancer: a critical review. Expert.Rev.Anticancer Ther., 8, 1399-1413.

Griffith, O. L., Chiu, C. G., Gown, A. M., Jones, S. J., & Wiseman, S. M. (2008). Biomarker panel diagnosis of thyroid cancer: a critical review. Expert.Rev.Anticancer Ther., 8, 1399-1413.

Hamburger, J. I., Husain, M., Nishiyama, R., Nunez, C., & Solomon, D. (1989). Increasing the accuracy of fine-needle biopsy for thyroid nodules. Arch.Pathol.Lab Med., 113, 1035-1041.

Hegedus, L. (2010). Can elastography stretch our understanding of thyroid histomorphology? J.Clin.Endocrinol.Metab, 95, 5213-5215.

Hegedus, L., Bonnema, S. J., & Bennedbaek, F. N. (2003). Management of simple nodular goiter: current status and future perspectives. Endocr.Rev., 24, 102-132.

Hoang, J. K., Lee, W. K., Lee, M., Johnson, D., & Farrell, S. (2007). US Features of thyroid malignancy: pearls and pitfalls. Radiographics, 27, 847-860.

Hong, Y., Liu, X., Li, Z., Zhang, X., Chen, M., & Luo, Z. (2009). Real-time ultrasound elastography in the differential diagnosis of benign and malignant thyroid nodules. J.Ultrasound Med., 28, 861-867.

Hong, Y. J., Son, E. J., Kim, E. K., Kwak, J. Y., Hong, S. W., & Chang, H. S. (2010). Positive predictive values of sonographic features of solid thyroid nodule. Clin.Imaging, 34, 127-133.

Huang, Y., Prasad, M., Lemon, W. J., Hampel, H., Wright, F. A., Kornacker, K. et al. (2001). Gene expression in papillary thyroid carcinoma reveals highly consistent profiles. Proc.Natl.Acad.Sci.U.S.A, 98, 15044-15049.

Hussain, M. U. (2012). Micro-RNAs (miRNAs): genomic organisation, biogenesis and mode of action. Cell Tissue Res., 349, 405-413.

Jarzab, B., Wiench, M., Fujarewicz, K., Simek, K., Jarzab, M., Oczko-Wojciechowska, M. et al. (2005). Gene expression profile of papillary thyroid cancer: sources of variability and diagnostic implications. Cancer Res., 65, 1587-1597.

Jin, J., Machekano, R., & McHenry, C. R. (2010). The utility of preoperative serum thyroid-stimulating hormone level for predicting malignant nodular thyroid disease. Am.J.Surg., 199, 294-297.

Jo, Y. S., Huang, S., Kim, Y. J., Lee, I. S., Kim, S. S., Kim, J. R. et al. (2009). Diagnostic value of pyrosequencing for the BRAF V600E mutation in ultrasound-guided fine-needle aspiration biopsy samples of thyroid incidentalomas. Clin.Endocrinol.(Oxf), 70, 139-144.

Jun, P., Chow, L. C., & Jeffrey, R. B. (2005). The sonographic features of papillary thyroid carcinomas: pictorial essay. Ultrasound Q., 21, 39-45.

Karger, S., Krause, K., Gutknecht, M., Schierle, K., Graf, D., Steinert, F. et al. (2012). ADM3, TFF3 and LGALS3 are discriminative molecular markers in fine-needle aspiration biopsies of benign and malignant thyroid tumours. Br.J.Cancer, 106, 562-568.

Kebebew, E., Weng, J., Bauer, J., Ranvier, G., Clark, O. H., Duh, Q. Y. et al. (2007). The prevalence and prognostic value of BRAF mutation in thyroid cancer. Ann.Surg., 246, 466-470.

Kelly, N. P., Lim, J. C., DeJong, S., Harmath, C., Dudiak, C., & Wojcik, E. M. (2006). Specimen adequacy and diagnostic specificity of ultrasound-guided fine needle aspirations of nonpalpable thyroid nodules. Diagn.Cytopathol., 34, 188-190.

Khurana, K. K., Truong, L. D., LiVolsi, V. A., & Baloch, Z. W. (2003). Cytokeratin 19 immunolocalization in cell block preparation of thyroid aspirates. An adjunct to fine-needle aspiration diagnosis of papillary thyroid carcinoma. Arch.Pathol.Lab Med., 127, 579-583.

Kim, H. G., Kwak, J. Y., Kim, E. K., Choi, S. H., & Moon, H. J. (2012). Man to man training: can it help improve the diagnostic performances and interobserver variabilities of thyroid ultrasonography in residents? Eur.J.Radiol., 81, e352-e356.

Kim, J. Y., Lee, C. H., Kim, S. Y., Jeon, W. K., Kang, J. H., An, S. K. et al. (2008). Radiologic and pathologic findings of nonpalpable thyroid carcinomas detected by ultrasonography in a medical screening center. J.Ultrasound Med., 27, 215-223.

Kim, M. J., Kim, E. K., Park, S. I., Kim, B. M., Kwak, J. Y., Kim, S. J. et al. (2008). US-guided fine-needle aspiration of thyroid nodules: indications, techniques, results. Radiographics, 28, 1869-1886.

Kim, S. K., Kim, D. L., Han, H. S., Kim, W. S., Kim, S. J., Moon, W. J. et al. (2008). Pyrosequencing analysis for detection of a BRAFV600E mutation in an FNAB specimen of thyroid nodules. Diagn.Mol.Pathol., 17, 118-125.

Knauf, J. A., Ma, X., Smith, E. P., Zhang, L., Mitsutake, N., Liao, X. H. et al. (2005). Targeted expression of BRAFV600E in thyroid cells of transgenic mice results in papillary thyroid cancers that undergo dedifferentiation. Cancer Res., 65, 4238-4245.

Krause, K., Eszlinger, M., Gimm, O., Karger, S., Engelhardt, C., Dralle, H. et al. (2008). TFF3-based candidate gene discrimination of benign and malignant thyroid tumors in a region with borderline iodine deficiency. J.Clin.Endocrinol.Metab, 93, 1390-1393.

Layfield, L. J., Cibas, E. S., Gharib, H., & Mandel, S. J. (2009). Thyroid aspiration cytology: current status. CA Cancer J.Clin., 59, 99-110.

Liu, F. T. & Rabinovich, G. A. (2005). Galectins as modulators of tumour progression. Nat.Rev.Cancer, 5, 29-41.

Manole, D., Schildknecht, B., Gosnell, B., Adams, E., & Derwahl, M. (2001). Estrogen promotes growth of human thyroid tumor cells by different molecular mechanisms. J.Clin.Endocrinol.Metab, 86, 1072-1077.

Marchetti, I., Lessi, F., Mazzanti, C. M., Bertacca, G., Elisei, R., Coscio, G. D. et al. (2009). A morpho-molecular diagnosis of papillary thyroid carcinoma: BRAF V600E detection as an important tool in preoperative evaluation of fine-needle aspirates. Thyroid, 19, 837-842.

McHenry, C. R. & Phitayakorn, R. (2011). Follicular adenoma and carcinoma of the thyroid gland. Oncologist., 16, 585-593.

Milas, M., Shin, J., Gupta, M., Novosel, T., Nasr, C., Brainard, J. et al. (2010). Circulating thyrotropin receptor mRNA as a novel marker of thyroid cancer: clinical applications learned from 1758 samples. Ann.Surg., 252, 643-651.

Mitchell, P. S., Parkin, R. K., Kroh, E. M., Fritz, B. R., Wyman, S. K., Pogosova-Agadjanyan, E. L. et al. (2008). Circulating microRNAs as stable blood-based markers for cancer detection. Proc.Natl.Acad.Sci.U.S.A, 105, 10513-10518.

Moon, W. J., Jung, S. L., Lee, J. H., Na, D. G., Baek, J. H., Lee, Y. H. et al. (2008). Benign and malignant thyroid nodules: US differentiation--multicenter retrospective study. Radiology, 247, 762-770.

Nam, S. Y., Han, B. K., Ko, E. Y., Kang, S. S., Hahn, S. Y., Hwang, J. Y. et al. (2010). BRAF V600E mutation analysis of thyroid nodules needle aspirates in relation to their ultrasongraphic classification: a potential guide for selection of samples for molecular analysis. Thyroid, 20, 273-279.

Namba, H., Rubin, S. A., & Fagin, J. A. (1990). Point mutations of ras oncogenes are an early event in thyroid tumorigenesis. Mol.Endocrinol., 4, 1474-1479.

Nikiforov, Y. E. (2002). RET/PTC rearrangement in thyroid tumors. Endocr.Pathol., 13, 3-16.

Nikiforov, Y. E., Ohori, N. P., Hodak, S. P., Carty, S. E., LeBeau, S. O., Ferris, R. L. et al. (2011). Impact of mutational testing on the diagnosis and management of patients with cytologically indeterminate thyroid nodules: a prospective analysis of 1056 FNA samples. J.Clin.Endocrinol.Metab, 96, 3390-3397.

Nikiforova, M. N., Biddinger, P. W., Caudill, C. M., Kroll, T. G., & Nikiforov, Y. E. (2002). PAX8-PPARgamma rearrangement in thyroid tumors: RT-PCR and immunohistochemical analyses. Am.J.Surg.Pathol., 26, 1016-1023.

Nikiforova, M. N., Chiosea, S. I., & Nikiforov, Y. E. (2009). MicroRNA expression profiles in thyroid tumors. Endocr.Pathol., 20, 85-91.

Nikiforova, M. N., Tseng, G. C., Steward, D., Diorio, D., & Nikiforov, Y. E. (2008). MicroRNA expression profiling of thyroid tumors: biological significance and diagnostic utility. J.Clin.Endocrinol.Metab, 93, 1600-1608.

Ohori, N. P., Nikiforova, M. N., Schoedel, K. E., LeBeau, S. O., Hodak, S. P., Seethala, R. R. et al. (2010). Contribution of molecular testing to thyroid fine-needle aspiration cytology of "follicular lesion of undetermined significance/atypia of undetermined significance". Cancer Cytopathol., 118, 17-23.

Papini, E., Guglielmi, R., Bianchini, A., Crescenzi, A., Taccogna, S., Nardi, F. et al. (2002). Risk of malignancy in nonpalpable thyroid nodules: predictive value of ultrasound and color-Doppler features. J.Clin.Endocrinol.Metab, 87, 1941-1946.

Park, C. S., Kim, S. H., Jung, S. L., Kang, B. J., Kim, J. Y., Choi, J. J. et al. (2010). Observer variability in the sonographic evaluation of thyroid nodules. J.Clin.Ultrasound, 38, 287-293.

Parkin, D. M., Bray, F., Ferlay, J., & Pisani, P. (2005). Global cancer statistics, 2002. CA Cancer J.Clin., 55, 74-108.

Peccin, S., de Castsro, J. A., Furlanetto, T. W., Furtado, A. P., Brasil, B. A., & Czepielewski, M. A. (2002). Ultrasonography: is it useful in the diagnosis of cancer in thyroid nodules? J.Endocrinol.Invest, 25, 39-43.

Prasad, M. L., Pellegata, N. S., Huang, Y., Nagaraja, H. N., de la Chapelle, A., & Kloos, R. T. (2005). Galectin-3, fibronectin-1, CITED-1, HBME1 and cytokeratin-19 immunohistochemistry is useful for the differential diagnosis of thyroid tumors. Mod.Pathol., 18, 48-57.

Propper, R. A., Skolnick, M. L., Weinstein, B. J., & Dekker, A. (1980). The nonspecificity of the thyroid halo sign. J.Clin.Ultrasound, 8, 129-132.

Raggio, E., Camandona, M., Solerio, D., Martino, P., Franchello, A., Orlandi, F. et al. (2010). The diagnostic accuracy of the immunocytochemical markers in the pre-operative evaluation of follicular thyroid lesions. J.Endocrinol.Invest, 33, 378-381.

Rago, T., Santini, F., Scutari, M., Pinchera, A., & Vitti, P. (2007). Elastography: new developments in ultrasound for predicting malignancy in thyroid nodules. J.Clin.Endocrinol.Metab, 92, 2917-2922.

Rago, T., Scutari, M., Santini, F., Loiacono, V., Piaggi, P., Di, C. G. et al. (2010). Real-time elastosonography: useful tool for refining the presurgical diagnosis in thyroid nodules with indeterminate or nondiagnostic cytology. J.Clin.Endocrinol.Metab, 95, 5274-5280.

Ries LAG, Melbert D, & Krapcho M. (2007). SEER Cancer Statistics Review.

Ref Type: Generic

Saleh, H. A., Feng, J., Tabassum, F., Al-Zohaili, O., Husain, M., & Giorgadze, T. (2009). Differential expression of galectin-3, CK19, HBME1, and Ret oncoprotein in the diagnosis of thyroid neoplasms by fine needle aspiration biopsy. Cytojournal., 6, 18.

Sanders, L. E. & Silverman, M. (1998). Follicular and Hurthle cell carcinoma: predicting outcome and directing therapy. Surgery, 124, 967-974.

Scognamiglio, T., Hyjek, E., Kao, J., & Chen, Y. T. (2006). Diagnostic usefulness of HBME1, galectin-3, CK19, and CITED1 and evaluation of their expression in encapsulated lesions with questionable features of papillary thyroid carcinoma. Am.J.Clin.Pathol., 126, 700-708.

Sebag, F., Vaillant-Lombard, J., Berbis, J., Griset, V., Henry, J. F., Petit, P. et al. (2010). Shear wave elastography: a new ultrasound imaging mode for the differential diagnosis of benign and malignant thyroid nodules. J.Clin.Endocrinol.Metab, 95, 5281-5288.

Serra, S. & Asa, S. L. (2008). Controversies in thyroid pathology: the diagnosis of follicular neoplasms. Endocr.Pathol., 19, 156-165.

Sheibani, K., Esteban, J. M., Bailey, A., Battifora, H., & Weiss, L. M. (1992). Immunopathologic and molecular studies as an aid to the diagnosis of malignant mesothelioma. Hum.Pathol., 23, 107-116.

Shen, R., Liyanarachchi, S., Li, W., Wakely, P. E., Jr., Saji, M., Huang, J. et al. (2012). MicroRNA signature in thyroid fine needle aspiration cytology applied to "atypia of undetermined significance" cases. Thyroid, 22, 9-16.

Stephen, J. K., Chitale, D., Narra, V., Chen, K. M., Sawhney, R., & Worsham, M. J. (2011). DNA methylation in thyroid tumorigenesis. Cancers.(Basel), 3, 1732-1743.

Takakura, S., Mitsutake, N., Nakashima, M., Namba, H., Saenko, V. A., Rogounovitch, T. I. et al. (2008). Oncogenic role of miR-17-92 cluster in anaplastic thyroid cancer cells. Cancer Sci., 99, 1147-1154.

Takano, T., Miyauchi, A., Yoshida, H., Kuma, K., & Amino, N. (2005). Decreased relative expression level of trefoil factor 3 mRNA to galectin-3 mRNA distinguishes thyroid follicular carcinoma from adenoma. Cancer Lett., 219, 91-96.

Takashima, S., Fukuda, H., Nomura, N., Kishimoto, H., Kim, T., & Kobayashi, T. (1995). Thyroid nodules: re-evaluation with ultrasound. J.Clin.Ultrasound, 23, 179-184.

Tallini, G. & Asa, S. L. (2001). RET oncogene activation in papillary thyroid carcinoma. Adv.Anat.Pathol., 8, 345-354.

Torregrossa, L., Faviana, P., Filice, M. E., Materazzi, G., Miccoli, P., Vitti, P. et al. (2010). CXC chemokine receptor 4 immunodetection in the follicular variant of papillary thyroid carcinoma: comparison to galectin-3 and hector battifora mesothelial cell-1. Thyroid, 20, 495-504.

van Heerden, J. A., Hay, I. D., Goellner, J. R., Salomao, D., Ebersold, J. R., Bergstralh, E. J. et al. (1992). Follicular thyroid carcinoma with capsular invasion alone: a nonthreatening malignancy. Surgery, 112, 1130-1136.

Vriens, M. R., Weng, J., Suh, I., Huynh, N., Guerrero, M. A., Shen, W. T. et al. (2012). MicroRNA expression profiling is a potential diagnostic tool for thyroid cancer. Cancer, 118, 3426-3432.

Wang, H. H. (2006). Reporting thyroid fine-needle aspiration: literature review and a proposal. Diagn.Cytopathol., 34, 67-76.

Weber, F., Teresi, R. E., Broelsch, C. E., Frilling, A., & Eng, C. (2006). A limited set of human MicroRNA is deregulated in follicular thyroid carcinoma. J.Clin.Endocrinol.Metab, 91, 3584-3591.

Xing, M. (2010). Genetic alterations in the phosphatidylinositol-3 kinase/Akt pathway in thyroid cancer. Thyroid, 20, 697-706.

Xing, M., Cohen, Y., Mambo, E., Tallini, G., Udelsman, R., Ladenson, P. W. et al. (2004). Early occurrence of RASSF1A hypermethylation and its mutual exclusion with BRAF mutation in thyroid tumorigenesis. Cancer Res., 64, 1664-1668.

Xing, M., Usadel, H., Cohen, Y., Tokumaru, Y., Guo, Z., Westra, W. B. et al. (2003). Methylation of the thyroid-stimulating hormone receptor gene in epithelial thyroid tumors: a marker of malignancy and a cause of gene silencing. Cancer Res., 63, 2316-2321.

Yip, L., Kelly, L., Shuai, Y., Armstrong, M. J., Nikiforov, Y. E., Carty, S. E. et al. (2011). MicroRNA signature distinguishes the degree of aggressiveness of papillary thyroid carcinoma. Ann.Surg.Oncol., 18, 2035-2041.

Yoo, C. B. & Jones, P. A. (2006). Epigenetic therapy of cancer: past, present and future. Nat.Rev.Drug Discov., 5, 37-50.

Yu, S., Liu, Y., Wang, J., Guo, Z., Zhang, Q., Yu, F. et al. (2012). Circulating microRNA profiles as potential biomarkers for diagnosis of papillary thyroid carcinoma. J.Clin.Endocrinol.Metab, 97, 2084-2092.

www.ingramcontent.com/pod-product-compliance
Lightning Source LLC
Chambersburg PA
CBHW050820220326
41598CB00006B/267